H.-J. Biersack F. Grünwald (Eds.)

Thyroid Cancer

2nd Edition

H.-J. Biersack F. Grünwald (Eds.)

Thyroid Cancer

Second Edition

With 62 Figures and 34 Tables

Springer

H.-J. BIERSACK, Professor Dr. med.
Klinik und Poliklinik für Nuklearmedizin
Rheinische Friedrich-Wilhelms-Universität
Sigmund-Freud-Strasse 25
53127 Bonn, Germany

F. GRÜNWALD, Professor Dr. med.
Klinik für Nuklearmedizin
Universität Frankfurt
Theodor-Stern-Kai 7
60590 Frankfurt am Main, Germany

Second Edition
ISBN-10 3-642-42413-9 Springer Verlag Berlin Heidelberg New York
ISBN-13 978-3-642-42413-7 Springer Verlag Berlin Heidelberg New York

First Edition
ISBN 3-540-20512-8 Springer Verlag Berlin Heidelberg New York

A catalog record for this book is available from Library of Congress.

Bibliographic information published by Die Deutsche Bibliothek.
Die Deutsche Bibliothek lists this publication in the Deutsche Nationalbibliographie; detailed bibliographic data is available in the Internet at http://dnb.ddb.de

Editor: Dr. Ute Heilmann, Heidelberg, Germany
Desk editor: Dörthe Mennecke-Bühler, Heidelberg, Germany
Production: PRO EDIT GmbH, Heidelberg, Germany
Cover-Design: Frido Steinen-Broo, eStudio Calamar, Spain
Typesetting: Satz-Druck-Service, Leimen, Germany
Printed on acid free paper 22/3151bg – 5 4 3 2 1 0

Preface to the Second Edition

One of the main reasons for publishing this second edition of "Thyroid Cancer" is the fact that the first edition has sold out. Furthermore, during the 4 years following the publication of the first edition in 2001, some progress, mainly in the basic sciences (molecular biology), has been made. The most prominent change in the clinical sciences has been the new classification of thyroid cancer, especially with relation to T1–T3 tumors. Now, tumors with a diameter of up to 2 cm are still classified T1. This new UICC classification (6th edition) follows the classification of the American Society of Pathology. These changes require a modification of the old guidelines. According to the Hedinger classification (1988) tumors with a diameter below 1 cm were classified as "papillary microcarcinoma of the thyroid". Only in those tumors was total or nearly total thyroidectomy deemed unnecessary and I-131 therapy not a prerequisite for treatment.

The majority of the chapters has been updated including references to many new publications. Two new chapters, on I-124 PET and dosimetry, have been added.

We strongly feel that this second edition of "Thyroid Cancer" is again a state-of-the-art overview of the diagnosis and treatment of thyroid cancer.

Bonn, Frankfurt am Main H.-J. Biersack, F. Grünwald

Preface to the First Edition

Thyroid cancer was first described at the end of the eighteenth century. For one and a half centuries surgery remained the only effective therapeutic option for this cancer, until in 1946 radioiodine therapy was performed for the first time. Radioiodine therapy was brought to Germany 4 years later, in 1950. In the intervening 50 years, the use of iodine-131 has proved able to cure the cancer and its metastases. Percutaneous radiation therapy had been added to the therapeutic armamentarium, but even now there is heated debate as to its potential. Suppressive L-thyroxine supplement is a prerequisite for successful treatment, while cytotoxic drugs are mainly used for palliation.

During the past 10 years, various new diagnostic and therapeutic approaches have been introduced. High-dose radioiodine therapy as well as redifferentiation therapy with retinoic acid seem beneficial. Diagnostic procedures such as magnetic resonance imaging (MRI), positron emission tomography (PET), as well as isonitriles (MIBI) and thallium (^{201}Tl), have proved useful for the follow-up of thyroid cancer.

Two special issues are also discussed in this book. Iodine supplementation in areas of iodine deficiency has led to a change in pathology insofar as papillary thyroid cancer (with a better prognosis) has become more frequent than follicular carcinoma. A special chapter is dedicated to thyroid cancer in Chernobyl children.

Medullary thyroid cancer remains a challenge for interdisciplinary diagnosis and therapy. The fate of the patient with medullary thyroid cancer is determined by surgery. Removal of all accessible lymph nodes and their metastases is mandatory. Percutaneous radiation therapy is usually not successful. The same holds true for cytotoxic medication. Nuclear medicine now provides new imaging procedures such as those taking advantage of ^{111}In-octreotide and ^{131}I-metaiodobenzylguanidine (mIBG) as well as ^{99m}Tc-dimercaptosuccinic acid (DMSA). mIBG and octreotide analogues may have therapeutic potential but have not yet been evaluated clinically in sufficiently large groups of patients.

Undifferentiated (anaplastic) thyroid cancer is not covered in such depth; therapy is still unsuccessful, and the 1-year survival rate is below 10%.

We strongly feel that the development of new imaging and therapeutic procedures during the past 10 years justifies the publication of a new survey. Almost 55 years have passed since the first successful radioiodine treatment of thyroid cancer, and many textbooks have appeared, but in our opinion the past 10 years have contributed enormously to the knowledge on diagnosis and treatment of this malignancy. Molecular biology will certainly enhance our knowledge further; recombinant TSH was one of the first steps. It may be speculated that molecular biology will help us to restore the sodium/iodine symporter, as is now achieved by retinoic acid. Recently published data on the existence of the sodium/iodine symporter in other malignant tissues give reason to hope that some successful therapeutic procedures in thyroid cancer can, at least in part, be transferred to other carcinomas.

While most cases of differentiated thyroid cancer have a relatively benign course, those patients whose cancer has lost the ability to accumulate radioiodine remain a therapeutic problem. We hope that this textbook may be helpful in such instances. All the abovementioned diagnostic and therapeutic procedures contribute to the nowadays very good prognosis of the majority of patients suffering from thyroid cancer.

Bonn, Frankfurt am Main H.-J. Biersack, F. Grünwald

Contents

Part I Basics

List of Contributors

W. BECKER, Prof. Dr. med.
Klinik für Nuklearmedizin
Georg-August-Universität
Robert-Koch-Strasse 40
37075 Göttingen, Germany

T.M. BEHR, Prof. Dr. med.
Klinik für Nuklearmedizin der Philipps-Universität Marburg
Baldingerstrasse
35043 Marburg/Lahn, Germany

M. BIERMANN, Dr. med.
Klinik und Poliklinik für Nuklearmedizin
Universitätsklinikum Münster
Zentralklinikum Ebene 03 Ost, Albert-Schweitzer-Strasse 30–33
48129 Münster, Germany

H.-J. BIERSACK, Prof. Dr. med.
Klinik und Poliklinik für Nuklearmedizin
Rheinische Friedrich-Wilhelms-Universität
Sigmund-Freud-Strasse 25
53127 Bonn, Germany

J. BIKO, Dr. med.
Klinik und Poliklinik für Nuklearmedizin
Universität Würzburg
Josef-Schneider-Strasse 2
97080 Würzburg, Germany

A. BOCKISCH, Prof. Dr. rer. nat., Dr. med.
Klinik für Nuklearmedizin
Universitätsklinikum Essen
45122 Essen, Germany

M.R. Carlisle, MD, PhD
Division of Nuclear Medicine
Department of Radiology and Medicine
Stanford University School of Medicine
Stanford, CA 94305, USA

E.P. Demidchik, MD
Center for Thyroid Tumors
Minsk, Belarus

M. Dietlein, Priv.-Doz., Dr. med.
Klinik und Poliklinik für Nuklearmedizin der Universität zu Köln
Joseph-Stelzmann-Strasse 9
50924 Köln, Germany

H. Dralle, Professor Dr. med.
Martin-Luther-Universität Halle-Wittenberg
Klinik für Allgemein-, Viszeral- und Gefäßchirurgie
Ernst-Grube-Strasse 40
06097 Halle/Saale, Germany

V. Drozd, MD
Research and Clinical Institute of Radiation Medicine
and Endocrinology
Minsk, Belarus

K. Frank-Raue, Dr. med.
Endokrinologische Gemeinschaftspraxis
Brückenstrasse 21
69120 Heidelberg, Germany

J. E. Freitas, MD
Dept. of Radiology
University of Michigan Medical School
Ann Arbor, MI, USA

L. S. Freudenberg, Dr. med.
Klinik für Nuklearmedizin
Universitätsklinikum Essen
45122 Essen, Germany

O. Gimm, Dr. med.
Martin-Luther-Universität Halle-Wittenberg
Klinik für Allgemein-, Viszeral- und Gefäßchirurgie
Ernst-Grube-Strasse 40
06097 Halle/Saale, Germany

R. Görges, Dr. med.
Universitätsklinikum Essen
Klinik und Poliklinik für Nuklearmedizin
Hufelandstrasse 55
45122 Essen, Germany

M.D. Gross, MD
Division of Nuclear Medicine
Department of Radiology
BIG 412 Box 0028
University of Michigan Health System
1500 East Medical Center Drive
Ann Arbor, MI 48109, USA

F. Grünwald, Prof. Dr. med.
Klinik für Nuklearmedizin
Universität Frankfurt
Theodor-Stern-Kai 7
60590 Frankfurt am Main, Germany

A. Heinecke, Dr. med.
Dept. of Biometrics
Universitätsklinikum Münster
Albert-Schweitzer-Strasse 30 – 33
48129 Münster, Germany

F. Hofstädter, Prof. Dr. med.
Institut für Pathologie der Universität Regensburg
Franz-Josef-Strauss-Allee 11
93042 Regensburg, Germany

W. Jentzen, Dr. med.
Klinik für Nuklearmedizin
Universitätsklinikum Essen
45122 Essen, Germany

I.R. McDougall, MD, PhD
Division of Nuclear Medicine, Room H-0101
Stanford University Medical Center
300 Pasteur Drive
Stanford, CA 94305-5281, USA

D. Moka, Priv.-Doz., Dr. med.
Klinik und Poliklinik für Nuklearmedizin der Universität zu Köln
Joseph-Stelzmann-Strasse 9
50924 Köln, Germany

M. K. Pixberg, Dr. med.
Klinik und Poliklinik für Nuklearmedizin
Universitätsklinikum Münster
Albert-Schweitzer-Strasse 30 – 33
48129 Münster, Germany

F. Raue, Prof. Dr. med.
Endokrinologische Gemeinschaftspraxis
Brückenstrasse 21
69120 Heidelberg, Germany

C. Reiners, Prof. Dr. med.
Klinik und Poliklinik für Nuklearmedizin
Universität Würzburg
Josef-Schneider-Strasse 2
97080 Würzburg, Germany

J.H. Risse, Priv.-Doz. Dr. med.
Gemeinschaftspraxis für Radiologie und Nuklearmedizin
Von-Stauffenberg-Strasse 9
53604 Bad Honnef, Germany

B. Saller, Priv.-Doz. Dr. med.
Pfizer GmbH, Abt. Endokrinologie & Diabetes
Pfizerstrasse 1
76139 Karlsruhe, Germany

H. Schicha, Prof. Dr. med.
Klinik und Poliklinik für Nuklearmedizin
der Universität zu Köln
Joseph-Stelzmann-Strasse 9
50924 Köln, Germany

T. Schilling, Priv.-Doz. Dr. med.
Abt. Innere Medizin I
Im Neuenheimer Feld 410
69120 Heidelberg, Germany

O. Schober, Dr. med.
Klinik und Poliklinik für Nuklearmedizin
Universitätsklinikum Münster
Albert-Schweitzer-Strasse 30–33
48129 Münster, Germany

Andreas Schuck, Dr. med.
Dept. of Radiooncology
Universitätsklinikum Münster
Albert-Schweitzer-Strasse 30 – 33
48129 Münster, Germany

P.-M. Schumm-Draeger, Prof. Dr. med.
3. Med. Abteilung
Städt. Krankenhaus München-Bogenhausen
Englschalkinger Str. 77
81925 München, Germany

B. Shapiro, MB
Division of Nuclear Medicine
Dept. of Radiology
University of Michigan Health System
1500 East Medical Center Drive
Ann Arbor, MI 48109, USA

D. Simon, Prof. Dr. med.
Evangelisches Krankenhaus Bethesda zu Duisburg GGmbH
Heerstrasse 219
47053 Duisburg, Germany

N. Willich, Prof. Dr. med.
Dept. of Radiooncology
Universitätsklinikum Münster
Albert-Schweitzer-Strasse 30 – 33
48129 Münster, Germany

R. Ziegler, Prof. Dr. med.
Abt. Innere Medizin I
Im Neuenheimer Feld 410
69120 Heidelberg, Germany

Part I

Basics

I

CHAPTER 1

The Changing Epidemiology of Thyroid Cancer 1

R. GÖRGES

1.1 Basic Epidemiological Problems in Thyroid Cancer

Two of the main features of thyroid malignancy are its rarity and its excellent prognosis in the overwhelming number of cases. On the other hand, these factors induce some specific difficulties in epidemiologic studies of thyroid cancer. Apart from special aspects for thyroid malignomas, the validity of epidemiological data in general depends on a number of factors, which may cause pitfalls. Each scientist who implements or analyzes studies in this field should bear in mind those fundamental difficulties, otherwise erroneous conclusions or fatal epidemiologic misinterpretations may be drawn. This chapter therefore opens with some basic methodological reflections.

Ideally, for epidemiological research, complete data on the entire population should be available. At least, it must be assured that the data sample is representative of the study population in every relevant aspect. For this aim, well-organized structures for data acquisition and transmission to centralized agencies are necessary. Mandatory reporting of all diagnosed malignancies, cancer deaths, routine autopsies, and comparison of these data with information from the official register of births and deaths by a centralized cancer registry would be beneficial for oncological epidemiology. This ideal situation does not exist, even in many industrial nations with highly developed health care systems, due in part to ethical considerations as well as concerns about the protection of privacy. For example, in Germany, not until 1995 was legislation passed to allow physicians to report newly diagnosed malignancies to the registry (however, reporting is not mandatory). Meanwhile, most German federal states have established central cancer registries, but even at present the registration is not nationwide. In the USA, the National Cancer Data Base (NCDB) records approximately 60% of all cancer cases but, again, the majority of the information is provided on a voluntary basis.

Due to the limitations of centrally acquired data or even their complete absence in many countries, epidemiological studies are often based on clinical data, which are flawed by selection biases. The continual improvement of diagnostic modalities is another factor complicating data comparison, e.g., the improved sensitivity of ultrasonography since the 1980s makes the historical comparison of incidence data highly problematic. The reported increasing incidence of thyroid cancer, especially in the early stages, is at least in part due to improved diagnostic techniques, which lead to earlier detection [69].

The slow growth rate of thyroid carcinomas causes another difficulty for epidemiological research. There are often decades between tumor induction and clinical manifestation, and in a substantial number of cases the disease remains undetected during life, and tumor mortality is generally low. In 1998 for example, in the United States 17,200 new cases of thyroid cancer from a total of 1,228,600 new cancer cases were estimated, with a male:female ratio of 1:3.7. In contrast, only 1,200 deaths from thyroid cancer were estimated [101]. For this reason, in contrast to highly malignant tumors such as lung or pancreatic cancer, mortality statistics do not reflect the incidence of thyroid cancer and statistics of the incidence of clinically manifest tumors do not describe the prevalence in the population.

Data from such mortality rates, incidence rates or survival rates of malignomas such as thyroid cancer should be described in terms of "age-standardized rates" rather than "crude rates". The "age-standardized mortality" describes the expected number of deaths per 100,000 for a reference population of a given age and sex distribution. Due to the age dependence of cancer incidence and mortality, comparison of those data in populations with different age distributions, e.g., in different regions or even within the same region are not possible without age standardization, since the age structure of the population changes over time. The reported age-standardized figures depend on the individual reference population, which may underlie regional or historical variations. For thyroid cancer in Wales/United Kingdom (1985–1996, all ages) for example, the crude incidence rates were 1.04 for males and 2.94 for females. The corresponding figures underlying the European age-standardized rates (EASR) were 0.97 and 2.52, and underlying the world age-standardized rates (WASR) 0.75 and 2.06, respectively [92].

Data on the frequency of thyroid cancer can be obtained by systematic thyroid diagnostics in large representative populations. However, the incidence of thyroid nodules in endemic goiter areas is substantially greater than the incidence of thyroid cancer: up to 30–50% nodules, of which only 5–10% are malignant [65, 87]. Adequate further examination (i.e., scintigraphy, cytology and histology) of all detected nodules is of critical importance, but due to the immense resources and costs such studies have remained scarce. Serial autopsy studies are another means of providing prevalence data for thyroid cancer, especially for clinically occult carcinomas; however, the data obtained from those studies do not represent the rate of clinically apparent and relevant malignancy.

The quality of all diagnostic data is also of critical importance. It is dependent on the technical equipment and the experience of the clinician and the training of the pathologist in the challenging task of classifying the subtypes of thyroid tumors. Classification schemes used for clinical staging as well as histological typing are important for making comparisons. In cancer registry data banks, epidemiological data (e.g., for incidence and mortality) are often only available following the International Classification of Disease (ICD) code, where all types of thyroid cancer are encoded with one common code number. Thus, no statements could be given concerning the considerable epidemiological differences for the individual histological subtype on the basis of those data banks. Since the classification of tumors and staging have repeatedly changed historically, appropriate reclassification is necessary for any comparison of current with older data, if the epidemiology of histological subtypes is examined.

The current histological World Health Organization (WHO) classification was published 1988 (2nd edition) and superseded the 1st edition published in 1974 [53, 54]. The decision in the 1st edition to regard a tumor with even minor papillary component as a papillary carcinoma (despite the presence of follicular patterns) has been upheld. In previous schemes, the predominant formation determined the final classification of the tumor, leading to a larger number of follicular carcinomas in these older reports. Differences between the 1st and the 2nd edition are: the removal of the subtypes of undifferentiated carcinomas, a revision of the nonepithelial and miscellaneous tumors, and the recognition that the great majority of tumors previously diagnosed as "small-cell carcinomas" of the thyroid are malignant lymphomas. Like the 1st edition, the 2nd edition does not consider certain subtypes as tumor entities in their own right (e.g., tall cell, columnar cell, diffuse sclerosing or diffuse follicular variant of papillary carcinoma, insular carcinoma, Hürthle cell carcinoma), although they show substantial epidemiological differences from the classic types of papillary and follicular carcinomas.

The tumor–node–metastasis (TNM) classification has also been revised repeatedly. The differences between the 3rd and the 4th edition [126] also influence the prognostic scoring in risk-group stages, which is derived from the TNM system. Lateralization and multicentricity of the primary tumor were abandoned in favor of tumor size, and the regional lymph node (N) classification was simplified. After a 2nd revision in 1992 of the 4th edition and a supplement in 1993, the 5th edition was published in 1997. It reconciled the systems of the American Joint Committee on Cancer (AJCC) and the Union International Contre Cancer (UICC) [115]. Another change was the definition of "occult papillary carcinoma" or "papillary microcarcinoma": older publications allow a maximal diameter of 1.5 cm, and the 5th edition of the TNM classification defined tumors smaller than 1 cm as T1 carcinomas. In 2002, the 6th edition was introduced [116]. It implies considerable modifications (e.g., borders for the T-stage classification, dependency of the T4 state from clinical information from the surgeon, lymph node level) and is not compatible with the former TNM classification, which is why previous study data involving TNM stages cannot be transformed. Even a recently published supplement [135] could not completely eliminate these criticisms.

Data quality concerning the prognosis of a given thyroid cancer and the prognosis itself not only depend on the tumor biology or the properties of the individual patient, but also on the quality and duration of aftercare of the patients (especially on the sensitivity of diagnostic methods for detection of recurrences), on demographic factors and on the therapy carried out. Due to the overall favorable prognosis of differentiated thyroid carcinoma, slight variations of relapse-free intervals or survival rates between different histological subtypes, stages or special risk-groups and changes of these factors in the time course or due to new forms of therapy can only be evaluated if large patient groups are observed over a long time period. On this point, the existence of long-term follow-up programs with adequate data documentation is of benefit.

1.2 General Epidemiological Data for Thyroid Cancer

Clinically recognized thyroid carcinoma is a rare malignancy, accounting for less than 1% of human malignant neoplasms. In the endocrine system however, it is the most common malignancy and is responsible for more deaths than all other endocrine cancers combined. The incidence shows a predominance in females with a male:female ratio about 1:1.5 to 1:3 in most countries. In contrast to the marked higher incidence and prevalence of clinically recognized thyroid cancer in females, the prevalence of occult thyroid carcinoma is not higher in women. The annual incidence rate of thyroid carcinoma in Iceland, for example, as published by the Icelandic Cancer Registry for the period 1955–1984, is high, at 4.4/100,000 for men and 11.7/100,000 for women, whereas the prevalence in autopsy series is 7.5% in males and 5.1% in females [123].

Whereas thyroid nodules in general are common in the population, their malignancy rate is low, especially in iodine-deficient areas with a high prevalence of nodular goiter. It has been estimated from the Framingham database, that the lifetime risk of developing a thyroid nodule is between 5 and 10%, and females were afflicted four times more frequently than males [129]. The importance of these population data rests with the fact that less than 15% of all clinically detected nodules will, in fact, contain cancer [65, 77]. Abu-Eshy et al. [2] in Saudi Arabia found similar results detecting a malignancy rate of 8% in multinodular goiters and of 15.2% in thyroid glands with a solitary nodule. In contrast, large autopsy studies have revealed single or multiple thyroid nodules in up to 50% of adults [83], these data have been recently corroborated using high-resolution ultrasonography [56] and have been increased through improvement of diagnostic sensitivity. The distribution of fine-needle biopsy has led to a 75% reduction of the frequency of nodules that have to undergo surgery for histologic examination, corresponding to a two–threefold increase in the malignancy rate in the actually operated patients.

In most countries, data for the annual incidence of thyroid cancer per 100,000 individuals range from 0.9 to 2.6 in men and from 2.0 to 5.9 in women [91]. Yet, considerable differences exist in incidence, in the male:female ratio or in the histological subtypes for some countries, and for individual regions, ethnic populations and age-groups within the same country (for data survey see Table 1.1). Countries in which the incidence rates of thyroid cancer exceed 3.0 in males and/or 4.0 in females (i.e., approximately twice the average) are as follows: Iceland (6.2 in males and 8.3 in females), the Jewish population in Israel, Columbia, and a few registries in the United States, Canada, Japan, Norway and Finland [37]. Exceptionally high incidence rates were reported for Hawaii, particularly in Chinese (8.1 in males and 11.3 in females) and in Filipino (6.6 in males and 24.2 in females) populations. Amazingly, the incidence rate is higher in each ethnic group in Hawaii than in their country of origin [45]. Furthermore, the

Table 1.1. World age-standardized incidence rates (per 100,000) for thyroid cancer in various countries (Franceschi and La Vecchia [37], Black et al. [14], Paterson et al. [92])

Country (region, populations)	Observed time period	Men	Women	Ratio men:women
United States (white)	1988–1992	2.5	6.4	1:2.6
United States (Hawaii, Chinese)	1983–1987	8.1	11.3	1:1.4
United States (Hawaii, Filipino)	1983–1987	6.6	24.2	1:3.7
United States (Hawaii, Hawaiian)	1983–1987	5.4	9.6	1:1.8
Columbia	1983–1987	1.8	6.6	1:3.7
Japan (Osaka)	1988–1992	1.1	3.5	1:3.2
India (Bombay)	1983–1987	0.8	1.5	1:1.9
Israel (Jewish)	1983–1987	2.5	5.9	1:2.4
Israel (non-Jewish)	1983–1987	1.0	2.6	1:2.6
New Zealand (non-Maori)	1983–1987	1.1	3.0	1:2.7
New Zealand (Maori)	1983–1987	1.6	4.0	1:2.5
European Community (EU)	1990	1.3	2.4	1:1.8
Austria	1990	1.8	4.0	1:2.2
Belgium	1990	1.9	1.8	1:0.9
Denmark	1990	0.6	1.9	1:3.2
Finland	1990	1.5	6.1	1:4.1
France	1990	1.7	1.9	1:1.1
Germany	1990	2.1	2.4	1:1.1
Greece	1990	0.4	1.5	1:3.8
Iceland	1983–1987	6.2	8.3	1:1.3
Ireland	1990	0.9	1.3	1:1.4
Italy	1990	1.1	3.6	1:3.3
Luxembourg	1990	1.9	2.0	1:1.1
Netherlands	1990	0.9	2.2	1:2.4
Norway	1988–1992	1.7	4.7	1:2.8
Portugal	1990	0.7	2.2	1:3.1
Spain	1990	0.7	2.2	1:3.1
Sweden	1990	1.3	3.4	1:2.6
UK	1990	0.8	1.7	1:2.2
UK (Wales)	1985–1996	0.8	2.1	1:2.6

Japanese and Chinese living in the USA have an elevated incidence of thyroid cancer (twice that of their country of origin), whereas it is a less common lesion in African-American patients [120].

Those differences may be due not only to genetic, but also to environmental factors (mainly dietary habits) and in part to the different standards of medicine. It is not possible to transfer epidemiological data for thyroid cancer from areas with iodine sufficiency (such as the USA or Japan) to iodine-deficient countries (such as Germany or Central Asia). In adults, the incidence of thyroid cancer in general tends to increase with age. In the USA the peak age at diagnosis has been reported as 30–39 years for papillary, 30–49 years for follicular, and over 70 years for anaplastic carcinoma [58]. In Europe the mean age of patients with thyroid cancer in general at diagnosis ranged from 44 to 58 years [110]. Analyzing data from 1,017 patients whose primary therapy took place in our department of nuclear medicine (University Hospital Essen, Germany) from 1978 to 1998, the peak age was the 3rd to the 5th decade for papillary, the 4th to the 5th decade for follicular, and the 5th decade for Hürthle cell carcinoma. In both sexes thyroid cancer ranges with less than 0.5% behind the 20 most frequent causes of cancer death. In most countries mortality due to thyroid cancer is 1½ to two times higher in females than in males. The mortality rate of a cancer type reflects its frequency and its prognosis. For the period 1990–1994, the age-standardized overall mortality rates for all histological types of thyroid cancer together in 27 European countries were in the mean 0.4 for men and 0.6 for women, with a range from 0.17 (Albania and Belgium) to 0.93 (Iceland) for men and from 0.21 (Albania) to 1.15 (Iceland) for women [71]. In Germany, the average age-standardized, overall mortality rate was 0.54 for men and 0.65 for women for the same period [71]. For the period 1985–1989, the average world age-standardized mortality rates for thyroid cancer for men compared with women were 0.2:0.3 in the USA, 0.2:0.4 in Australia, 0.3 (both sexes) in Canada, 0.3:0.5 in Japan, 0.4:0.5 in New Zealand, 0.6:0.7 in Israel, and 0.8 (both sexes) in Singapore [37], 0.56:0.70 in West Germany and 0.49:0.69 in East Germany.

Concerning the proportions of histological subtypes of epithelial thyroid malignomas, remarkable differences exist between different countries. The data from the United States National Cancer Database (53,856 thyroid cancer cases during the period 1985–1995) reveal 79% papillary, 13% follicular, 2.9% Hürthle cell, 3.6% medullary and 1.7% undifferentiated or anaplastic thyroid carcinomas [58]. In 1,103 patients treated in our department (University Hospital Essen, Germany, an area with endemic iodine deficiency) 1985–1998 with the initial diagnosis of thyroid carcinoma (papillary microcarcinoma excluded), the proportions were: 61% papillary, 24% follicular, 7% Hürthle cell, 5% medullary and 3% anaplastic thyroid carcinomas. According to the WHO histological classification of thyroid tumors, where Hürthle cell cancer does not appear as a separate entity but mostly is assigned to the group of follicular carcinomas,

Table 1.2. Proportions of various histologic types of epithelial thyroid cancer (incidental autopsy cases excluded)

Authors	Country	Time period	No. of patients	Papillary	Follicular	Medullary	Anaplastic
Ezaki et al. [34]	Japan	1977–1986	10,973*	78.4%	17.2%	1.4%	2.7%
Freitag et al. [40]	Germany	1982–1997	239	70.3%	18.4%	6.3%	5.0%
Levi et al. [70]**	Switzerland	1974–1987	308	61%	31%	5.7%	2.3%
Christensen et al. [26]	Sweden	1660–1977	104	65%	21%	4%	12%
Shah et al. [112]**	Pakistan	1995–1997	8541	72%	12%	10%	6%

*Approximately 27% of all Japanese thyroid cancer cases; **recalculated after exclusion of non-epithelial malignomas

the following ranges of proportions are reported in most literature: 40–80% for papillary, 10–40% for follicular, 1–10% for medullary and 2–14% for anaplastic carcinoma [37, 86]. Table 1.2 summarizes the data from various countries.

In general, subtype patterns from autopsy studies are similar to data from clinical incident thyroid malignancies, whereas data about prevalence and sex distribution differ. Thorough examination of complete thyroid glands from 500 autopsies in a Swedish population revealed in 8.6% carcinomas; 74% were papillary, 16% follicular and 9% medullary [15]. The male:female ratios of the main histological subtypes are reported with 1:3 in papillary and 1:2 in follicular carcinoma [37]. In Japan, where age-adjusted incidence rates of all thyroid cancer types in the year 1985 were 1.1/100,000 for men and 3.1/100,000 for women (with higher rates for Hiroshima and Nagasaki), the male:female ratio was 1:6 in papillary and follicular and 1:2 in medullary and anaplastic carcinomas, in contrast to the above-mentioned proportions [66].

In childhood and adolescence thyroid cancer is even rarer than in adults (incidence rates about 0.05/100,000) and accounts for 0.5–1.5% of all malignancies [21, 48]. The percentage of histological subtypes has been reported as 68–87% for papillary, 2.7–22% for follicular and 11–17% for medullary carcinoma in this age group [35, 44, 48]. In general, the male:female ratio for differentiated thyroid cancer is comparable to that in adults (about 1:2 for follicle cell derived carcinomas and 1:2–3 for medullary thyroid cancer), with the exception of puberty. The frequency of tumor cases reveals an increase with age, with a remarkable peak for females in puberty (especially pronounced for papillary thyroid carcinoma).

1.3 Prognosis

The overall prognosis for patients with thyroid cancer is one of the best among all cancers. It is therefore difficult to demonstrate a beneficial effect of diagnostic and therapeutic measures unless very large cohorts are studied over several decades. No such long-term prospective, randomized clinical trials have been done, and virtually all presently existing views of the efficacy of different treatments are based on retrospective studies [75]. Like data for incidence, histologic subtype pattern and mortality, data concerning prognosis differ from country to country.

Evaluation of 53,856 thyroid carcinoma cases from the National Cancer Database from the USA during the time period 1985–1995 revealed 5- and 10-year overall survival rates of 96 and 93% for patients with papillary carcinoma, 91 and 85% for follicular, 91 and 76% for Hürthle cell, 80 and 75% for medullary and 14% for undifferentiated/anaplastic carcinoma [58]. Data on the survival rates for undifferentiated/anaplastic carcinoma from this study were criticized as being overestimated, since no clear-cut distinction between poorly differentiated and anaplastic carcinomas had been performed [113]. In a population-based study of 15,698 cases from the Surveillance, Epidemiology and End Results (SEER) program in the USA during the time period 1973–1991, the following 5- and 10-year survival rates were reported [43]: 99 and 98% for papillary thyroid carcinoma (males 99 and 99% and females 99 and 98%), 95 and 92% for follicular thyroid carcinoma (males 95 and 90% and females 94 and 93%), 11% for anaplastic thyroid carcinoma (males 13% and females 11%), and 85 and 80% for medullary carcinoma (males 78 and 68% and females 89 and 87%). Apart from differences between the sexes and between tumor stages, markedly variations for different age and ethnic groups were obvious: increasing age was associated with lower relative survival for each histologic type.

The EUROCARE database does not contain data that make a calculation of survival rates for separate histological types possible. In general, the prognosis is significantly better in females than in males. The mean age-standardized, 5-year relative survival of adults diagnosed during 1990–1994 in the examined European countries for all age-groups was 74% for men and 85% for women, and was highest amongst young patients. In the age-group 15–44 years, the rate was 94% for men and 98% for women [110]. In contrast, much lower rates and substantial intercountry variation were seen among the two oldest age-groups (65–74 years and >75 years), with 58%/63% and 42%/37% for men/women, respectively. In Germany, the relative 5-year survival rates for females have been reported as 73.0% and 71.7% (West and East Germany) and for males, 54.5% and 63.9% [11]. Evaluating data from 337 patients with thyroid carcinoma during the time period 1960–1992 in the southeastern Netherlands [67], the following relative survival rates were calculated: 80% (males 76 and females 81%) for 5-year, 75% (males 72 and females 78%) for 10-year-, and 75% (males 70 and females 77%) for 20-year survival. According to the histological type, the relative 5-, 10-, 20-year survival rates were: 95%, 94%, 94% for papillary, 82%, 80%, 79% for papillary, 87%, 85%, 84% for medullary, and 5%, 0% for anaplastic carcinoma in this study.

Marked differences concerning the prognosis between the United States and European countries are evident. Even though the proportion of histologic types and some demographic data differ and also the medical standards may have been still lower in some European countries, a more aggressive tumor pattern in the European countries compared with the USA can be suggested. In Europe the mean 5-year survival rates between 1985 and 1989 for all thyroid cancer types together have been estimated with 67% (range between the countries: 57%

Table 1.3. Influence of tumor stage and age at diagnosis on the relative survival rates of differentiated thyroid cancer in the USA (from Gilliland et al. [43])

Stage at diagnosis	Papillary carcinoma		Follicular carcinoma	
	5-year	10-year	5-year	10-year
Local	100%	100%	100%	98%
Regional	97%	97%	89%	87%
Distant	82%	81%	60%	45%
Age <20 years	99%	99%	98%	99%
Age 40–49 years	99%	98%	98%	99%
Age ∅70 years	89%	86%	79%	70%

in Estonia to 100% in Austria) for men and 78% (range between the countries: 66% in Poland to 90% in Iceland) for women [122]. In comparison with these European data, the relative 5-year survival rate in the USA (mean from both sexes) is reported as 94% for the time period 1980–1982 and with 96% for the time period 1986–1993 [101]. The hypothesis that if the proportion of papillary carcinomas in a given country is high, the survival rate would also be higher than in countries with a lower proportion, did not always hold true. In fact, Iceland and Switzerland do have a high ratio of papillary/follicular carcinomas (4.2 and 2.9) and also higher than average survival rates. Yet, in the Netherlands a low papillary/follicular ratio but a high survival rate occurs [122].

Apart from histologic type and patient age, the most important prognostic factors in differentiated thyroid carcinoma are tumor size, tumor extension, tumor differentiation, the presence of metastases, and the treatment modalities. In the population-based study of 15,698 cases from the SEER program [43], stage at diagnosis, tumor differentiation, and histology were strong independent predictors of risk, although the relative effect varied by histologic type (some examples are given in Table 1.3). Comparing follicular and papillary carcinoma, prognosis was found to be more strongly determined by stage at diagnosis, age, and tumor differentiation than by the follicular or papillary histology. In contrast, studies are not consistent regarding the prognostic importance of sex in papillary and follicular carcinoma [43]. A number of prognostic scoring systems have been introduced for thyroid cancer, such as EORTC, AGES, AMES, MACIS, OSU, and SKMMC (AACE 1997); however, in a comparative study none of these scoring systems showed clear advantages over the TNM scoring system of the AJCC and the UICC [19].

1.4 Thyroid Malignancies with Special Features

Some subentities of follicle cell-derived thyroid cancer types such as Hürthle cell carcinoma, poorly differentiated (insular) carcinoma, and special variants of papillary carcinoma (like tall-cell, columnar cell, diffuse sclerosing, or diffuse follicular variant) are assigned to the group of papillary or follicular thyroid carcinomas, applying the current WHO histological classification. Therefore, in most statistics they do not appear as separate entities, although they differ from the usual follicular and papillary carcinomas in several epidemiological features. Medullary and non-epithelial thyroid malignomas also show some differences in epidemiology. For that reason, some special subentities are treated separately in this section.

1.4.1 Papillary Microcarcinoma

Initially, Woolner et al. [136] defined the term "occult papillary carcinoma" for a tumor with maximum diameter of 1.5 cm or less. This has been replaced by the term papillary microcarcinoma with a maximum diameter of 1.0 cm or less according to the WHO definition and the pT1 stage of the TNM classification (5th edition).

The low metastatic potential of these lesions is shown by their high prevalence as incidental findings in autopsy studies, 6 to 9% being recorded in the United States, Canada, Japan, Germany, Portugal, Poland and Sweden [16, 42, 68, 109, 117], 18% in Hiroshima and Nagasaki [107], 24% in Honolulu and in the Japanese population in Hawaii [41, 42], and maximum 35% in Finland [39, 49]. The determined frequencies depend on the thickness and completeness of slices microscopically examined. The more closely the gland is studied, the more frequently such lesions are found. When serial sections are examined, the prevalence of microscopic thyroid cancer is as high as 13% in the United States [88] and 29% in Japan [106]. In nearly 37% of cases, papillary microcarcinoma occurs in multicentric fashion, frequently in both thyroid lobes. The evaluation of various studies revealed an average frequency of clinical occult lymph node metastases of 28%. Lymph node metastases particularly occur in multicentric microcarcinomas [108], their prevalence further depends on size and ultrastructural features of the tumor. Distant metastases are extremely rare [121].

In the majority of autopsy studies, no significant difference in the prevalence rate of occult papillary microcarcinoma has been demonstrated between the sexes [17], in sharp contrast to clinically apparent papillary carcinoma, which is more common in women. Furthermore, most autopsy studies have demonstrated no age-related difference in prevalence of papillary microcarcinoma [17]. The incidence of clinically apparent papillary carcinoma is not proportional to the prevalence of papillary microcarcinomas between different countries. In Japan for example, the prevalence of papillary microcarcinoma but not the incidence of clinical apparent papillary carcinoma is higher than in the USA or in Germany.

These epidemiological data support the hypothesis that the majority of papillary microcarcinoma constitutes a separate entity with very low morbidity and mortality. Referring to the reported prevalence data, Sampson [106] calculated a number of 28,400 expected cases of occult papillary microcarcinoma in the 100,000 people of the JNIH-ABCC Life Span Study in Japan. In contrast, within 15 years of follow-up only 90 cases of thyroid carcinoma became clinically apparent and only 5 tumor-caused deaths occurred in this collective. In a recently published Japanese study on 178 patients with papillary microcarcinoma, the cause-specific 10-year survival rate was reported as 96% [121].

1.4.2 Hürthle Cell Carcinoma

With reference to the current WHO histological classification [52], Hürthle cell (oxyphilic) carcinomas of the thyroid are mostly assigned to the group of follicular carcinoma, accounting for about 15–20% of follicular carcinomas. Oxyphilic variants of papillary thyroid carcinoma are even rarer, their frequency is reported at about 2% [118]. In most publications with large patient groups, the contribution of Hürthle cell carcinoma on all thyroid carcinomas is reported at only about 3–6% [28, 46, 47, 124, 132].

The overall manifestation age ranges between the fourth and seventh decade, with a mean age in the fifth decade. As with other thyroid malignancies, there is a predominance of this lesion in women, with a male:female ratio of 1:2–7. Patients with this tumor entity have a poorer prognosis than patients with papillary and follicular carcinoma. The overall 5-year survival rate is in the range of 85% and the 10-year survival rate in the range of 70% [46, 47, 61]. The rate of relapses and metastases is reported as being up to 50% [76]. If distant metastases are present, the 5-year survival rate decreases to the range of 60% [61, 102]. In most patients with metastases, radioiodine accumulation is absent or insufficient for therapeutic effects.

1.4.3 Histological Variants of Papillary Thyroid Cancer

About two-thirds of all papillary thyroid carcinomas are assigned to the classic type, and one-third are variants which have in part special epidemiological features (e.g., concerning frequency, age, and sex distribution). Regarding the prognosis of the subtypes mentioned below, most authors agree that it is worse than in the classic type, whereas Wenig et al. [134] and Akslen and LiVolsi [4] argue that subclassification of papillary carcinoma has only a minor prognostic impact if histological staging and grading are taken into consideration.

The *tall-cell variant* of papillary thyroid carcinoma is associated with a higher incidence of recurrence and mortality as compared with the "classic" papillary carcinomas [62, 81, 127]. Hawk and Hazard [51] first described this entity as "well differentiated papillary thyroid cancer in which the cells were columnar shaped and twice as high as they were wide". Referring to Johnsson et al. [62], the tall-cell variant is defined as a papillary thyroid cancer of the thyroid in which a minimum of 30% of the cells have a height at least twice their width, indicating a more aggressive pattern of growth. A histologic re-examination of the operative specimen from 162 patients with papillary thyroid carcinomas [103] revealed 11 cases (6.8%) of tall-cell variant underlying Johnsson's criteria and 9% underlying Hawk's criteria; prior to re-examination, only 3 cases (1.9%) of tall-cell variant were described. The mean patient age is 57 years (compared to 30–39 years for the "classic" papillary carcinoma). In many studies of differentiated thyroid cancer no tall-cell variants at all have been reported, indicating that its identification is difficult.

One to seven percent of papillary carcinomas belong to the *columnar-cell variant* [4, 79, 84]. As an exception to the rule among thyroid papillary carcinomas, men are significantly more affected than women by this subtype. Other forms with aggressive clinical behavior are the *diffuse sclerosing* and the *diffuse follicular variant*, each comprising about 1–2% of all papillary carcinomas in most series [4, 60, 82]. The latter differs significantly from the classic type of papillary carcinoma in targeting younger patients and in exhibiting a prevalence of multicentricity, extrathyroid extension, and vascular invasion [60].

1.4.4 Poorly Differentiated (Insular) Thyroid Carcinoma

Poorly differentiated (insular) thyroid carcinoma is a rare entity, situated morphologically and biologically between well differentiated (papillary or follicular) carcinoma and anaplastic thyroid carcinoma. Its histopathologic criteria were first defined by Carcangiu et al. [22]. The frequency is described as 4–6% of all carcinomas of follicular cell origin [7, 22, 127] and appears to be higher in some parts of Europe and South America than in the United States. There are relatively more males (41%) affected than in well-differentiated thyroid carcinomas, and the average age of manifestation is quite high at 49 years. Coexistence of well-differentiated tumor parts with anaplastic areas as well as a mix of tall-cell and insular carcinoma can occur within the same lesion [127]. Metastases frequently arise in lymph nodes and in distant organs. Like in the tall-cell variant of papillary thyroid carcinoma, the most undifferentiated part of the tumor determines the prognosis. The overall prognosis is worse than in differentiated follicular carcinoma, especially in those frequently observed cases, in which radioiodine accumulation of metastases is absent. The 5- and 10-year overall survival rates have been reported with 30-65% and 25-35%, respectively [131].

1.4.5 Anaplastic Carcinoma

The frequency of anaplastic carcinoma of the thyroid is reported as 1% to 14% of primary malignant thyroid neoplasms [3, 58, 86, 105]. The reported higher frequencies are probably due to the inaccurate distinction between poorly differentiated and classic anaplastic carcinoma in some studies [3, 100, 113]. The mean male:female ratio is 1:1.3–3.5 with a peak in the seventh decade of life [23, 119]. Concomitant well-differentiated thyroid carcinoma is found in 35–55% [30, 73, 99, 119, 130], supporting the hypothesis that anaplastic carcinoma arises from pre-existing well-differentiated carcinoma. In countries where the endemic iodine deficiency has been compensated, a marked decrease of the undifferentiated and anaplastic thyroid carcinoma types chargeable to the differentiated (especially papillary) types was registered.

The mean duration of survival is 2–12 months, and the 2- and 5-year survival rates have been reported as no more than 4–5% [30, 73, 130]. Published higher survival rates may be due to inaccurate distinction between poorly differentiated and anaplastic carcinomas [113]. Patients selected for surgical resection, absence of distant metastases at presentation, young age, and tumor size less than 6 cm were associated with an increased survival time [73].

1.4.6 Medullary Thyroid Carcinoma

Medullary carcinoma was first recognized as a separate entity in 1959 [52]; until then it had been assigned to the group of undifferentiated thyroid carcinoma. It accounts for 5–12% of all thyroid cancers [97, 112]. Whereas the contribution of hereditary forms was previously believed to be about 20%, it is now estimated as 30% [27, 97], which is probably due to the improved registration of familial forms and progress in molecular genetic diagnostics. The familial form of medullary thyroid carcinoma (MTC; as only a manifestation or as part of MEN II) is transmitted in autosomal dominant manner with a high degree (>90%) of penetrance. Among all thyroid malignomas, the exact genetic mechanisms (*RET* proto-oncogene) are best understood in MTC.

The average annual incidence of MTC is reported to be 0.1–0.2/100,000 [12, 55]. The age-standardized incidence rate in Sweden 1959–1981 was 0.18 for males and 0.23 for females [12]. Its frequency among all thyroid malignomas has been reported to be about 2–10% in various countries: as 2% for Italy 1977–1981 and Switzerland 1974–1987 [10, 70], 3.7% in the USA 1985–1990 and 3.5% in the USA 1991–1995 [58], 3.6% in Norway 1956–1978 [55], 4% in Sweden 1960–1977 [26], and 10% in Great Britain 1985–1996 [92]. In children and teenagers, the frequency was 10.8% [44]. In Germany, the mean age at diagnosis for all patients was 43.9±17.0 years [97]. The age-specific incidence of sporadic medullary carcinoma increases markedly with age (peaking in the fourth decade), whereas no significant rise was found after age 20 for familial disease [12]. The overall male:female ratios are 1:1.3–1.6 [18, 80, 97]. The male:female ratios in Germany are 1:1.4 for sporadic forms, 1:2.2 for MEN IIb and familial MTC and 1:1.0 for MEN IIa [97].

The overall survival rates for patients with MTC are reported to be 80–87% at 5 years, and 65–78% at 10 years [13, 25, 80, 97]. The worst prognostic factors are: extensive tumor and higher tumor stages, male sex, age older than 45 years, and sporadic MTC [13, 97]. Modigliani et al. [80] calculated a 10-year survival rate of 98% in "biochemically cured" patients (postoperative normalized calcitonin levels) and 70% in non-cured patients.

1.4.7 Thyroid Lymphoma

After the above-mentioned epithelial tumors, lymphomas are the most frequent primary thyroidal malignomas. Primary lymphomas of the thyroid account for approximately 2% of extranodal lymphomas and far less than 5% of all thyroid malignancies. The most common histological type is non-Hodgkin's lymphoma, accounting for 93%, especially the large-cell variant [114]. The mean age is 73 years for men and 63 years for women, and the mean male:female ratio is about 1:4–6 [93, 95].

Eighty-three percent of the patients have evidence of chronic lymphocytic thyroiditis, indicated by antithyroid antibodies and histology [6]. In a Japanese study, thyroid lymphoma was increased 80 fold in patients with pre-existing chronic thyroiditis compared to the expectation in the general population [64]. The overall cause-specific 5-year survival is published as 46–82%, and the influence of whether patients are treated with external radiotherapy alone or with combined radiotherapy and chemotherapy on these rates is discussed controversial [63, 93, 95, 125]. Unfavorable prognostic factors are tumor bulk, infiltration of the perithyroidal tissue, high stage of disease and (to a lesser extent) older age of the patient, whereas the histological subtype appears not to be a significant determinant of prognosis [63, 95, 125].

1.4.8 Secondary Tumors

Whereas clinically detected metastasis to the thyroid gland is rare, it has been shown in some autopsy series to be more common than primary thyroid malignancy (with the exception of occult papillary microcarcinoma). The overall incidence in autopsy series varies between 1.25 and 2.8% in unselected autopsy studies to 24% in patients with widespread malignant neoplasms [36, 85]. In most autopsy series, breast and lung carcinomas are the two most frequent metastatic diseases to the thyroid gland. In contrast, renal cell carcinoma is usually the most frequent source of metastasis in clinical series [50]. On the other hand, only a small number of patients with renal cell carcinoma present with metastasis to the thyroid gland, although in 60–70% of patients metastases develop in the course of the disease [90, 128]. Whereas 80% of overall metastases in the thyroid present within 3 years of primary tumor resection, in renal cell cancer time intervals of up to one or two decades are not uncommon [24, 85].

1.5 Changes in Epidemiology

In a number of cancer registries, an increased incidence of overall thyroid cancer has been observed during the past decades, including the USA, Canada (males), Japan, Germany, UK, east European and Nordic countries [37]. The time course of this increase and the proportion of histologic subtypes, sexes and age groups differ from country to country. This increase cannot be explained only with improvements in diagnostic sensitivity and capture of cancer data, though these factors indeed exert an influence. Devesa et al. [31] assessed incidence trends among the white population of six geographical areas in the USA, including data from the SEER program; they reported an increase in thyroid cancer incidence of more than 75% in both sexes from the late 1940s to the late 1970s, with stabilization thereafter until 1983/1984 (end of the observed period). In males, the most evident increases occurred in the age group 60 years and older, whereas in females an earlier peak occurred in the age group 20–39 years [31, 133]. In contrast, the age-specific mortality curves for both sexes increase with age, but the overall mortality rates declined during the period of the study.

In another study from the USA, Zheng et al. [139] analyzed epidemiological changes in Connecticut during the period 1935–1992. Again, they calculated an overall increase of age-standardized incidence rate of all thyroid cancer types, from 0.3 (in 1935–1939) to 2.77 (in 1990–1992) in males and from 1.30 (in 1935–1939) to 5.78 (in 1990–92) in females, mainly due to papillary carcinoma. Their birth cohort analyses indicated that the increase occurred among the cohorts born between 1915 and 1945, whereas a decreasing incidence was calculated for those born since the 1945 cohort. Results from age-period-cohort modeling revealed a strong birth cohort effect of increase in incidence, which closely follows the introduction of X-radiation therapy for benign conditions of the head and neck in childhood between 1920 and the 1950s in the USA. In England and Wales during the time period 1962–1984, a significant increase in thyroid carcinoma was also observed for both sexes [32]. The observed peak of cancer risk in women born in 1952–1955 was hypothesized to be a carcinogenic effect of fallout radiation from atmospheric nuclear weapon tests in the late 1950s and early 1960s when these women were children.

An analysis of thyroid cancer cases registered at the Japanese Cancer Registry revealed gradually increased incidence rates for both sexes over the study period 1959–1985, but no significant change in the histological subtype distribution [66]. In the Swiss canton of Vaud, the incidence rates for men compared with women were 1.36 and 4.28 in the time period 1974–1980 and 1.74 and 4.51 in the time period 1981–1987 [70]. In a study from Slovakia, examining data from 1968 to 1990, an increase of thyroid cancer over this period from approximately 1.5 to 2.5/100,000 has been reported [96]. This increase concerns predominantly women, younger age groups and papillary carcinomas. In a study of 10,736 biopsy specimens presenting diverse thyroid gland pathology from Bulgaria over the time period 1974–1993 [78], an increase of frequency for malignancy from 4.03% in the first to 6.63% in the second decade has been reported with a peak in the period 1986–1993 (again particularly for women, younger age groups and papillary carcinomas), indicating that not only the incidence but also the prevalence of thyroid cancer increases. Yeole [138] found an increasing trend in age-adjusted incidence rate in both sexes for the area of Bombay in the period under review 1964–1993, but this increase was found to be statistically significant only in males.

In Germany, continuous incidence data since 1970 were only available from the cancer registries of the state Saarland and of the former German Democratic Republic. Calculating the mean world age-standardized incidence rates of the time periods 1970–1979 and 1980–1989 based on the available data, a tendency of increase for both sexes is obvious: in males from 1.12 (1970–1979) up to 1.63 (1980–1989) and from 0.79 up to 1.17 (Saarland compared with former GDR), in females from 2.58 (1970–1979) up to 3.60 (1980–1989) and from 1.56 up to 2.60 (Saarland compared with former GDR). Studying the incidence pattern of 4,691 thyroid cancer cases in Norway 1955–1989, Akslen et al. [5] reported about a twofold increase for both sexes, but a decline especially among females during the last 5-year period. Similarly, Hrafnkelsson et al. [57], examining thyroid cancer in Iceland 1955–1984, noted a considerable increase in the incidence around 1965, but a subsequent decrease in the last 5 years of the study report.

The mean size of the cancer nodules at diagnosis decreased and survival rates of patients improved, leading to nearly constant mortality rates during this 30-year period. Pettersson et al. [94] examined trends in thyroid cancer incidence in Sweden during the period 1958–1981 (5,838 clinically apparent cases) and observed a mean annual increase in the age-standardized incidence rates of 1.2% in males and 1.9% in females.

In a number of countries, the observed trend of increase for thyroid cancer incidence seems to continue through the 1990s. For the USA, the data of the NCDB show an overall increase in reported thyroid carcinoma cases, but the proportional representation of the histological subtypes varies only slightly comparing the time periods 1985–1990 and 1991–1995 [58]. In Germany, incidence rates for the entire national territory are not yet available. Combining the data from the cancer registry of the German state Saarland – which have been available for the last three decades – in 5-year intervals, the mean world age-standardized incidence rates (per 100,000 per year) show a continuous increase from the period 1971–1975 (0.9 in men and 2.14 in women) up to a peak in the period 1991–1995 (2.29 in men and 5.71 in women); however, this trend will not necessarily continue in the future, because the rates for the period 1996–2000 show a slight decrease (1.78 in men and 4.35 in women).

A distinct epidemiological situation has resulted from the Chernobyl nuclear power plant accident in 1986. By 4 years after the accident, a significant rise of thyroid cancer incidence (in about 95% papillary carcinoma) had been observed in the radioiodine-contaminated regions of the former USSR (southern Belarus, northern Ukraine, and southwestern Russia). The incidence further increased in the mid-1990s and has not yet returned to normal [59, 89]. In the largest proportion, the increase concerns subjects of both sexes who were less than 5 years old at the time of exposure. The maximum increase occurred in Belarus and has been reported to be 75-fold in children, about 10-fold in adolescents, and about 3.5-fold in adults, while the incidence in this region before 1990 was low and comparable with other European countries or the USA. Artificial effects on these data due to intensified screening have been proved to be of minor importance, as demonstrated by a recent case-control study [8]. Chapter 16 of this book is dedicated especially to thyroid cancer in Chernobyl children.

Outside the abovementioned regions, epidemiological consequences for thyroid cancer cannot be finally assessed at present. Mangano [74] has reported a minor, but significant post-Chernobyl rise in some states of the USA (Connecticut, Iowa, and Utah). In Connecticut, the age-adjusted incidence rate increased from 0.16 (1985–1989) to 0.31/100,000 (1990–1992) among children aged under 15 years, and from 0.35 to 0.43/100,000 for all age-groups; after 10 years there was no change. However, Sali et al. [104] have found no evidence of a major epidemiological change in countries of Europe outside the former USSR, and a recently published study from Turkey could not demonstrate significant effects, too [33].

Concerning the distribution of histological types, the worldwide predominantly observed trend is an increased frequency of papillary carcinoma, and, in parallel, a decrease of anaplastic carcinoma. In a German study, Freitag et al. [40] compared the proportions of histologic subtypes thyroidectomized in a department of general surgery between 1982–1989 and 1990–1997 and reported a significant increase of papillary carcinoma from 50% to 75% in combination with a decrease of anaplastic carcinoma from 14% to 3%. In a study from Italy, the ratio of papillary to follicular carcinoma even varied from 0.60 in the time period 1974–1976 to 6.88 in 1992–1994 [29]. In a Swedish study on changes in thyroid cancer epidemiology during the period 1958–1981 [94], the annual increase in the age-standardized incidence was predominant in papillary carcinoma (average 2.1% in males and 4.9% in females) and less pronounced in follicular carcinoma (average 2.1% in males and 0.9% in females). In the same time period, an annual decrease in the age-standardized incidence rates was observed for anaplastic carcinomas (average –2.1% in males and –1.0% in females). In iodine-deficient areas, the risk of papillary and anaplastic carcinoma was lower while follicular cancer risk (for men only) was twice as high in these areas.

Swiss studies demonstrated in the 1970s, that the introduction of iodine prophylaxis in a region with prevalent iodine-deficiency led to a shift in the proportion of histologic subtypes resulting in more papillary and fewer anaplastic carcinomas [20]. More recent studies from Austria [9, 72, 111] support this hypothesis and demonstrate that not only the relative contribution but also the incidence of papillary carcinoma increases following supplementation of iodine deficiency. In the area of Tyrol (iodized salt prophylaxis since 1963, elevated since 1992), the absolute incidence rate of thyroid carcinoma rose from 3.07 (period 1957–1970) to 7.8 (1990–1994). During this time, the proportion of papillary carcinoma increased from 21% to 55%, follicular carcinoma remained constant with 37.8%, and the proportion of anaplastic carcinoma decreased from 28.4% to 3.5%. In parallel, a shift to less advanced tumor stages was obvious. These changes significantly improved the prognosis (current 5-year survival rate of 90.7%, compared with 73% in the 1960s). The net effect is a stabilization or even a decrease of mortality rates, observing long-term trends from the period 1956–1965 to 1985–1989: in Switzerland from 1.4 to 0.7 in males and 1.6 to 0.7 in females, and in Austria from 1.2 to 0.6 in males and from 1.7 to 0.8 in females [37].

Even in countries with less pronounced differences in the development of iodine intake during the last decades, the overall mortality rates have tended

Table 1.4. Age-standardized mortality rates for overall cancer and for thyroid cancer in Germany (from Becker and Wahrendorf [10])

Sex	West Germany Male	Female	East Germany Male	Female
1955	Overall cancer 152.8	Overall cancer 128.0	–	–
	Thyroid cancer 0.5	Thyroid cancer 0.9	–	–
1983	Overall cancer 182.2	Overall cancer 113.4	Overall cancer 165.8	Overall cancer 104.1
	Thyroid cancer 0.6	Thyroid cancer 0.8	Thyroid cancer 0.6	Thyroid cancer 0.8
1995	Overall cancer 169.4	Overall cancer 104.4	Overall cancer 182.0	Overall cancer 104.3
	Thyroid cancer 0.6	Thyroid cancer 0.6	Thyroid cancer 0.4	Thyroid cancer 0.7

to decrease, in contrast to the increasing trend for thyroid cancer incidence. In the USA, a continuous, statistically significant trend towards improved survival rates has been registered for thyroid cancer: the 5-year relative survival rate in the white population was 83% in the years 1960–1963 and increased to 96% in the years 1986–1993 [101]. In Europe, the EUROCARE II study showed consistent improvements of the 5-year relative survival rates between 1978 and 1989 only in Denmark (for men), Sweden (for men) and Scotland (for both sexes), whereas in Finland, England and Italy survival was largely unchanged [122]. Regarding the expanded time period from 1955 to 1994, mortality rates for thyroid cancer declined in most European countries, except Hungary and Spain [37, 71]. It is not yet clear in which proportions this reflects improvements in diagnosis and treatment of thyroid neoplasms, including better control of benign thyroid disease (which are the proven strongest risk factor for thyroid cancer, apart from radiation during childhood [38]), or changes of the pattern in favor of less aggressive tumor types.

For Germany, age-standardized and sex-specific mortality rates for thyroid cancer have been available since 1955 (West Germany) and since 1983 (East Germany). Regarding all available data (extracts in Table 1.4), the rates in men vary between 0.4 and 0.7 without significant trend; in women there has been a decrease since the 1980s, from previously about 0.9 to up to 0.6 [11]. The recent available German data derive from the year 2000, displaying a world age-standardized mortality rate of 0.43 for men and 0.45 for women [98].

In their study from Japan, Yamashita et al. [137] focussed on changing prognostic trends for 2,423 patients with papillary carcinoma during the observation period 1965–1990. The prognosis continuously improved, reflected by an increase in the 10-year disease-specific survival rate from 95.5% in the group thyroidectomized in 1965–1973 to 98.2% in the group thyroidectomized in 1983–1990. In the same time period, the mean tumor size decreased, which was explained by earlier tumor diagnosis, and the patient's age increased.

1.6 Summary

Clinically recognized thyroid cancer accounts for less than 1% of human malignancies. In the mean, females are affected 1.5–3 times more often than males. The prevalence of occult thyroid malignancy is up to a factor of 10^4 higher than the incidence of clinical recognized thyroid cancer, and the cause-specific mortality rate is, for its part, about 3–10 times lower than the average incidence rate (about 1.5/100,000 per year in men and 3/100,000 per year in women). The rarity and favorable prognosis of clinically recognized thyroid cancer cause specific problems for epidemiological studies. There is a lack of long-term prospective, randomized clinical trials with large cohorts, which would be necessary to demonstrate changes in epidemiology and effects of environmental factors or improvements of medical methods on this data. Currently, the majority of available data on thyroid cancer derive from retrospective studies or from cancer registry databases. Additionally, the wider use and the improvement in sensitivity of diagnostic methods (especially ultrasound) influence epidemiologic data such as prevalence and incidence and complicate the comparison with historical data.

Despite these problems in obtaining valid epidemiological data, the following trends are obvious in the majority of countries:

- The overall incidence of thyroid cancer has increased in both sexes during the past decades, but the latest available data do not indicate whether this trend will further continue.
- This increase is mainly due to papillary thyroid cancer, whereas anaplastic carcinoma has become rarer.
- Especially in countries where preexisting iodine deficiency has been supplemented, the above-mentioned current trend can be observed: not only the relative contribution, but also the incidence of papillary carcinoma has increased markedly.
- In contrast, the overall cause-specific mortality has remained constant or even declined, reflecting the growing proportion of less aggressive cancer types and the medical improvements leading to tumor detection at earlier stages.

References

1. AACE (1997) Clinical practical guidelines for the management of thyroid carcinoma. Endocr Pract 3:60–71
2. Abu-Eshy SA, Khan AR, Khan GM, al-Humaidi MA, al-Shehri MY, Malatani TS (1995) Thyroid malignancy in multinodular goitre and solitary nodules. J R Coll Surg Edinb 40:310–312
3. Agrawal S, Rao RS, Parikh DM, Parikh HK, Borges AM, Sampat MB (1996) Histologic trends in cancer 1969–1993: a clinico-pathologic analysis of the relative proportion of anaplastic carcinoma of the thyroid. J Surg Oncol 63:251–255
4. Akslen LA, LiVolsi VA (2000) Prognostic significance of histological grading compared with subclassification of papillary thyroid carcinoma. Cancer 88:1902–1908
5. Akslen LA, Haldorsen T, Thoresen SO, Glattre E (1993) Incidence pattern of thyroid cancer in Norway: influence of birth cohort and time period. Int J Cancer 53:183–187
6. Aozasa K, Inoue A, Tajima K, Miyauchi A, Matsuzuka F, Kuma K (1986) Malignant lymphomas of the thyroid gland. Analysis of 79 patients with emphasis on histological prognostic factors. Cancer 58:100–104
7. Ashfaq R, Vuitch F, Delgado R, Albores-Saavedra J (1994) Papillary and follicular thyroid carcinomas with an insular component. Cancer 73:416–423
8. Astakhova LN, Anspaugh LR, Beebe GW, et al (1998) Chernobyl-related thyroid cancer in children of Belarus: a case-control study. Radiat Res 150:349–356
9. Bacher-Stier C, Riccabona G, Totsch M, Kemmler G, Oberaigner W, Moncayo R (1997) Incidence and clinical characteristics of thyroid carcinoma after iodine prophylaxis in an endemic goiter country. Thyroid 7:733–741
10. Baroni CD, Manente L, Maccallini V, Di Matteo G (1983) Primary malignant tumors of the thyroid gland. Histology, age and sex distribution and pathologic correlations in 139 cases. Tumori 69:205–213
11. Becker N, Wahrendorf J (1998) Atlas of cancer mortality in the Federal Republic of Germany 1981–1990, 3rd edn. Springer, Berlin Heidelberg New York
12. Bergholm U, Adami HO, Telenius-Berg M, Johansson H, Wilander E (1990) Incidence of sporadic and familial medullary thyroid carcinoma in Sweden 1959 through 1981. A nationwide study in 126 patients. Swedish MCT Study Group. Acta Oncol 29:9–15

13. Bergholm U, Bergström R, Ekbom A (1997) Long-term follow-up of patients with medullary carcinoma of the thyroid. Cancer 79:132–138
14. Black RJ, Bray F, Ferlay J, Parkin DM (1997) Cancer incidence and mortality in the European Union: cancer registry data and estimates of national incidence for 1990. Eur J Cancer 33:1075–1107
15. Bondeson L, Ljungberg O (1981) Occult thyroid carcinoma at autopsy in Malmö, Sweden. Cancer 47:319–323
16. Bondeson L, Ljunberg O (1984) Occult papillary thyroid carcinoma in the young and the aged. Cancer 53:1790–1792
17. Bramley MD, Harisson BJ (1996) Papillary microcarcinoma of the thyroid gland. Br J Surg 83:1674–1683
18. Brierley J, Tsang R, Simpson WJ, Gospodarowicz M, Sutcliffe S, Panzarella T (1996) Medullary thyroid cancer: analyses of survival and prognostic factors and the role of radiation therapy in local control. Thyroid 6:305–310
19. Brierley JD, Panzarella T, Tsang RW, Gospodarowicz MK, O'Sullivan B (1997) A comparison of different staging systems predictability of patient outcome: thyroid carcinoma as an example. Cancer 79:2414–2423
20. Bubenhofer R, Hedinger C (1977) Schilddrüsenmalignome vor und nach Einführung der Jodsalzprophylaxe. Schweiz Med Wochenschr 107:733–741
21. Bucsky P, Parlowsky T (1997) Epidemiology and therapy of thyroid cancer in childhood and adolescence. Exp Clin Endocrinol Diabetes 105 [Suppl 4]:70–73
22. Carcangiu ML, Zampi G, Rosai J (1984) Poorly differentiated („insular") thyroid carcinoma. A reinterpretation of Langhans „wuchernde Struma." Am J Surg Pathol 8:655–668
23. Chang TC, Liaw KY, Kuo SH, Chang CC, Chen FW (1989) Anaplastic thyroid carcinoma: review of 24 cases, with emphasis on cytodiagnosis and leukocytosis. Taiwan I Hsueh Hui Tsa Chih 88:551–556
24. Chen H, Nicol TL, Udelsman R (1999) Clinically significant, isolated metastatic disease to the thyroid gland. World J Surg 23:177–180
25. Chong GC, Beahrs OH, Sizemore GW, Woolner LH (1975) Medullary carcinoma of the thyroid gland. Cancer 35:695–704
26. Christensen SB, Ljungberg O, Tibblin S (1984) A clinical epidemiological study of thyroid carcinoma in Malmö, Sweden. Curr Probl Cancer 8:1–49
27. Cohen R, Modigliani E (1993) Medullary thyroid carcinoma: 25 years on. Cancer J 6:59–64
28. Cooper DS, Schneyer CR (1990) Follicular and Hürthle cell carcinoma of the thyroid. Endocrinol Metab Clin North Am 19:577–591
29. Deandrea M, Gallone G, Veglio M, et al (1997) Thyroid cancer histotype changes as observed in a major general hospital in a 21-year period. J Endocrinol Invest 20:52–58
30. Demeter JG, Jong SA de, Lawrence AM, Paloyan E (1991) Anaplastic thyroid carcinoma: risk factors and outcome. Surgery 110:956–961
31. Devesa SS, Silverman DT, Young JL Jr, et al (1987) Cancer incidence and mortality trends among whites in the USA, 1947–1984. J Natl Cancer Inst 79:701–770
32. Dos Santos Silva I, Swerdlow AJ (1993) Thyroid cancer epidemiology in England and Wales: time trends and geographical distribution. Br J Cancer 67:330–340
33. Emral R, Bastemir M, Güllü S, Erdogan G (2003) Thyroid consequences of the Chernobyl nuclear power station accident on the Turkish population. Eur J Endocrinol 148:497–503
34. Ezaki H, Ebihara S, Fujimoto Y (1992) Analysis of thyroid carcinoma based on material registered in Japan during 1977–1986 with special reference to predominance of papillary type. Cancer 15:808–814
35. Farahati J, Parlowsky T, Mäder U, Reiners C, Bucsky P (1998) Differentiated thyroid cancer in children and adolescents. Langenbecks Arch Surg 383:235–239
36. Fleischmann A, Hardmeier T (1999) A normal thyroid gland upon autopsy: a relatively uncommon finding. Schweiz Med Wochenschr 129:873–882

37. Franceschi S, La Vecchia C (1994) Thyroid cancer. Cancer Surv 19–20:393–422
38. Franceschi S, Preston-Martin S, Maso L dal, et al (1999) A pooled analysis of case-control studies of thyroid cancer. IV. Benign thyroid diseases. Cancer Causes Control 10:583–595
39. Franssila KO, Harach HR (1985) Occult papillary carcinoma of the thyroid in children and young adults. A systemic autopsy study in Finland. Cancer 58:715–719
40. Freitag T, Baier A, Dewitz D (1999) Alters- und Geschlechtsverteilung beim primären Schilddrüsenmalignom in Abhängigkeit vom Tumortyp. Zentrabl Chir 124:331–335
41. Fukunaga FH, Lockett LJ (1971) Thyroid carcinoma in the Japanese in Hawaii. Arch Pathol 92:6–13
42. Fukunaga FH, Yatani R (1975) Geographic pathology of occult thyroid carcinomas. Cancer 36:1095–1099
43. Gilliland FD, Hunt WC, Morris DM, Key CR (1997) Prognostic factors for thyroid carcinoma: a population-based study of 15,698 cases for the Surveillance, Epidemiology and End Results (SEER) program 1973–1991. Cancer 79:564–573
44. Goepfert H, Dichtel WJ, Samaan NA (1984) Thyroid cancer in children and teenagers. Arch Otolaryngol 110:72–75
45. Goodman MT, Yoshizawa CN, Kolonel LN (1988) Descriptive epidemiology of thyroid cancer in Hawaii. Cancer 61:1272–1281
46. Hamann A, Gratz KF, Soudah B, Fritsch RS, Georgii A, Hundeshagen H (1992) The clinical course of oxyphilic carcinoma of the thyroid. Nuklearmedizin 31:230–238
47. Har-El G, Hadar T, Segal K, Levy R, Sidi J (1986) Hürthle cell carcinoma of the thyroid gland. A tumor of moderate malignancy. Cancer 57:1613–1617
48. Harach HR, Williams ED (1995) Childhood thyroid cancer in England and Wales. Br J Cancer 72:777–783
49. Harach HR, Franssila KO, Wasenius VM (1985) Occult papillary carcinoma of the thyroid: A "normal" finding in Finland: a systematic autopsy study. Cancer 56:531–538
50. Haugen BR, Nawaz S, Cohn A et al (1994) Secondary malignancy of the thyroid gland: a case report and review of the literature. Thyroid 4:297–300
51. Hawk W, Hazard J (1976) The many appearances of papillary carcinoma of the thyroid. Cleve Clin Q 43:207
52. Hazard JB, Hawk WA, Crile G Jr (1959) Medullary (solid) carcinoma of the thyroid, a clinico-pathologic entity. J Clin Endocrinol 19:152–161
53. Hedinger C, Sobin LH (1974) Histological typing of thyroid tumors. (International histological classification of tumours, no. 11) World Health Organisation, Geneva
54. Hedinger C, Williams ED, Sobin LH (1988) Histological typing of thyroid tumors, 2nd edn. (International histological classification of tumours, no 11) World Health Organisation. Springer, Berlin Heidelberg New York
55. Hoie J, Jorgensen OG, Stenwig AE, Langmark F (1988) Medullary thyroid cancer in Norway. A 30-year experience. Acta Chir Scand 154:339–343
56. Horlocker TT, Hay ID, James EM, et al (1986) Prevalence of incidental nodular thyroid disease detected during high-resolution parathyroid ultrasonography. In: Medeiros-Neto G, Gaitan E (eds) Frontiers of thyroidology, vol 2. Plenum, New York, pp 1309–1312
57. Hrafnkelsson J, Jonasson JG, Sigurdsson G, Sigvaldason H, Tulinius H (1988) Thyroid cancer in Iceland 1955–1984. Acta Endocrinol (Copenh) 118:566–572
58. Hundahl SA, Fleming ID, Fremgen AM, Menck HR (1998) A national cancer database report on 53,856 cases of thyroid carcinoma treated in the US, 1985–1995. Cancer 82:2638–2648
59. Ivanov VK, Gorsky AI, Tysb AF, Maksyutov MA, Rastopchin EM (1999) Dynamics of thyroid cancer incidence in Russia following the Chernobyl accident. J Radiol Prot 19:305–318
60. Ivanova R, Soares P, Castro P, Sobrinho-Simoes M. (2003) Diffuse (or multinodular) follicular variant of papillary thyroid carcinoma: a clinicopathologic and immunohisto-

chemical analysis of ten cases of an aggressive form of differentiated thyroid carcinoma. Virchows Arch 440:418–424
61. Janser JC, Solis C, Rodier JF, Ghnassia JP (1996) Oncocytic cancers of the thyroid. Hürthle cell cancers. Chirurgie 121:28–36
62. Johnsson T, Lloyd R, Thompson N, Beierwaltes W, Sisson J (1988) Prognostic implications of the tall cell variant of papillary thyroid carcinoma. Am J Surg Pathol 12:22
63. Kanetake H, Toda M, Kawamoto Y (1993) Prognostic factors in primary lymphoma of the thyroid-a review of 74 cases. Nippon Jibiinkoka Gakkai Kaiho 96:1105–1111
64. Kato I, Tajima K, Suchi T, et al (1985) Chronic thyroiditis as a risk factor of B-cell lymphoma in the thyroid gland. Jpn J Cancer Res 76:1085–1090
65. Klein M, Aubert V, Weryha G, Leclere J (1996) Classification and epidemiology of thyroid tumors. Rev Prat 46:2288–2295
66. Koike A, Naruse T (1991) Incidence of thyroid cancer in Japan. Semin Surg Oncol 7:107–111
67. Kuijpens JL, Hansen B, Hamming JF, Ribot JG, Haak HR, Coebergh JW (1998) Trends in treatment and long-term survival of thyroid cancer in southeastern Netherlands, 1960–1992. Eur J Cancer 34:1235–1241
68. Lang W, Borrusch H, Bauer L (1988) Occult carcinomas of the thyroid. Evaluation of 1,020 sequential autopsies. Am J Clin Pathol 90:72–76
69. Leenhardt L, Bernier MO, Boin-Pineau MH, Conte Devolx B, Marechaud R, Niccoli-Sire P, Nocaudie M, Orgiazzi J, Schlumberger M, Wemeau JL, Cherie-Challine L, De Vathaire F (2004) Advances in diagnostic practices affect thyroid cancer incidence in France. Eur J Endocrinol 150:133–139
70. Levi F, Franceschi S, Te VC, Negri E, La Vecchia C (1990) Descriptive epidemiology of thyroid cancer in the Swiss Canton of Vaud. J Cancer Res Clin Oncol 116:639–647
71. Levi F, Lucchini F, Negri E, Boyle P, La Vecchia C (1999) Cancer mortality in Europe, 1990–1994, and an overview of trends from 1955 to 1994. Eur J Cancer 35:1477–1516
72. Lind P, Langsteger W, Molnar M, Gallowitsch HJ, Mikosch P, Gomez I (1998) Epidemiology of thyroid diseases in iodine sufficiency. Thyroid 8:1179–1183
73. Lo CY, Lam KY, Wan KY (1999) Anaplastic carcinoma of the thyroid. Am J Surg 177:337–339
74. Mangano JJ (1996) A post-Chernobyl rise in thyroid cancer in Connecticut, USA. Eur J Cancer Prev 5:75–81
75. Mazzaferri EL (1996) Radioiodine and other treatments and outcomes. In: Braverman LE, Utiger RD (eds) Werner and Ingbar's the thyroid: a fundamental and clinical text, 7th edn. Lippincott-Raven, Philadelphia, pp 922–943
76. McDonald MP, Sanders LE, Silverman ML, Chan HS, Buyske J (1996) Hürthle cell carcinoma of the thyroid gland: prognostic factors and results of surgical treatment. Surgery 120:1000–1005
77. Mellemgaard A, From G, Jorgensen T, Johansen C, Olsen JH, Perrild H (1998) Cancer risk in individuals with benign thyroid disorders. Thyroid 8:751–754
78. Mikhailov I, Petkov R, Gavrailov M et al (1995) The incidence and morphological aspects of thyroid cancer. Khirurgiia (Sofia) 48:15–17
79. Mizukami Y, Nonomura A, Michigishi T, Noguchi M, Nakamura S, Hashimoto T (1994) Columnar cell carcinoma of the thyroid gland: a case report and review of the literature. Hum Pathol 25:1098–1101
80. Modigliani E, Cohen R, Campos JM et al (1998) Prognostic factors for survival and biochemical cure in medullary thyroid carcinoma: results in 899 patients. The GETC Study Group. Clin Endocrinol (Oxf) 48:265–273
81. Moreno Egea A, Rodriguez Gonzales JM, Sola PJ, Soria CT, Parilla PP (1993) Prognostic value of the tall cell variety of papillary cancer of the thyroid. Eur J Surg Oncol 19:517–521

82. Moreno Egea A, Rodriguez Gonzalez JM, Sola Perez J, Soria T, Parrilla Paricio P (1994) Clinicopathological study of the diffuse sclerosing variety of papillary cancer of the thyroid. Presentation of 4 new cases and review of the literature. Eur J Surg Oncol 20:7–11
83. Mortensen JD, Woolner LB, Bennett WA (1955) Gross and microscopic findings in clinically normal thyroid gland. J Clin Endocrinol Metab 15:120–128
84. Muzaffar M, Nigar E, Mushtaq S, Mamoon N (1998) The morphological variants of papillary carcinoma of the thyroid: a clinico-pathological study – AFIP experience. J Pak Med Assoc 48:133–137
85. Nakhjavani MK, Gharib H, Goellner JR, Van Heerden JA (1997) Metastasis to the thyroid gland. A report of 43 cases. Cancer 79:574–578
86. Negri E, Ron E, Franceschi S (1999) A pooled analysis of case-control studies of thyroid cancer. I. Methods. Cancer Causes Control 10:131–142
87. Nielsen B, Zetterlund B (1985) Malignant thyroid tumors at autopsy in a Swedish goitrous population. Cancer 55:1041–1043
88. Nishiyama RH, Ludwig GK, Thompson NW (1977) The prevalence of small papillary thyroid carcinomas in 100 consecutive necropsies in an American population. In: DeGroot LJ, Frohman LA, Kaplan EL, Refetoff S (eds) Radiation-associated thyroid carcinoma. Grune and Stratton, New York, pp 123–135
89. Pacini F, Vorontsova T, Demidchik EP et al (1997) Post-Chernobyl thyroid carcinoma in Belarus children and adolescents: comparison with naturally occurring thyroid carcinoma in Italy and France. J Clin Endocrinol Metab 82:3563–3569
90. Palazzo FF, Bradpiece HA, Morgan MW (1999) Renal cell carcinoma metastasizing to the thyroid gland. Scand J Urol Nephrol 33:202–204
91. Parkin DM, Muir CS, Whelan SL, Gao YT, Fenlay J, Powell J (1992) Cancer incidence in five continents, vol 6. (IARC scientific publication 120) International Agency for Research on Cancer, Lyon
92. Paterson IC, Greenlee R, Adams Jones D (1999) Thyroid cancer in Wales 1985–1996: a cancer registry-based study. Clin Oncol (R Coll Radiol) 11:245–251
93. Pedersen RK, Pedersen NT (1996) Primary non-Hodgkin's lymphoma of the thyroid gland: a population based study. Histopathology 28:25–32
94. Pettersson B, Adami HO, Wilander E, Coleman MP (1991) Trends in thyroid cancer incidence in Sweden, 1958–1981, by histopathologic type. Int J Cancer 48:28–33
95. Pledge S, Bessell EM, Leach ICH, et al (1996) Non-Hodgkin's lymphoma of the thyroid: a retrospective review of all patients diagnosed in Nottinghamshire from 1973–1992. Clin Oncol (R Coll Radiol) 8:371–375
96. Plesko I, Macfarlane GJ, Obsitnikova A, Vlasak V, Kramarova E (1994) Thyroid cancer in Slovakia, 1968–1990: incidence, mortality and histological types. Eur J Cancer Prev 3:345–349
97. Raue F and the German MTC/MEN Study Group (1998) German medullary thyroid carcinoma/multiple endocrine neoplasia registry. Langenbecks Arch Surg 383:334–336
98. Robert Koch-Institut, Germany (2004) Aktuelle Daten zur Inzidenz und Mortalität (individuelle Auswahl). http://www.rki.de. Cited 4 October 2004
99. Rodriguez JM, Pinero A, Ortiz S, et al (2000) Clinical and histological differences in anaplastic thyroid carcinoma. Eur J Surg 166:34–38
100. Rosai J, Saxen EA, Woolner L (1985) Undifferentiated and poorly differentiated carcinoma. Semin Diagn Pathol 2:123–136
101. Rosenthal DS (1998) Changing trends. CA Cancer J Clin 48:3–23
102. Ruegemer JJ, Hay ID, Bergstrahl EJ, et al (1988) Distant metastases in differentiated thyroid carcinoma. J Clin Endocrinol Metab 67:501–508
103. Rüter A, Nishiyama R, Lennquist S (1997) Tall-cell variant of papillary thyroid cancer: disregarded entity? World J Surg 21:15–21
104. Sali D, Cardis E, Sztanyik L, et al (1996) Cancer consequences of the Chernobyl accident in Europe outside the former USSR: a review. Int J Cancer 67:343–352

105. Samaan NA, Ordonez NG (1990) Uncommon types of thyroid cancer. Endocrinol Metab Clin North Am 19:637–648
106. Sampson RJ (1977) Prevalence and significance of occult thyroid carcinoma. In: DeGroot LJ, Frohman LA, Kaplan EL, Refetoff S (eds) Radiation-associated thyroid carcinoma. Grune and Stratton, New York, pp 137–153
107. Sampson RJ, Key CR, Buncher CR, Iijima S (1969) Thyroid carcinoma in Hiroshima and Nagasaki. I. Prevalence of thyroid carcinoma at autopsy. JAMA 209:65–70
108. Sampson RJ, Oka H, Key CR, Buncher CR, Iijima S (1970) Metastases from occult thyroid carcinoma. Cancer 25:803–811
109. Sampson RJ, Woolner LB, Bahn RC, Kurland LT (1974) Occult thyroid carcinoma in Olmsted County, Minnesota: Prevalence at autopsy compared with that in Hiroshima and Nagasaki, Japan. Cancer 34:2072–2076
110. Sant M, Aareleid T, Berrino F, Bielska Lasota M, Carli PM, Faivre J, Grosclaude P, Hedelin G, Matsuda T, Moller H, Moller T, Verdecchia A, Capocaccia R, Gatta G, Micheli A, Santaquilani M, Roazzi P, Lisi D, EUROCARE Working Group (2003) EUROCARE-3: survival of cancer patients diagnosed 1990–94: results and commentary.Ann Oncol 14 [Suppl 5]:61–118
111. Segovia IG, Gallowitsch HJ, Kresnik E, Kumnig G, Igerc I, Matschnig S, Stronegger WJ, Lind P (2004) Descriptive epidemiology of thyroid carcinoma in Carinthia, Austria: 1984–2001. Histopathologic features and tumor classification of 734 cases under elevated general iodination of table salt since 1990: population-based age-stratified analysis on thyroid carcinoma incidence. Thyroid 14:277–286
112. Shah SH, Muzaffar S, Soomro IN, Hasan SH (1999) Morphological pattern and frequency of thyroid tumors. J Pak Med Assoc 49:131–133
113. Shaha AR (1998) The National Cancer Data Base report on thyroid carcinoma. Reflections of practice patterns. Cancer 83:2434–2436
114. Shaw JH, Holden A, Sage M (1989) Thyroid lymphoma. Br J Surg 76:895–897
115. Sobin LH, Wittekind C (eds) (1997) International Union Against Cancer (UICC). TNM classification of malignant tumors, 5th edn. Wiley, New York
116. Sobin LH, Wittekind C (eds) (2002) International Union Against Cancer (UICC). TNM classification of malignant tumors, 6th edn. Wiley, New York
117. Sobrinho-Simões MA, Sambade MC, Gonçalves V (1979) Latent thyroid carcinoma at autopsy: a study from Oporto, Portugal. Cancer 43:1702–1706
118. Sobrinho-Simões MA, Neland JM, Hohn R, Sambade MC, Johannessen JV (1985) Hürthle cell and mitochondrion-rich papillary carcinomas of the thyroid gland: an ultra-structural and immunocytochemical study. Klin Wochenschr Pathol 8:131–142
119. Spires JR, Schwartz MR, Miller RH (1988) Anaplastic thyroid carcinoma. Association with differentiated thyroid cancer. Arch Otolaryngol Head Neck Surg 114:40–44
120. Spitz MR, Sider JG, Katz RL, Pollack ES, Newell GR (1988) Ethnic patterns of thyroid cancer incidence in the USA, 1973–1981. Int J Cancer 42:549–553
121. Sugitani I, Fujimoto Y (1999) Symptomatic versus asymptomatic papillary thyroid microcarcinoma: a retrospective analysis of surgical outcome and prognostic factors. Endocr J 46:209–216
122. Teppo L, Hakulinen T and the Eurocare Working Group (1998) Variation in survival of adult patients with thyroid cancer in Europe. Eur J Cancer 34:2248–2252
123. Thorvaldsson SE, Tulinius H, Bjornsson J, Bjarnason O (1992) Latent thyroid carcinoma in Iceland at autopsy. Pathol Res Pract 188:747–750
124. Tollefsen HR, Shah JP, Huvos AG (1975) Hürthle cell carcinoma of the thyroid. Am J Surg 130:390–394
125. Tsang RW, Gospodarowicz MK, Sutcliffe SB, Sturgeon JF, Panzarella T, Patterson BJ (1993) Non-Hodgkin's lymphoma of the thyroid gland: prognostic factors and treatment outcome. The Princess Margaret Hospital Lymphoma Group. Int J Radiat Oncol Biol Phys 27:599–604

126. UICC (1987,1992) TNM classification of malignant tumors. Hermanek P, Sobin LH (eds) 4th edn, 1987; 2nd revision 1992. Springer, Berlin Heidelberg New York
127. Van den Brekel MWM, Hekkenberg RJ, Asa SL, et al (1997) Prognostic features in tall cell papillary carcinoma and insular thyroid carcinoma. Laryngoscope 107:254–259
128. Van der Poel HG, Roukema JA, Horenblas S, Geel AN van, Debruyne FM (1999) Metastasectomy in renal cell carcinoma: a multicenter retrospective analysis. Eur Urol 35:197–203
129. Vander JB, Gaston EA, Dawber TR (1968) The significance of nontoxic thyroid nodules: final report of a 15 year study of the incidence of thyroid malignancy. Ann Intern Med 69:537–540
130. Venkatesh YS, Ordonez NG, Schultz PN, Hickey RC, Goepfert H, Samaan NA (1990) Anaplastic carcinoma of the thyroid. A clinicopathologic study of 121 cases. Cancer 66:321–330
131. Volante M, Landolfi S, Chiusa L, et al (2004) Poorly differentiated carcinomas of the thyroid with trabecular, insular, and solid patterns: a clinicopathological study of 183 patients. Cancer 100:950–957
132. Watson RG, Brennan MD, Goellner JR, Heerden JA van, McConahey WM, Taylor WF (1984) Invasive Hürthle cell carcinoma of the thyroid: natural history and management. Mayo Clin Proc 59:851–855
133. Weiss W (1979) Changing incidence of thyroid cancer. J Natl Cancer Inst 62:1137–1142
134. Wenig BM, Thompson LD, Adair CF, Shmookler B, Heffess CS (1998) Thyroid papillary carcinoma of columnar cell type: a clinicopathologic study of 16 cases. Cancer 82:740–753
135. Wittekind C, Greene FL, Henson DE, et al (2003) TNM supplement. A commentary on uniform use, 3rd edn. Wiley, New York
136. Woolner LB, Lemmon ML, Beahrs OH, Black BM, McConahey WM, Keating FR (1960) Occult papillary carcinoma of the thyroid gland: a study of 140 cases observed in a 30-year period. J Clin Endocrinol Metab 20:89–105
137. Yamashita H, Noguchi S, Yamashita H, et al (1998) Changing trend and prognoses for patients with papillary cancer. Arch Surg 133:1058–1065
138. Yeole BB (1998) Descriptive epidemiology of thyroid cancer in greater Bombay. Indian J Cancer 35:57–64
139. Zheng T, Holford TR, Chen Y, et al (1996) Time trend and age-period-cohort effect on incidence of thyroid cancer in Connecticut, 1935–1992. Int J Cancer 67:504–509

Chapter 2

Histopathology, Immunohistochemistry, and Molecular Biology 2

F. Hofstädter

2.1 Introduction

The pathology of thyroid carcinoma is characterized by a defined histopathological classification system that has only undergone minor changes in the past few years, which is the basis of clinical diagnostic and treatment modalities as well as by a rapid progress of application of new methods and increasing knowledge of basic mechanisms in molecular pathology. However, at least in the field of C-cell carcinoma, thyroid pathology represents an impressive example of the successful application of molecular pathology in clinical practice. The aim of this review is to summarize the principles of clinical histopathology in thyroid carcinoma followed by a brief analysis of recent work in molecular pathology concentrating on original recent articles on surgical material and revealing some correlations to the questions of diagnostic clinical histopathology.

2.2 Principles of Histopathological Diagnosis and Classification

2.2.1 The Rules and Their Problems

According to the World Health Organization classification (Fig. 2.1) malignant tumors of the thyroid are subdivided into thyroid-specific, which are unique to the thyroid (for example follicular, papillary, and medullary carcinoma), and tumors commonly found also in other organs, but still have some particular characteristics when they occur in the thyroid gland (for example lymphoma, some types of sarcoma). Thyroid-specific tumors are thought to be derived from follicle cells (follicular and papillary carcinoma) and from parafollicular, calcitonin-producing C cells (medullary carcinoma). Interestingly, and in contrast to other organ systems, each of these tumors has its own rules of histopathological diagnosis, referring not only to the subclassification, but also to the histopathological establishment of malignancy. Interestingly, a change has been noted in the distribution of the subtypes of differentiated carcinoma, with a relative increase in papillary carcinoma in several countries, thought to be a consequence of altered iodine uptake [27, 59].

WHO classification of thyroid carcinoma[a]

1	Epithelial tumors		
1.1.	Benign		
1.1.1.	Follicular adenoma		8330/0
1.1.2.	Others		
1.2.	Malignant		
1.2.1.	Follicular carcinoma	Minimally invasive (encapsulated) Widely invasive Oxyphilic cell type Clear cell variant	8330/3
1.2.2.	Papillary carcinoma	Papillary microcarcinoma Encapsulated variant Follicular variant Diffuse sclerosing variant Oxyphilic cell type	
1.2.3.	Medullary (C-cell) carcinoma	Mixed medullary-follicular carcinoma	
1.2.4.	Undifferentiated (anaplastic) carcinoma		8020/3
1.2.5.	Others		
2	Nonepithelial tumors		
3	Malignant lymphomas		
4	Miscellaneous tumors		
5	Secondary tumors		
6	Unclassified tumors		
7	Tumor-like lesions		

[a] Hedinger Chr. (1998): Histological typing of thyroid tumours. Springer, Heidelberg New York

Fig. 2.1. World Health Organization classification of thyroid carcinoma [54]

2.2.2 Papillary Carcinoma

Papillary carcinoma is the most frequent type of follicle cell-derived carcinoma. The histopathological diagnosis was originally based on microscopic detection of papillae. These are delicate stalks of epithelial cells situated on basal membranes covering stromal fibers and thin capillaries. Often the tumors contain round laminated calcifications (psammoma bodies). The papillary structures often have a follicular pattern. These tumors have been called "mixed carcinomas". Since these tumors show a clinicopathological behavior identical to that of pure papillary carcinoma, the histostructural component of the papilla has been replaced as the primary criterion of this tumor type, and nuclear characteristics have been defined, which are now the main tool used for diagnosis. These nuclei (ground-glass nuclei) are enlarged, round-to-oval structures, with a pale karyoplasm condensing continuously to the nuclear membrane. This is an optical phenomenon caused by cytoplasmatic pseudoinclusions. The nuclei are densely arranged and often overlap each other (shingle roof pattern). The occurrence of ground-glass nuclei is the main criterion for diagnosing papillary carcinoma. For technical reasons this phenomenon cannot be detected in frozen material, i.e., frozen sections or paraffin sections after frozen section procedures. The nuclear criterion of ground-glass nuclei overrules the histoarchitectural structure (follicular/papillary) in the differential diagnosis of follicle cell-derived tumors and so-called mixed tumors. Additionally, the papillary carcinomas have specific features, which may further substantiate the diagnosis. They are often accompanied by a lymphocytic-type thyroiditis, a phenomenon that may give rise to analyses both to pathogenetic mechanisms and to prognostic implications (see the respective chapters). The surrounding stroma may show a dense fibrosis (with or without coexisting lymphocytic thyroiditis). This phenomenon can be seen regularly in the group of small (>10 mm, mostly 1- to 3-mm) papillary carcinomas (occult sclerosing papillary carcinoma [71] or papillary microcarcinoma [53]), which are frequent incidental findings in surgical specimens removed for reasons unrelated to malignancy (e.g., multinodular goiter) but also in large, clinically overt carcinomas with a diffuse type of sclerosis. This fibrotic reaction of the stroma also gives rise to investigations into both pathogenetic mechanism and prognostic factors. Papillary microcarcinoma may occur in a familial form and these tumors show more aggressive clinical behavior than sporadic cases [83].

Papillary carcinoma may be encapsulated, i.e., surrounded by a collagenous capsule, often with large venous vessels inside and outside the capsule. The carcinoma may infiltrate the capsule or may diffusely infiltrate the surrounding parenchyma without any capsule formation. Additionally, it may infiltrate the surrounding veins, but this is not a necessary basis for the diagnosis of malignancy in this tumor type. This is in sharp contrast to follicular carcinoma, where vascular infiltration is one of the main criteria of malignancy.

Comparable with follicular carcinoma, papillary carcinoma of the thyroid can show variations of the cytoplasm of the tumor cells. These are the oncocytic cell type (Hürthle or eosinophilic cell) based upon an enormous increase in the number of mitochondria (or in rare cases rough endoplasmatic reticulum) in the cytoplasm, or rare, clear-cell types with an increase in lipid (or other) vacuoles. The oncocytic-cell type of papillary carcinoma causes diagnostic problems because it obscures the pattern of ground-glass nuclei. Nuclei of oncocytes are hyperchromatic, often with condensed chromatin structures. Therefore, diagnosis cannot depend only on nuclear criteria in oncocytic-cell variation, but must depend on papillary structure and/or infiltrating growth. However, papillary structures are difficult to detect in highly cellular oncocytic tumors because of very similar technical artifacts in microfollicular adenomas. Several specific subtypes of papillary carcinoma have been investigated and described in recent years. They are be discussed in a separate chapter.

2.2.3 Follicular Carcinoma

Second in frequency of occurrence is follicular carcinoma. Nuclear characteristics do not play a role in the diagnosis of follicular carcinoma apart from the exclusion of ground-glass nuclei. The diagnosis of follicular carcinoma is based on the histopathological demonstration of infiltrative growth. There are two criteria: (1) true infiltration of the venous vessels outside the tumor capsule, and (2) fungus-like infiltration through the tumor capsule into the surrounding parenchyma. There is intensive debate among pathologists as to how indisputable vessel infiltrations can be demonstrated. The staining of vascular components (elastic fibers, endothelial cells) may be helpful in difficult cases. It is not easy to discern follicular proliferations adjacent to enlarged (originally perifollicular) capillaries and seemingly infiltrating the capillary lumen. As a rule, the infiltrated vessel must be a vein and must be situated outside the tumor capsule. Also the interstitial infiltrative growth into the surrounding parenchyma may be difficult to evaluate. The vessels have to be separated from artificial clefts at the tumor capsule made during surgical or pathological preparation. Therefore, intracapsular (tumor capsule) enucleated tumor specimens cannot be analyzed histopathologically for infiltrative growth characteristics. There is ongoing debate in the literature as to whether infiltrative growth alone without vascular infiltration is sufficient for the diagnosis of malignancy. The criteria for histopathological vascular infiltration analysis were described precisely by Schmid et al. [122].

Cytoplasmatic variations also raise specific diagnostic problems in follicular carcinoma. The most frequent – as in papillary carcinoma – is the oncocytic variant (Hürthle-cell type, eosinophilic-cell type). Eosinophilic cells usually show low cytoplasmatic coherence and thus are artificially disseminated into the surrounding parenchyma. This phenomenon may create problems, particularly in intraoperative frozen sections. Additionally, there are two main questions discussed in the literature concerning the oncocytic-type tumors: firstly, are large oncocytic (follicular structured) tumors malignant even without vascular/parenchymal infiltration? Secondly, is the prognosis of eosinophilic carcinoma equal to, worse than or better when compared with their follicular counterparts with regular cytoplasm? These questions will be discussed in the chapter concerning prognosis. A second cytoplasmic subtype is the clear-cell variant [59, 123].

The rules of histopathological diagnosis in the field of follicular carcinoma described above clearly point toward a problem in clinical pathology of the thyroid: the evaluation of capsular infiltration (better extracapsular extension) and venous infiltration of the tumor presupposes the investigation of the whole tumor capsule, when infiltrating growth is not detectable by gross examination. Intraoperative frozen sections therefore cannot rely on classic cytological features such as nuclear atypia to rule out an infiltrative growth pattern. This may be difficult in cases of encapsulated follicular tumors, because the whole capsule is not available in the intraoperative situation in large tumor specimens. Therefore, the vascular infiltration may be missed during frozen sectioning. This problem has raised the problem of whether frozen sections on the whole should be performed for follicular tumors. This will be discussed later.

For follicular carcinoma – as for papillary carcinoma – several subtypes have been described which differ from the main type regarding prognosis. These subtypes are situated mainly at the border with anaplastic carcinoma as poorly differentiated carcinoma and will be described in detail.

2.2.4
Anaplastic (Undifferentiated) Carcinoma

Anaplastic carcinoma is mostly detected by the pathologist by fine-needle aspiration biopsy (FNAB) or tumor reduction specimen. Complete resection specimens are rare. The diagnosis of malignancy is evident by cytological polymorphism and histological dedifferentiation. Most tumors show large areas of necrosis; in cases of hemorrhagic necrosis, hemangioendothelioma has to be excluded. Some cases of anaplastic carcinoma show remnants of differentiated (mostly follicular) carcinomas, indicating a dedifferentiation pathway from differentiated to anaplastic carcinoma. Histopathologically the tumors are solid sheets of highly anaplastic cells or spindle cells with morphologically sarcoma-like areas and frequent appearance of giant cells. There is now general agreement that these tumors represent carcinomas and true sarcomas are rare in the thyroid.

Small-cell anaplastic carcinomas were diagnosed frequently many years ago but now there is general agreement that most cases of "small-cell carcinoma" are in fact non-Hodgkin lymphomas. Curative treatment of anaplastic carcinoma is extremely rare [80], but there are reports including patients with 5-year survival after R0 resection [104]. Even in this highly aggressive tumor, statistically independent prognostic factors have been elucidated [147].

2.2.5
Medullary (C-Cell) Carcinoma

The histopathological hallmarks of medullary thyroid carcinoma are more variable than originally supposed. Characteristically the tumor is composed of solid nests and infiltrating formations of polygonal or spindle-shaped cells. Amyloid deposits within the stroma are found in about the half of the tumors. Several subtypes have been described, demonstrating a large variety of this tumor type. These include papillary, giant-cell, squamous differentiation or classic carcinoid patterns. Even mucus production and melanin pigmentation have been observed [2]. According to general agreement, no preexisting adenoma exists; all tumors exceeding 50 cells are considered malignant and separate from C-cell hyperplasia. Immunohistochemistry is strongly indicated for all cases of solid tumors without typical features of papillary or follicular carcinoma to prevent underdiagnosis of medullary carcinoma. Thyroid paraganglioma [75], hyalinizing trabecular adenoma, and metastatic neuroendocrine tumor are typical differential diagnoses.

T[a]	Primary tumor
TX	Primary tumor cannot be assessed
T0	No evidence of primary tumor
T1	Tumor 2 cm or less maximum dimension, limited to the thyroid
T2	Tumor more than 2 cm but not more than 4 cm maximum dimension, limited to the thyroid
T3	Tumor more than 4 cm maximum dimension limited to the thyroid or any tumor with minimal extrathyroid extension (e.g., extension to sternothyroid muscle or perithyroid soft tissues
T4a[b]	Tumor of any size extending beyond the thyroid capsule to invade subcutaneous soft tissues, larynx, trachea, esophagus, or recurrent laryngeal nerve
T4b[b]	Tumor invades prevertebral fascia or encases carotid artery or mediastinal vessels
N[a]	Regional lymph nodes
NX	Regional lymph nodes cannot be assessed
N0	No regional lymph node metastasis
N1	Regional lymph node metastasis
N1a	Metastasis to level VI (pretacheal, paratracheal, and prelaryngeal/Delphian lymph nodes)
N1b	Meastasis to unilateral, bilateral, or contralateral cervical or superior mediastinal lymph nodes
M[a]	Distant metastasis
MX	Distant metasasis cannot be assessed
M0	No distant metastasis
M1	Distant metastasis

Fig. 2.2 TNM classification of thyroid carcinoma

2.3 Histopathology and Prognosis

The histopathological classification into the main types of thyroid carcinoma (papillary, follicular, medullary and anaplastic) has been shown to be the most powerful prognostic factor concerning overall survival, disease-free survival, recurrence and metastasis rate [43]. To improve the accuracy of prognosis and to allow specific treatment modalities histopathology has been combined with other prognostic factors to establish a more individual scoring system. Additionally, within the histopathological classification system, several subtypes have been described which are proposed to have prognostic implications. However, these studies are often based on a small number of cases and most studies are performed retrospectively.

2.3.1 Histopathology and Prognostic Scores

Several clinical staging and prognostic scoring systems have been proposed and all of them include the histopathological type as a major component. The tumor

Stage grouping[c]				
Papillary or follicular carcinoma				
Under	Stage I	Any T	Any N	M0
45 years	Stage II	Any T	Any N	M1
45 years and	Stage I	T1	N0	M0
older	Stage II	T2	N0	M0
	Stage III	T3	N0	M0
		T1	N1a	M0
		T2	N1a	M0
		T3	N1a	M0
	Stage IVA	T4a	N0	M0
		T4a	N1a	M0
		T1	N1b	M0
		T2	N1b	M0
		T3	N1b	M0
		T4a	N1b	M0
	Stage IVB	T4b	Any N	M0
	Stage IVC	Any T	Any N	M1
Medullary	Stage I	T1	N0	M0
carcinoma	Stage II	T2	N0	M0
	Stage III	T3	N0	M0
		T1	N1a	M0
		T2	N1a	M0
		T3	N1a	M0
	Stage IVA	T4a	N0	M0
		T4a	N1a	M0
		T1	N1b	M0
		T2	N1b	M0
		T3	N1b	M0
		T4a	N1b	M0
	Stage IVB	T4b	Any N	M0
	Stage IVC	Any T	Any N	M1
Anaplastic	Stage IVA	T4a	Any N	M0
carcinoma[d]	Stage IVB	T4b	Any N	M0
	Stage IVC	Any T	Any N	M1

[a] All categories may be subdivided: (a) solitary tumor; (b) multifocal tumor (the largest determines the classification)

[b] All anaplastic carcinomas are considered T4 tumors: T4a intrathyroidal anaplastic carcinoma – surgically resectable; T4b extrathyroidal anaplastic carcinoma – surgically unresectable

[c] Separate stage groupings are recommended for papillary or follicular, medullary, and anaplastic (undifferentiated carcinoma)

[d] All anaplastic carcinomas are considered Stage IV

Fig. 2.2 Continued

node metastasis (TNM) system [129] (Fig. 2.2) of thyroid carcinoma follows a strategy differing from that of other tumors: there is a general classification schedule (T1–4, N, M) applying to all four histological main types (follicular, papillary, medullary, anaplastic). The specific influence of cell types and other prognostic factors (age >45 years) are taken into consideration at the specific tumor stage grouping. Thus, independent from the specific T (or N, M) category each anaplastic carcinoma is considered as stage IV. Most other staging systems refer only to differentiated follicular/papillary (EORTC [14]; AMES [15]; Ohio State University [85]) or to papillary carcinoma (AGES [51]; MACIS [52]; University of Chicago [28]) and include size (except EORTC), age (except University of Chicago and Ohio State University), sex (EORTC and AMES), and lymph-node metastasis (University of Chicago and Ohio State University, TNM depending on age). Extrathyroid extension and distant metastasis are considered in all scoring systems, completeness of resection only by MACIS and TNM by the use of R category. The TNM classification has been shown to be useful in distinguishing patients with different prognostic outcomes, but in large retrospective series its value for therapy decisions is diminished by the relatively small proportion of patients in stages other than stage I [82]. TNM principally recommends the application of grading, but there is agreement that a general differentiation grading such as that for squamous carcinoma in the head and neck region is not applicable to thyroid carcinoma. Some subtypes of follicle-cell tumors (Chap. 3) as defined by their infiltration or differentiation type may be candidates for grading steps between well-differentiated and anaplastic carcinoma, but presently they do not fit into the TNM definition. Brierley et al. [12] compared the discriminating ability of ten different staging systems on 382 patients and recommended the use of the TNM classification.

Major changes in the new TNM classification system include: (1) new metrical dimensions in the T category, with an increase from 1 to 2 cm in the smallest tumor category and new definitions for local tumor growth beyond the thyroid capsule; (2) new definitions for lymph node metastasis; (3) anaplastic carcinomas are subdivided into resectable and unresectable ones; (4) regrouping of papillary and follicular carcinomas of patients aged 45 years or older. The new classification has been critized and therefore it seems important to state the exact tumor diameter in the pathological report, as well as giving a correlation with the old classification to avoid misunderstanding.

Additional prognostic factors have been detected also in medullary carcinoma patients. Age and stage (especially extrathyroidal extension) have been shown to be important variables in all recent series [40, 44]. Several histological findings have been shown to be prognostically relevant, such as lack of amyloid and heterogeneous calcitonin staining [124] and necrosis, focal squamous pattern and presence of oxyphilic cells [38]. In the specific group of sporadic medullary microcarcinoma (<1 cm), the preoperative calcitonin level and clinical symptoms are predictors of an unfavorable outcome [47].

2.3.2 Histological Subtypes Influencing Prognosis

In both the papillary and the follicular carcinoma groups, several subtypes or variants have been described. The most frequent and first-described variant is the Hürthle-cell carcinoma. The diagnostic problems of the oncocytic variant of papillary carcinoma are described above. Berho and Suster [11] described 15 cases of unquestionable oncocytic papillary carcinomas and concluded that these tumors do not appear to behave more aggressively than usual papillary carcinomas. In follicular oncocytic carcinomas, Khafif et al [68] demonstrated that the prognosis of Hürthle-cell carcinoma did not differ from that of pure follicular carcinoma.

In a large series of patients, McDonald et al. [87] showed that the behavior of Hürthle-cell carcinoma follows the rules of prognostic scores such as AMES risk stratification used by the authors. Papotti et al. [102] have investigated a series of 60 cases of Hürthle-cell carcinomas and defined a subgroup with predominant solid or trabecular pattern resembling variants of poorly differentiated follicular carcinoma. This group showed a significantly worse clinical outcome than cases with a predominantly follicular structure. The results of this study also show that the prognostic factors of the general classification (specifically the histostructural differentiation) are valid within the group of oncocytic carcinomas.

Both follicular and papillary carcinoma can be subdivided concerning the degree of invasive growth into an encapsulated (minimally invasive) or widely invasive type. However, in both cases the exact differentiation between the two types is under discussion and not fully standardized. In most studies that use this criterion, the prognosis of encapsulated follicular carcinoma is excellent [76, 122]. Goldstein et al. [45] used a semiquantitative approach to quantify the number of vascular infiltrations and/or complete capsular penetrations in metastatic encapsulated follicular and Hürthle-cell thyroid carcinoma. They find no differences either between follicular and Hürthle-cell carcinoma or between metastatic and nonmetastatic carcinomas.

There are correlations between widely invasive follicular carcinomas and insular carcinoma as described by Carcangiu et al. [19]. These tumors are characterized by infiltrating, but well-defined nests of small, uniform cells with frequent areas of necrosis and resemble the "*wuchernde Struma Langhans*" [77]. Pilotti et al. [106] compared 27 cases of insular carcinoma with 29 widely invasive follicular carcinomas and found statistically more frequent extrathyroidal extension and lymph-node metastasis in the group of insular carcinomas. However, the survival data were identical between the two groups investigated. Interestingly, both tumor groups share a frequent point mutation at codon 61 of the *ras* gene. Sasaki et al. [119] identified insular components both in follicular and papillary carcinomas. Besides age, tumor size, vascular invasion, necrosis and capsule formation, the insular component was an independent prognostic marker both in follicular and papillary carcinoma. This correlates well with earlier series indicating a group of poorly differentiated carcinomas (with both elements of follicular and papillary carcinomas), indicating prognosis midway between differentiated and anaplastic carcinoma [86, 118, 142]. Nishida et al. [98] subdivided poorly differentiated carcinoma into diffuse and focal types and found significant differences in the outcome of patients concerning frequency of tumor relapse and overall survival.

Several subtypes have also recently been described in the papillary group of carcinomas. Tall-cell variant was originally described by Hawk and Hazard

[50]. The tumor cells covering the papillary stalks are by definition twice as tall as they are wide. There is some overlap [125] with the columnar-cell variant described by Evans [33]. The nuclei show striking stratification and lack typical cytomorphological features such as the ground-glass appearance. Ostrowski and Merino [100] showed by immunohistochemical analyses that the tall-cell variant is phenotypically different from classical papillary carcinoma. The immunohistochemical overexpression of *p53* has been shown to be significantly more frequent in the tall-cell variant than in age- and sex-matched common papillary carcinomas [117]. Yunta et al. [155] and Evans [34] stressed the importance of a tumor capsule in columnar-cell carcinoma. This raises the question of whether the worse prognosis in tall-cell and columnar variants reflects interrelationships with other relevant prognostic findings or represents an independent prognostic factor. Also, extensive lymphocytic infiltration seems to influence the prognosis [101] as it is under discussion in the common types of papillary carcinoma. In contrast to these variants, which are suggested to worsen the patient's prognosis, the macrofollicular variant implies a good prognosis even when accompanied by a small, insular component [3].

The influence of concomitant thyroiditis on the pathogenesis or prognosis of thyroid tumors has been discussed. Whereas severe lymphocytic thyroiditis is now accepted as a disease pathogenetically related to non-Hodgkin's lymphoma of the thyroid, the pathogenetic influence on papillary carcinoma has not been proved. However, an influence has been shown of lymphocytic infiltration and fibrous reaction on the prognosis of papillary carcinoma. Coexisting lymphocytic thyroiditis has been shown to be associated with lower pT stages in 153 thyroid carcinomas [121]. By means of a multivariate approach Kashima et al. [66] showed that apart from age (45 years or more), vascular invasion, and lymph-node metastasis, the absence of chronic thyroiditis represents an independent prognostic indicator both for relapse-free and overall survival.

This has been confirmed by Loh et al. [81] in a retrospective study on a large series of patients. However, a diffuse lymphocytic infiltration combined with extensive fibrosis (diffuse sclerosing variant according to Vickery et al., [146] has been shown to have worse prognostic signs (lymph-node metastasis, pulmonary metastasis). Albareda et al. [1] also found a greater degree of lymph-node metastases in this group of patients, but the authors found no difference for overall survival. In recent years variants with exuberant fibrosis (nodular fasciitis-like) have been described and correlated with increased transforming growth factor (TGF)-beta production [140]. An interesting theory was contributed by Mitsiades et al. [90], who showed that the expression of the apoptosis-inducing FAS ligand was correlated with a more aggressive phenotype of papillary thyroid carcinoma, suggesting that these tumors induce apoptosis of infiltrating lymphocytes and escape immune surveillance.

2.4 Histo-/Cytopathology in Preoperative and Intraoperative Diagnosis (Problem of Frozen Section)

As can be clearly seen from the microscopy principles discussed above, a preoperative diagnosis of thyroid carcinoma by FNAB is affected by two thyroid-specific phenomena: Firstly, many of the tumors are clinically small, indolent tumors (occult carcinoma) or carcinomas arising in multinodular goiter. Therefore, FNAB in such cases cannot be guaranteed to show the relevant cellular material. This is mainly a problem of the clinical detection systems. However, Sugino et al. [133], in their series of 112 patients with papillary microcarcinoma (10 mm or less), were able to confirm the diagnosis in 100 patients (89.3%). The second problem is based exclusively on microscopic factors: Whereas papillary, medullary and anaplastic carcinomas show well-defined, clearly detectable cytological findings in most cases, follicular carcinomas are by definition characterized by their infiltrative growth pattern not detectable in FNAB specimens and causing problems even in intraoperative frozen sections, when only a limited number of sections of the tumor capsule are available for analysis.

There has been much controversy in the literature about the diagnostic impact of intraoperative histopathologic diagnosis by frozen sectioning [73, 113]. Intraoperative cytology may be an additional help especially in cases of encapsulated papillary carcinoma [8, 145]. The size of the respective lesion has been shown to be predictive of malignancy in Hürthle-cell neoplasms [23], but not in the general differential diagnosis between follicular adenoma and follicular carcinoma [42]. Even concerning cost-effectiveness the results are contradictory. Whereas McHenry et al. [88] found frozen-section examination to change the intraoperative management in only 3% of patients and therefore not to be cost-effective, Paphavasit et al. [103] found in 1,023 patients with follicular and Hürthle-cell neoplasms that intraoperative frozen section evaluation was highly accurate and cut costs considerably by reducing the number of two-stage operations. We agree with Rosai et al. [112] that frozen sections are helpful in widely invasive follicular carcinoma, papillary carcinoma, anaplastic carcinoma and medullary carcinoma. In cases of conspicuous follicular structured lesions, the diagnosis of a follicular lesion has to be made and the diagnosis has to be deferred to permanent sections of paraffin-embedded tissues. This has to be performed within 3 days for surgical reasons. Perhaps new fixation techniques may significantly shorten this time period until final diagnosis [109].

2.5 Auxiliary Techniques (Cytometry, Immunohistochemistry, Molecular Pathology)

Beyond classic histopathology and cytopathology additional techniques have been developed in tumor pathology and have been used for thyroid carcinoma specimens to improve both the accuracy of preoperative cytological diagnosis and the precision of prediction of the biological behavior of the respective tumors. These techniques include morphometric and cytometric as well as immunohisto-/cytochemical and molecular pathology approaches.

2.6 Preoperative Diagnosis (Fine-Needle Aspiration Biopsy)

Descriptive cytomorphometric approaches [29, 94] and DNA cytophotometry have been investigated for several years for their ability to assist in the differential diagnosis of follicular adenoma and follicular carcinoma in FNAB specimens. More recently Horii et al. [60] have combined DNA cytometry (ploidy pattern) with Ki67 staining and found an accuracy of over 80%, but their work was performed on surgical material. Also AgNOR staining has been shown to be of some discriminatory value [115]. Immunostaining of both FNAB specimens and the corresponding surgical material with antibodies against galectin-3 (a carbohydrate-binding protein involved in cell-cell and cell-matrix interactions) has been shown by Orlandei et al. [99] to be highly discriminative with positive staining of all follicular carcinoma specimens but galectin-3 expression in only 3 of 29 follicular adenomas. An interesting approach has been used by Winzer et al. [152] with the successful application of reverse transcription polymerase chain reaction (RT-PCR) on FNAB specimens detecting mRNA in cell numbers as small as ten for some genes and opening the possibility for molecular genetic analyses for preoperative diagnosis on such specimens. Also by RT-PCR from FNAB, Zeiger et al. [156] were able to demonstrate the expression of telomerase transcriptase in 2 out of 3 follicular carcinomas but not in 3 follicular adenomas and 5 hyperplastic nodules. For all specimens they achieved predictive values of more than 90%. In contrast, Haugen et al. [49], by using a telomeric repeat amplification protocol (TRAP) on surgical material, found no telomerase activity in three follicular carcinomas, but a positive reaction in 10 of 14 papillary carcinomas.

Although papillary carcinoma has – in contrast to well-differentiated follicular carcinoma – clearly defined cytomorphologic patterns detectable in FNAB specimens, there are also some problems in making a differential diagnosis between papillary hyperplasia in nodular goiter; therefore, new techniques have been used to solve this problem. Immunocytochemistry with antibodies against CD 57 [69] and CD 44 [25] have been shown to be of diagnostic value. Takano et al. [135] have used a real-time quantitative RT-PCR technique to measure the copy number of oncofetal fibronectin mRNA in FNAB specimens and found significant differences between papillary carcinomas and adenomatous goiter. The expression of *MAGE-1* and *GAGE-1/-2* genes in FNAB has been shown by Ruschenburg et al. [116] to give additional information to delineate papillary carcinoma from papillary hyperplasia.

These molecular techniques may be the basis of a clinically useful method to solve this diagnostic problem that hampers the application of FNAB in presurgical decision making.

2.7 Prognosis

Several attempts have been made to improve the accuracy of prognosis beyond the scope of classic histopathology and its combinations with clinicopathological scoring systems. These attempts refer to cell-biological mechanisms such as cellular proliferation or differentiation and tumor-stromal interaction (or combinations thereof). Nuclear morphometry and cytometry (both image cytometry and flow cytometry) have been used for many years. Recently, Sturgis et al. [131] readdressed this method and showed that DNA image cytometry on fine-needle aspirates from 26 primary and metastatic papillary thyroid carcinomas by the detection of aneuploidy predicts distant metastasis and death from the tumor. Tseleni et al. [143] showed a correlation of descriptive nuclear morphometric patterns (such as area, perimeter, axis length and roundness) with clinical prognostic factors (age, tumor size, and thyroid capsule infiltration). More precisely defined proliferation markers have been studied by several authors. The antibody against proliferating cell nuclear antigen (PCNA) has given contradictory results. Ando et al. [4] found a correlation of PCNA staining index with age and sex, but Moreira Leite et al. [92] found PCNA to be independent from the prognostic MACIS score.

The best standardized proliferation marker *Ki67* (or *Mib1*) has also been used alone or in combination with other cell biological markers. Tallini et al. [137] compared the immunohistochemical expression of *Ki67/Mib1* and cyclin-dependent kinase inhibitor *p27/KIP1* with morphologically based prognostic groups (well-differentiated papillary or follicular carcinoma, papillary or follicular carcinoma with unfavorable pathologic features: poorly differentiated or tall-cell variant, and undifferentiated carcinomas). Whereas both tested parameters showed a clear correlation with the histological groups and with some clinical prognostic factors, no significant association could be found within any of the histological groups. Resnick et al. [110] came to similar conclusions, but in contrast to Tallini et al. [137] they found different levels of p27 staining between papillary and follicular carcinoma. In the papillary microcarcinoma group, Sugitani et al. [134] demonstrated that besides bulky lymph-node metastases, *Ki67* and TGF beta3 labeling indices may be indicators of a worse outcome for the patients. Also, p53 overexpression and growth factor receptors (such as epidermal growth factor receptor [EGFR]) have been shown to be correlated with classic prognostic factors [22]. CD97 originally found on the cell surface of leukocytes has been shown to be a marker of dedifferentiation in thyroid carcinoma [5]. Two pathogenetically interesting groups of papillary carcinoma have been analyzed as to whether they represent prognostic specific entities: carcinomas with sporadic ret oncogene rearrangement and carcinomas arising in patients with familial adenomatous polyposis. Soares et al. [128] demonstrated ret rearrangement by Southern blot analysis in 24.2% of sporadic papillary carcinomas and found no correlation with several pathological and clinical parameters, but with significantly younger age and lower proliferation rate.

Interesting results have been obtained by investigations on mechanisms of cellular interactions. Walgenbach et al. [149] showed that the immunohistochemical downregulation of E-cadherin was associated with advanced

T categories and higher rates of lymph-node involvement and distant metastasis and represents a significant prognostic factor for worse survival. CD44-v6 was shown by Kurozumi et al. [74] to be correlated with lymph-node metastasis. Angiogenesis, as a promising field of research, has also been investigated in thyroid carcinoma by several groups. Ishiwata et al. [61] demonstrated that the counting of factor VIII-related antigen-stained microvessels represents an independent prognostic factor in papillary thyroid carcinomas. Accordingly, Dhar et al. [30] found that microvessel density was significantly correlated with recurrence-free survival. In contrast, Fontanini et al. [37] found an association between newly formed vessels and survival in medullary carcinoma patients but not in the groups with well-differentiated or undifferentiated carcinomas. These discrepancies may also be influenced by methodology aspects: Wong et al. [153] showed, by differentiation between systematic measurements across one dimension of the tumor (systematic field analysis) and assessment from the three most vascularized fields of the tumor (hot spot analysis) that only hot-spot analysis was correlated with prognosis in cases of follicular carcinoma. In contrast, vascularity was not correlated with outcome in cases of papillary carcinoma, regardless of the method of assessment. However, Miki et al. [89], using an immunohistochemical approach, showed a higher expression in clinically evident tumors than in occult carcinomas and higher expression in tumors with extrathyroidal extension and concluded that the *ret/PTC* oncogene may be involved in the local invasion of papillary carcinomas. The second molecular pathological pathway also under investigation for specific prognostic characteristics is the rare but well-documented occurrence of papillary carcinoma at the familial adenomatous polyposis (FAP) syndrome. These tumors frequently show cribriform structures and multicentricity and bilateral disease and occur at young age, but the long-term prognosis is good according to Perrier et al. [105].

2.8 Pathogenesis

Molecular biology and pathology have supported us with an enormous arsenal of molecular tools and mechanisms to study thyroid cancer and to evolve solutions to many of the problems in clinical pathology. These new data enable us to analyze the anatomical and molecular histogenesis of the tumors, the cytogenetic development from benign tumors to highly aggressive neoplasms and complex regulation systems of cellular growth and differentiation, including thyroidcarcinoma-specific interactions with stromal elements. Some of these data are represented where close associations with clinical pathology are obvious.

2.8.1
Anatomical Histogenesis

Tumors with both follicular and C-cell differentiation have been recognized for several years [48]. Trapping of thyroglobulin-positive preexisting follicles within the tumor areas has always been a problem. Recently, neuroendocrine differentiation in follicle-cell thyroid carcinoma has been observed by several authors, comparable with similar observations in other nonneuroendocrine organ tumors [64]. Tseleni-Balafouta et al. [143] found a statistically significant correlation between very frequent (46.6%) focal neuroendocrine differentiation of papillary carcinomas and some prognostically relevant factors such as old age, tumor size, infiltration of the tumor capsule, or lymph-node involvement.

2.8.2
Molecular Pathogenesis

2.8.2.1
Genetics

Medullary thyroid carcinoma in its inherited form (about 20% of all thyroid C-cell carcinomas) is now one of the best accepted and standardized examples of the application of molecular tumor pathology. It occurs in three distinct clinical syndromes [MEN 2a, MEN 2b and familiar medullary carcinoma (FMTC)] and is based upon germline mutations of the *RET* proto-oncogene. The entity of FMTC was criticized by Moers et al. [91], who found that the specific type of the respective germline mutation rather than the actual predominating phenotype should be the basis of classification. By screening a large family with FMTC over a long period of time, the authors found a similar phenotypic course of the disease with MEN 2a families with the same mutation of the *RET* oncogene (Cys 618), but different results from that in families with a Cys634 mutation. Prophylactic thyroidectomy is justified in gene carriers. Hinze et al. [56] investigated the thyroids of patients at risk of hereditary medullary carcinoma after prophylactic thyroidectomy. The youngest patient with carcinoma was 6 years, the youngest with lymph-node metastasis, 17 years. Kebebew et al. [67] presented three cases of children who underwent preventive total thyroidectomy who had no evidence of medullary carcinoma or C-cell hyperplasia. According to their review of the literature, 3.4% of patients have normal glands, indicating that the intervention occurred before the appearance of hyperplasia.

Interestingly, a proportion of sporadic medullary carcinomas are associated with somatic mutations of the *ret* proto-oncogene indistinguishable from the MEN 2b syndrome (codon-918, and very rarely codon 883). Eng et al. [32] detected codon 918 mutations in 80% of sporadic medullary carcinomas in at least one subpopulation of the tumor.

Both papillary and follicular carcinoma may also occur in a familial form. Papillary carcinoma is a rare manifestation of familiar adenomatous polyposis and occurs in about 1–2% of patients. These tumors have been shown to present "unusual" histology in the majority of cases [105]. Comparable histological findings were described in non-FAP cases by Cameselle-Teijeiro and Chan [17], suggesting that this cribriform-molecular variant may represent the sporadic counterpart of FAP-associated carcinoma. Cetta et al. [21], in a large series of patients with FAP-associated thyroid carcinomas, found germline mutations of the *APC* gene frequently in exon 15 in the genomic area associated with congenital hypertrophy of the retinal pigment epithelium (CMPE). Interesting types of familial carcinoma have been described by Canzian et al. [18], with the mapping of a gene site on chromosome *19p* and with cellular oxyphilia of the tumors. Lupoli et al. [83] described a familial papillary microcarcinoma with unfavorable behavior. The occurrence of follicular carcinoma in patients with Cowden's disease has long been well known. Recently, *PTEN* gene germline mutations have been detected and *PTEN* inactivation in transgenic mice developed spontaneous thyroid tumors besides tumors at other sites [31].

2.8.2.2 Malignant Transformation

In papillary carcinoma the *ret* proto-oncogene activation has been intensively studied. The *PTC/ret* oncogene arises through an intrachromosomal inversion or translocation of the tyrosine-kinase domain of the *ret* proto-oncogene with different activating genes. Three transforming fusion proteins are known (rcVPTC 1–3). The *ret/PTC 1* rearrangement has been shown to occur in children suffering from Chernobyl-associated papillary thyroid carcinomas in 29% [107]. Nikiforov et al. [96] compared the ret oncogene rearrangements and histomorphology in post-Chernobyl papillary carcinomas in children with children without history of radiation exposure. Both the histopathology and molecular findings showed interesting differences. Whereas in the sporadic group a typical papillary pattern was prevalent, among radiation-induced tumors solid variants of papillary carcinoma were found in 37% and typical papillary carcinoma only in 18%. Among radiation-induced tumors the distribution pattern of the *ret* oncogene subtypes (pTC1-3) was 16.2 and 58%, whereas in the sporadic group 47% showed PTC1 and only 18% pTC3. The NTRKI tyrosine kinase/tropomyosin (TPM) rearrangement has been found in only 5 of 81 tumors without *ret* rearrangement from children after the Chernobyl reactor accident [9]. Waldmann and Rabes [148] demonstrated that, in contrast to thyroid neoplasia in adults, *G(s) alpha* gene mutations do not play a role in the development of childhood thyroid tumors. Nikiforov et al. [97] have investigated the breakpoints of the two genes involved in the fusion of the *ret/PTC3* oncogene in radiation-induced post-Chernobyl papillary thyroid carcinomas (*ELEI* and *RET*) and found them distributed in a relatively random fashion, except for clustering in the ALU region of ELEI. The alignment of *ELEI* and *RET* introns in the opposite orientation showed that the position of the break in one gene corresponded to the break in the other gene. Their suggestion is that a single radiation track could produce concerted breaks in both genes leading to inversion and fusion due to reciprocal exchange via end-joining of the gene fragments. Animal models have been used to study the pathogenetic mechanisms of ret oncogene activation leading to papillary carcinoma. Cho et al. [26] demonstrated increased follicle-cell proliferation rate, distorted follicle formation, and reduced radioiodide-concentrating activity after targeted expression of *RET/PTC 1* in the thyroid gland in transgenic mice. Interestingly, Fischer et al. [36] were able to demonstrate by the use of a *RET/PTC* retroviral construct infection of human thyroid epithelial cells, that the *RET/PTC*-infected cells showed an altered nuclear morphology with an irregular nuclear contour and a euchromatic appearance similar to papillary carcinoma in vivo. The growth pattern was also changed in vitro following infection with *RET/PTC*. In a large series from 27 regions of the Ukraine, Tronko et al. [141] in agreement with molecular pathology data, have shown a high frequency of papillary carcinomas with solid growth pattern, lymph-node metastasis, and extrathyroidal spread. In contrast, in sporadic papillary carcinoma in adult patients, *ret/PTC* activation did not correlate with clinical markers of increased morbidity (large tumor size, extrathyroidal extension, and metastases) [136].

Besides these thyroid-specific mechanisms the role of many oncogenes and growth-regulating proteins also active in other tumors has been investigated. *Ras* point mutations have been shown to occur very early in tumorigenesis (reviewed by Wynford-Thomas [154]). Even follicular adenomas have revealed one of the three known point mutations in up to 33%. In contrast, by the use of a highly sensitive single-stranded conformation polymorphism (SSCP) approach combined with DNA sequencing, Ezzat et al. [35] found one H *ras* mutation (codon 13) and two discrete alterations on codon 17, and 22 N61 mutations in two papillary carcinomas and one follicular adenoma. K *ras* mutations were not present in any of the tumors examined (n=45). Bartolone et al. [7] have investigated the frequency of activating mutations of the three ras mutations in thyroid tumors from patients from a iodine-deficient and from a relatively iodine-sufficient area and found no mutations at the three known mutation spots. Sugg et al. [132] have compared the appearance of H, N, K *ras* mutations with *ret/PTC* rearrangement and *erbB- 2/neu* mutations. They also found a relatively low frequency of *ras* mutation in papillary carcinoma. *ErbB-2/neu* gene amplification and activating mutations have not been detected, but elevated mRNA levels have. The lack of correlation among the three oncogenes was interpreted as suggesting that they are not cumulative factors in the pathogenesis of papillary carcinoma. A comparative analysis of c-erbB-2, bcl-2, p53 and p21 was performed by Soda et al. [130] by immunohistochemical staining. Bel-2 was expressed only in well-differentiated tumors, with only some poorly differentiated tumors staining positive. p21 was detected in about the half of the tumors and p53 in 10% with strong reaction in poorly differentiated tumors. Bel-2 and Bax as apoptosis-repressing and -promoting proteins were also investigated by Manetto et al. [84]. In their immunohistochemical and Western blot analysis, the authors have shown Bcl-2 expression in benign lesions and well-differentiated carcinomas, expression of both proteins in cases of tall-cell variant papillary carcinoma and poorly differentiated carcinoma, and sole Bax expression in anaplastic carcinoma.

2.8.2.3 Mechanisms of Invasion and Metastasis

The *met* oncogene encodes for a protein with tyrosine kinase activity, which serves as a receptor for hepatocyte growth factor/scatter factor, which stimulates cell motility and invasion in particular. This complex has been investigated especially in papillary carcinoma. Ruco et al. [114] found Met protein expression immunohistochemically in 77% of papillary carcinomas. By functional in vitro investigations on primary cultures of papillary carcinomas, the same group has demonstrated the involvement of the HGF/*Met* system in the invasiveness of tumor cells. Another mechanism of invasion investigated is cathepsin B activity. Shuja et al. [126] found a ninefold increase of cathepsin B in papillary carcinoma. Altered patterns of immunohistochemical staining and additional protein bands on Western blots led to the suggestion that Cathepsin B may play a role in invasion and metastasis. Inactivation of E-cadherin, a suppressor of invasion and metastasis has been shown by Graff et al. [46] to be caused not by mutations but by hypermethylation of the 5 CpG island frequently in papillary carcinoma. Beta-catenin mutations were frequently detected in anaplastic carcinomas by Garcia-Rostan et al. [41]. The role of integrins in particular in bone metastasis has been investigated. Smit et al. [127] demonstrated an effect of synthetic RGD peptides on the attachment of cell lines of primary and metastatic follicular carcinomas in vitro. The attachment could be inhibited by anti-integrin antibodies. Bellahcene et al. [10] demonstrated the expression of bone sialoprotein in the majority thyroid carcinomas with significantly higher expression in poorly differentiated carcinomas. Bone sialoprotein is found physiologically in the mineral compartment of the developing bone. Interestingly, this protein is expressed ectopically in tumors known to metastasize to the skeleton. The proto-oncogene ets-1, a transcription factor controlling a number of genes involved in remodeling of the extracellular matrix, was detected in the majority of thyroid carcinomas, but also in 40% of follicular adenomas by Nakayama et al. [95].

2.8.2.4 Cell Cycle Regulation

Many cell cycle regulators have been investigated in thyroid carcinoma. By semiquantitative immunohistochemical staining of follicular adenomas and follicular variants of papillary carcinomas Wang et al. [150] demonstrated similar staining results of cyclin DI and E, but a significant increase in staining intensity of p27 in adenomas when compared with papillary carcinoma (follicular variant). Muro-Cacho et al. [93] found an increase in cyclin D1 and down regulation of p27kip by immunohistochemical staining of papillary carcinomas. This was explained by functional abnormalities in type 11 receptors of transforming growth factor beta. In contrast, Baldassarre et al. [6] found an abnormal cytoplasmic localization of p27, which was explained by overexpression of cyclin D3. These mechanisms were analyzed by in vitro transfection of a mutant p27 devoted to its nuclear localization signal and thereby intermitting the interaction with nuclear cyclin-dependentkinase 2. The Axl protein as a new family of receptor tyrosine kinase has been shown to play a crucial role in regulating thyroid-cell growth and differentiation. The respective ligand Gas6, a protein S-related molecule, is a mitogenic factor for thyroid follicle cells. Ito et al. [63] have demonstrated increased Axl expression by immunohistochemistry and mRNA in situ hybridization in papillary and anaplastic carcinomas.

The frequency of p53 mutations is generally low in differentiated thyroid carcinoma. Ho et al. [57] combined immunohistochemical staining of *p53* with genotypic analyses and found nuclear overexpression only in poorly differentiated (10.5%) and undifferentiated carcinomas (25%). Mutations occurred in 4.35% of well-differentiated carcinomas and in 17.2% of poorly differentiated carcinomas. The mutation rate in undifferentiated carcinoma is high [62].

2.8.2.5 Cytogenetics and Clonality

Chromosomal and cytogenetic studies are of interest both for diagnostic and basic reasons apart from analyses of the known genes. Clonality was studied by Kim et al. [70] using a PCR assay in the X-linked human androgen receptor (*HUMARA*) gene by random X chromosome inactivation in women. All papillary carcinomas and follicular adenomas investigated were monoclonal, but also 3 of 13 follicular nodules from nodular goiters were monoclonal. This technique was successfully applied by Kakudo et al. [64] to the differentiation between aberrant thyroid tissue (tongue and bilateral neck lymph nodes) from true metastases of thyroid carcinoma. On a chromosomal level, Califano et al. [16] investigated 30 papillary carcinomas for loss of heterozygosity (LOH) and found LOH in 15 cases with frequent loci at 4q, 5p, 7p and 11p suggesting putative tumor-suppressor genes at these chromosomal arms. Polysomies of chromosomes 7 and 12 were detected by Roque et al. [111] by conventional and fluorescence in situ hybridization (FISH) cytogenetic studies. With the FISH technique they found gains with increasing frequency from goiters to adenomas and follicular carcinomas (18.2%, 52.4% and 66%). By comparative genomic hybridization (CGH) analyses, Hemmer et al. [55] found mostly gains in adenomas (chromosomes 7, 5, 12, 14, X, 18, 17) but losses in follicular carcinomas (chromosome 22, 1). Loss of chromosome 22 has been shown to be common in widely invasive follicular carcinoma. In Hürthle-cell neoplasms Tallini et al. [136], by the use of CGH, found two separate groups of tumors, one with gains of chromosomes 5 and 7, the other by loss of chromosome 2. Pathological and clinical features were similar in the two groups and the chromosomal unbalance was found to be independent from the ras-mutation (only one case in this series with a balanced karyotype). Recently Wilkens et al. [151] have used FISH and CGH and found aberrations of *5p*, *8p* and *8q* to play a role in the development of anaplastic thyroid carcinoma, whereas Komoike et al. [72] also found frequent loss of 16p by CGH techniques on tumor-cell lines. Microsatellite instability was detected by Lazzereschi et al. [78] in 21.5% of thyroid tumors and tumor He lesions investigated, including 9.8% of cases with instability at three or more loci. Instability was significantly more frequent in follicular adenoma and carcinoma than in papillary carcinoma. In the group of familial nonmedullary thyroid cancer (FNMTC) Canzian et al. [18] mapped a chromosomal gene locus to chromosome 19p by linkage analyses.

2.8.2.6 Receptor Activation

Mutations of the TSH receptor have been shown to be a major cause of toxic adenoma of the thyroid. Tonacchera et al. [139] demonstrated activating mutations in 12 of 15 hyperfunctioning thyroid adenomas. In one adenoma, which was negative for *TSH-R* mutations, a mutation of the *Gs alpha* gene was identified. In contrast, in nonfunctioning adenomas (and including two cases with malignant transformation) no mutations of the *TSH-R* or the *Gs alpha* gene could be identified. In a larger series of carcinomas, the same group has corroborated these data and suggested that clonal somatic mutations of the *THS-R* gene do not play a role in the pathogenesis of differentiated thyroid carcinoma [20]. The insulin receptor has been demonstrated by immunohistochemistry and functional assays [39] to be significantly increased in follicular and papillary thyroid carcinoma, but also in nonfunctioning benign adenoma.

2.8.2.7 Telomerase

Much interest has been concentrated on telomerase in thyroid neoplasms. Some of the diagnostic aspects have been discussed above. Brousset et al. [13] detected telomerase activity in 20% of papillary carcinomas and 4 of 6 follicular and 2 of 3 undifferentiated carcinomas. One case out of 12 adenomas was positive. Similar results were reported by Cheng et al. [24]. They found 52% of papillary carcinomas and 91% of follicular carcinomas to be positive by the use of telomeric repeat amplification protocol and 4 out of 14 adenomas. The cancers negative for telomerase activity were mostly in the early stages.

References

1. Albareda M, Puig-Domingo M, Wengrowicz S, Soldevila ,J, Matias-Guiu X, Caballero A, Chico A, De Leiva A (1998) Clinical forms of presentation and evolution of diffuse sclerosing variant of papillary carcinoma and insular variant of follicular carcinoma of the thyroid. Thyroid 8:385–391
2. Albores-Saavedra J, LiVolsi VA, Williams ED (1985) Medullary carcinoma. Semin Diagn Pathol 2:137–146
3. Albores-Saavedra J, Housine I, Vuitch F, Snyder VM (1997) Macrofollicular variant of papillary thyroid carcinoma with minor insular component. Cancer 80:1110–1116

4. Ando H, Funahashi H, Ito M, Imai T, Takagi H (1996) Proliferating cell nuclear antigen expression in papillary thyroid carcinoma. J Clin Pathol 49:657–659
5. Aust G, Eichler W, Laue S, Lehmann I, Heldin NE, Lotz O, Scherbaum WA, Dralle H, Hoang-Vu C (1997) Cd97: a dedifferentiation marker in human thyroid carcinomas. Cancer Res 57:1798–1806
6. Balsassarre G, Belletti B, Bnnü P, Bocia A, Trapasso F, Pentimalli F, Barone MV, Chiapetta G, Vento MT, Spiezia S, Fusco A, Viglietto G (1999) Overexpressed cyclin D3 contributes to retaining the growth inhibitor p27 in the cytoplasm of thyroid tumor cells. J Clin Invest 104:865–874
7. Bartolone L, Vermiglio F, Finocchiaro MD, Violi MA, French D, Pontecorvi A, Trimarchi F, Benvenga S (1998) Thyroid follicle oncogenesis in iodine deficient and iodine-sufficient areas: search for alterations of the ras, met and BFGF oncogenes and of the Rb anti-oncogene. J Endocrinol Invest 21:680–687
8. Basolo F, Baloch ZW, Baldanzi A, Miccoli P, LiVolsi VA (1999) Usefulness of Ultrafast Papanicolaou- stained scrape preparations in intraoperative management of thyroid lesions. Mod Pathol 12:653–657
9. Beimfohr C, Klugbauer S, Demidchik EP, Lengfelder E, Rabes HM (1999) NTKRI re-arrangement in papillary thyroid carcinomas of children alter the Chernobyl reactor accident. Int J Cancer 80:842–847
10. Bellahcene A, Albert V, Pollina L, Basolo F, Fisher LW, Castronovo V (1998) Ectopic expression of bone sialoprotein in human thyroid cancer. Thyroid 8:637–641
11. Berho M, Suster S (1997) The oncocytic variant of papillary carcinoma of the thyroid: a clinicopathologic study of 15 cases. Hum Pathol 28:47–53
12. Brierley JD, Panzarella T, Tsang RW, Gospodarowicz MK, O'Sullivan B (1997) A comparison of different staging systems predictability of patient's outcome. Thyroid carcinoma as an example. Cancer 79:2414–2423
13. Brousset P, Chaouche N, Leprat F, Branet-Brousset F, Trouettc II, Zenou RC, Merlio JP, Delsol G (1997) Tclomerase activity in human thyroid carcinomas originating from the follicular cells. J Endocrinol Metab 82:4214–4216
14. Byar DP, Green SB, Dor P, Williams ED, Colo J, van Gilse HA, Mayer M, Sylvester RJ, van Glabbeke M (1979) A prognostic index for thyroid carcinoma. A study of the E.O.R.T.C. thyroid cancer cooperative Group. Eur J Cancer 15:1033–1041
15. Cady B, Rossi R (1988) An expanded view of risk-group definition in differentiated thyroid carcinoma. Surgery 104:947–953
16. Califano JA, Johns MM, Westra WH, Lango MN, Eisele D, Saji M, Zeiger MA, Udelsman R, Koch WM, Sidransky D (1996) An allelotype of papillary thyroid cancer. Int J Cancer 69:442–444
17. Cameselle-Teijeiro J, Chan JK (1999) Cribriform-morular variant of papillary carcinoma: a distinctive variant representing the sporadic counterpart of familial adenomatous polyposis-associated thyroid carcinoma? Mod Pathol 12:400–411
18. Canzian F, Amati P, Harach W, Kraimps JL, Lesueur F, Barbier J, Levillain P, Remeo G, Bonneau D (1998) A gene predisposing to familiar thyroid tumors with cell oxyphilia maps to chromosome 19p13.2. Am J Hum Genet 63:1743–1748
19. Carcangiu ML, Zampi G, Rosai J (1984) Poorly differentiated ("insular") thyroid carcinoma. A reinterpretation of Langhans' "wuchernde Struma". Am J Surg Pathol 8:655–668
20. Cetani F, Tonacchera M, Pinchera A, Barsacchi R, Basolo F, Miccoli P, Pacini F (1999) Genetic analysis of the TSH receptor gene in differentiated human thyroid carcinomas. J Endocrinol Invest 22:273–278
21. Cetta F, Montalto G, Gori M, Curia MC, Cama A, Olschwang S (2000) Germline mutations of the APC gene in patients with familial adenomatous polyposis-associated thyroid carcinoma: results from a European cooperative study. J Clin Endocrinol Metab 85:286–292
22. Chen BK, Ohtsuki Y, Furihata M, Takeuchi T, lwata J, Liang SB Sonobe H (1999) Co-overexpression of p53 protein and epidermal growth factor receptor in human papillary

thyroid carcinomas correlated with lymph node metastasis, tumor size and clinicopathologic stage. Int J Oncol 15:893–898
23. Chen H, Nicol TL, Zeiger MA, Dooley WC, Ladenson PW, Cooper DS, Ringel M, Parkerson S, Allo M, Udelsman R (1998) Hurtle cell neoplasms of the thyroid: Are there factors predictive of malignancy? Ann Surg 227:542–546
24. Cheng AJ, Lin JD, Chang T, Wang TC (1998) Telomerase activity in benign and malignant human thyroid tissues. Br J Cancer 77:2177–2180
25. Chieng DC, Ross JS, McKenna BJ (1997) CD 44 immunostaining of thyroid fine-needle aspirates differentiates thyroid papillary carcinoma from other lesions with nuclear grooves and inclusions. Cancer 81:157–162
26. Cho JY, Sagartz JE, Capen CC, Mazzaferri EL, Jhiang SM (1999) Early cellular abnormalities induced by RET/PTC 1 oncogene in thyroid-targeted transgenic mice. Oncogene 18:3659–3665
27. Deandrea M, Gallone G, Veglio M, Balsamo A, Grassi A, Sapelli S, Rossi C, Nasi PG, Porcellana V, Varvello G, Capussotti L, Taraglio S, Ravarino N, Torchio B, Fonzo D (1997) Thyroid cancer histotype changes as observed in a major general hospital in a 21-year period. J Endocrinol Invest 20:52–58
28. DeGroot LJ, Kaplan EL, McCormick M, Straus FH (1990) Natural history, treatment, and course of papillary thyroid carcinoma. J Clin Endocrinol Metab 71:414–424
29. Deshpande V, Kapila K, Sai KS, Venna K (1997) Follicular neoplasms of the thyroid. Decision tree approach using morphologic and morphometric parameters. Acta Cytol 41:369–376
30. Dhar DK, Kubota H, Kotoh T, Tabara H, Watanabe R, Tachibana M, Kohno H, Nagasue N (1998) Tumor vascularity precincts recurrence in differentiated thyroid carcinoma. Am J Surg 176:442–447
31. Di Cristofano A, Pesce B, Cordon-Cardo C, Pandolfi PP (1998) Pten is essential for embryonic development and tumor suppression. Nat Genet 19:348–355
32. Eng C, Thomas GA, Neuberg DS, Mulligan LM, Healey CS, Houghton C, Frilling A, Raue F, Williams ED, Ponder BA (1998) Mutation of the RET proto-oncogene is correlated with immunostaining in subpopulations of cells in sporadic medullary carcinoma. J Clin Endocrinol Metab 83:4310–4313
33. Evans HL (1986) Columnar-cell carcinoma of the thyroid. A report of two cases of an aggressive variant of thyroid carcinoma. Am J Clin Pathol 85:77–80
34. Evans HL (1996) Encapsulated columnar-cell neoplasms of the thyroid. A report of four cases suggesting a favorable prognosis. Am J Surg Pathol 20:1205–1211
35. Ezzat S, Zheng L, Kolenda J, Safarian A, Freeman JL, Asa SL (1996) Prevalence of activating ras mutations in morphologically characterized thyroid nodules. Thyroid 6:409–416
36. Fischer AH, Bond JA, Taysavang P, Battles OE, Wynford-Thomas D (1998) Papillary thyroid carcinoma oncogene (RET/PTC) alters the nuclear envelope and chromatin structure. Am J Pathol 153:1443–1450
37. Fontanini G, Vignati S, Pacini F, Pollina L, Basolo F (1996) Microvessel count: an indicator of poor outcome in medullary thyroid carcinoma but not in other types of thyroid carcinoma. Mod Pathol 9:636–641
38. Franc B, Rosenberg-Bourgin M, Caillou B, Dutrieux-Berger N, Floquet J, Houcke-Lecomte M, Justrabo E, Lange F, Labat-Moleur F, Le Bodic MF, Patey M, Beauchet A, Saint-Andre JP, Hejblum G, Viennet G (1998) Medullary thyroid carcinoma: search for histological predictors of survival (109 proband cases analysis). Hum Pathol 29:1078–1084
39. Frittitta L, Sciacca L, Catalfamo R, Ippolito R, Gangemi P, Pezzino V, Filetti V, Vigneri R (1999) Functional insulin receptors are overexpressed in thyroid tumors: is this an early event in thyroid tumorgenesis? Cancer 85:492–498
40. Fuchshuber PR, Loree TR, Hicks WL, Cheney RT, Shedd DP (1998) Medullary carcinoma of the thyroid: prognostic factors and treatment recommendations. Ann Surg Oncol 5:81–86

41. Garcia-Rostan G, Tallini G, Herrero A, D'Aquila TG, Carcangiu ML, Rimm DL (1999) Frequent mutation of beta-catenin in anaplastic thyroid carcinoma. Cancer Res 59:1811–1815
42. Gauger PG, Reeve TS, Delbridge LW (1999) Intraoperative decision making in follicular lesions of the thyroid: is tumor size important? J Am Coll Surg 189:253–258
43. Gilliland FD, Hunt WC, Morris DM, Key CR (1997) Prognostic factors for thyroid carcinoma. A population-based study of 15,698 cases from the Surveillance, Epidemiology and End Results (SEER) program 1973–1991. Cancer 79:564–573
44. Girelli ME, Nacamulli D, Pelizzo MR, De Vido D, Mian C, Piccolo M, Busnardo B (1998) Medullary thyroid carcinoma: clinical features and long-term follow-up of seventy-eight patients treated between 1969 and 1986. Thyroid 8:517–5.23
45. Goldstein NS, Czako P, Neill JS (2000) Metastatic minimally invasive (encapsulated) follicular and Hurthle cell thyroid carcinoma: a study of 34 patients. Mod Pathol 13:123–130
46. Graff M, Greenberg VE, Herman JG, Westra WH, Boghaert ER, Ain KB, Saji M, Zeiger MA, Zimmer SG, Baylin SB (1998) Distinct patterns of E-cadherin CpG island methylation in papillary, follicular, Hurthle's cell, and poorly differentiated thyroid carcinoma. Cancer Res 58:2063–2066
47. Green FL (2002) AJCC. Cancer staging handbook, 6th edn. TNM classification of malignant tumors. Springer, Berlin Heidelberg New York, pp 89–98
48. Guyetant S, Dupre F, Bigorgne JC, Franc B, Dutrieux-Berger N, Lecomte-Houcke M, Patey M, Caillou B, Viennet G, Guerin O, Saint-Andre JP (1999) Medullary thyroid microcarcinoma: a clinicopathological retrospective study of 38 patients with no prior familial disease. Hum Pathol 30:957–963
49. Hales M, Rosenau W, Okerlund MD, Galante M (1982) Carcinoma of the thyroid with a mixed medullary and follicular pattern: morphologic, immunohistochemical, and clinical laboratory studies. Cancer 50:1352–1359
50. Haugen BR, Nawaz S, Markham N, Hashizumi T, Shroyer AL, Werness B, Shroyer KR (1997) Telomerase activity in benign and malignant thyroid. Thyroid 7:337–342
51. Hawk WA, Hazard JB (1976) The many appearances of papillary carcinoma of the thyroid. Comparison with the common form of papillary carcinoma by DNA and morphometric analysis. Cleve Clin Q 43:207–215
52. Hay ID (1990) Papillary thyroid carcinoma. Endocrinol Clin North Am 19:658–718
53. Hay ID, Bergstralh EJ, Goellner M, Ebersold M, Grant CS (1993) Predicting outcome in papillary thyroid carcinoma: development of a reliable prognostic scoring system in a cohort of 1779 patients surgically treated at one institution during 1940 through 1989. Surgery 114:1050–1057
54. Hazard JB (1960) Small papillary carcinoma of the thyroid. A study with special reference to so-called nonencapsulated sclerosing tumor. Lab Invest 9:86–97
55. Hedinger C, Williams ED, Sobin LH (1988) Histological typing of thyroid tumors, 2nd edn. International histological classification of tumors, no 11. World Health Organization. Springer, Berlin Heidelberg New York
56. Hemmer S, Wasenius VM, Knuutila S, Joensuu H, Franssila K (1998) Comparison of benign and malignant follicular thyroid tumors by comparative genomic hybridization. Br J Cancer 78:1012–1017
57. Hinze R, Holzhausen HJ, Gimm O, Rath FW (1998) Primary hereditary medullary thyroid carcinoma-C-cell morphology and correlation with preoperative calcitonin levels. Virchows Arch 433:203–208
58. Ho YS, Tseng SC, Chin TY, Hsieh LL, Lin JD (1996) p53 gene mutation in thyroid carcinoma. Cancer Lett 103:57–63
59. Hofstaedter F (1980) Frequency and morphology of malignant tumors of the thyroid before and after the introduction of iodine-prophylaxis. Virchows Arch A 385:263–270
60. Hofstaedter F (1980) Electron microscopic investigations about the differentiation of thyroid carcinoma. Pathol Res Pract 169:304–322

61. Horii A, Yoshida J, Sakai, M Okamoto S, Honjo Y, Mitani K, Hattori K, Kubo T (1999) Ki-67 positive fractions m benign and malignant thyroid tumors: application of flow cytometry. Acta Otolaryngol 119:617–620
62. Ishiwata T, Iino Y, Takei H, Oyama T, Morishita Y (1998) Tumor angiogenesis as an independent prognostic indicator in human papillary thyroid carcinoma. Oncol Rep 5:1343–1348
63. Ito T, Seyama T, Mizuno T (1992) Unique association of p53 mutations with undifferentiated but not with differentiated carcinomas of the thyroid gland. Cancer Res 52:1369-1371
64. Ito T, Ito M, Naito S, Ohtsuru A, Nagayama Y, Kanematsu T, Yamashita S, Sekine I (1999) Expression of the Axi receptor tyrosine kinase in human thyroid carcinoma. Thyroid 9:563–567
65. Kakudo K, Shan L, Nakamura Y, Inoue D, Koshiyama H, Sato H (1998) Clonal analysis helps to differentiate aberrant thyroid tissue from thyroid carcinoma. Hum Pathol 29:187–190
66. Kargi A, Yorukoglu Aktas S, Cakalagaoglu E (1996) Neuroendocrine differentiation in non-neuroendocrine thyroid carcinoma. Thyroid 6:207–210
67. Kashima K, Yokoyama S, Noguchi S, Murakami N, Yamashita H, Watanabe S, Uchino S, Toda M, Sasaki A, Daa T, Nakayama I (1998) Chronic thyroiditis as a favorable prognostic factor in papillary thyroid carcinoma. Thyroid 8:197–202
68. Kebebew E, Tresler PA, Siperstein AE, Duh QY, Clark OH (1999) Normal thyroid pathology in patients undergoing thyroidectomy for finding a RET gene germline mutation: a report of three cases and review of the literature. Thyroid:127–131
69. Khafif A, Khafif RA, Attie JN (1999) Hurthle cell carcinoma: A malignancy of low-grade potential. Head Neck 21:506–511
70. Khan A, Baker SP, Patwardhan NA, Pullman JM (1998) CD 57 (Leu-7) expression is helpful in diagnosis of the follicular variant of papillary thyroid carcinoma. Virchows Arch 432:427–432
71. Kim H, Piao Z, Park C, Chung MTY, Park CS (1998) Clinical significance of clonality in thyroid nodules. Br J Surg 85:1125–1128
72. Klinck GH, Winship T (1955) Occult sclerosing carcinoma of the thyroid. Cancer 8:701–706
73. Komoike Y, Tamaki Y, Sakita I, Tomita N, Ohoue M, Sekimoto M, Miyazaki M, Kadota M, Masuda N, Ooka M, Ohnishi T, Nakano Y, Kozaki T, Kobayashi T, Matsuura N, Ikeda T, Horti A, Monden M (1999) Comparative genomic hybridization defines frequent loss on 16p in human anaplastic thyroid carcinoma. Int J Oncol 14:157–162
74. Kraemer BB (1987) Frozen section diagnosis and the thyroid. Semin Diagn Pathol 4:169–189
75. Kurozumi K, Nakao K, Nishida T, Nakahara M, Ogino N, Tsujimoto M (1998) Significance of biologic aggressiveness and proliferating activity in papillary thyroid carcinoma. World J Surg 22:1237–1242
76. LaGuette J, Matias-Guiu X, Rosai J (1997) Thyroid paraganglioma: A clinicopathologic and immunhistochemical study of three cases. Am J Surg Pathol 21:748–753
77. Lang W, Choritz H, Hundeshagen U (1986) Risk factors in follicular thyroid carcinomas. A retrospective follow-up study covering a 14-year period with emphasis on morphological findings. Am J Surg Pathol 10:246–255
78. Langhans T (1907) Über die epithelialen Formen der malignen Struma. Virchows Arch 189:69–188
79. Lazzereschi D, Palmirotta R, Rarnieri A, Ottini L, Veri MC, Cama A, Cetta F, Nardi F, Coletta G, Mariani-Costantini R (1999) Microsatellite instability in thyroid tumors and tumor-like lesions. Br J Cancer 79:340–345
80. Lindsay S (1960) Carcinoma of the thyroid gland. A clinical and pathological study of 293 patients at the university of California hospital. Thomas, Springfield, Ill

81. Lo CY, Lam KY, Wan KY (1999) Anaplastic carcinoma of the thyroid. Am J Surg 177:337–339
82. Loh KC, Greenspan FS, Gee L, Miller TR, Yeo PP (1997) Pathological tumor-node-metastasis (PTNM) staging for papillary and follicular carcinomas: a retrospective analysis of 700 patients. J Clin Endocr Metab 82:3553–3562
83. Loh KC, Greenspan FS, Dong F, Miller TR, Yeo PP (1999) Influence of lymphocytic thyroiditis on the prognostic outcome of patients with papillary thyroid carcinoma. J Clin Endocrinol Metab 84:458–463
84. Lupoli G, Vitale G, Caraglia M, Fittipaldi MR, Abbruzzese A, Tagliaferri P, Bianco AR (1999) Familial papillary thyroid microcarcinoma: a new clinical entity. Lancet 353:637–639
85. Manetto V, Lorenzini R, Cordon-Cardo C, Krajewski S, Rosai J, Reed JC, Eusebi V (1997) Bcl-2 and Bax expression in thyroid tumors. An immunohistochemical and Western blot analysis. Virchows Arch 430:125–130
86. Mazzaferri EL, Jhiang SM (1994) Long-term impact of initial surgical and medical therapy on papillary and follicular thyroid cancer. Am J Med 97:418–428
87. McConahey WM, Hay ID, Woolner LB, van Heerden JA, Taylor WF (1986) Papillary thyroid cancer treated at the Mayo Clinic, 1946 through 1970: initial manifestations, pathologic findings, therapy, and outcome. Mayo Clin Proc 61:978–996
88. McDonald MP, Sanders LE, Silverman ML, Chan HS, Buyske J (1996) Hurthle cell carcinoma of the thyroid gland: prognostic factors and results of surgical treatment. Surgery 120:1000–1004
89. McHenry CR, Raeburn C, Strickland T, Marty JJ (1996) The utility of routine frozen section examination for intraoperative diagnosis of thyroid cancer. Am J Surg 172:658–661
90. Miki H, Kitaichi M, Masuda E, Komaki K, Yamamoto Y, Monden Y (1999) ret/PTC expression may be associated with local invasion of thyroid papillary carcinoma. J Surg Oncol 71:76–81
91. Mitsiades N, Poulaki V, Mastorakos G, Tseleni-Balafouta ST, Kotoula V, Koutras DA, Tsokos M (1999) Fas ligand expression in thyroid carcinomas: a potential mechanism of immune evasion. J Clin Endocrinol Metab 84:2924–2932
92. Moers AM, Lansvater RM, Schaap C, Jansen-Schillhorn van Veen JM, de Valk IA, Blijham GH, Hoppener JW, Vroom TM, van Amstel HK, Lips CJ (1996) Familial medullary thyroid carcinoma: not a distinct entity? Genotype-phenotype correlation in a large family. Am J Med 101:635–641
93. Moreira Leite KR, de Araujo VC, Rezende Meirelles MI, Lopes Costa AD, Camara-Lopes LH (1999) No relationship between proliferative activity and the MACIS prognostic scoring system in papillary thyroid carcinoma. Head Neck 21:602–605
94. Muro-Cacho CA, Munoz-Antonia T, Livingston S, Klotch D (1999) Transforming growth factor beta receptors and p27kip in thyroid carcinoma. Arch Otolaryngol Head Neck Surg 125:76–81
95. Nagashima T, Suzuki M, Oshida M, Hashimoto FL Yagata H, Shishikura T, Koda K, Nakajima N (1998) Morphometry in the cytological evaluation of thyroid follicular lesions. Cancer 84:115–118
96. Nakayama T, Ito M, Ohtsuru A, Naito S, Nakashima M, Sekine I (1999) Expression of the ets-1 proto-oncogene in human thyroid tumor. Mod Pathol 12:61–68
97. Nikiforov YE, Rowland JM, Bove KE, Monforte-Munoz H, Fagin JA (1997) Distinct pattern of rot oneogene rearrangements in morphological variants of radiation-induced and sporadic thyroid papillary carcinomas in children. Cancer Res 57:1690–1694
98. Nikiforov YE, Koshoffer A, Nikiforova M, Stringer J, Fagin JA (1999) Chromosomal breakpoint positions suggest a direct role for radiation in inducing illegitimate recombination between the ELEI and RET genes in radiation-induced thyroid carcinomas. Oncogene 18:6330–6334
99. Nishida T, Katayama S, Tsujimoto M, Nakamura J, Matsuda U (1999) Clinicopathological significance of poorly differentiated thyroid carcinoma. Am J Surg Pathol 23:205–211

100. Orlandei F, Saggiorato E, Pivano G, Puligheddu B, Ternine A, Cappia S, De Giuli P, Angeli A (1998) Galectin-3 is a presurgical marker of human thyroid carcinoma. Cancer Res 58:3015–3020
101. Ostrowski ML, Merino MJ (1996) Tall cell variant of papillary thyroid carcinoma: a reassessment and immunohistochemical study with comparisons to the usual type of papillary carcinoma of the thyroid. Am J Surg Pathol 20:964–974
102. Ozaki O, Ito K, Mimura T, Sugino K, Hosoda Y (1996) Papillary carcinoma of the thyroid. Tall cell variant with extensive lymphocytic infiltration. Am J Surg Pathol 20:695–698
103. Papotti M, Torchio B, Grassi, L, Favero A, Bussolati G (1996) Poorly differentiated oxyphilic (Hurthle cell) carcinomas of the thyroid. Am J Surg Pathol 20:686–694
104. Papahavasit A, Thompson GB, Hay ID, Grant CS, van Heerden JA, Ilstrup DM, Schleck C, Goellner JR (1997) Follicular and Hurthle cell neoplasms. Is frozen-section evaluation worthwhile? Arch Surg 132: 674-678
105. Passler C, Scheuba, C, Prager G, Kaserer K, Flores JA, Vierhappen H, Niederle B (1999) Anaplastic (undifferentiated) thyroid carcinoma (ATC): a retrospective analysis. Langenbecks Arch Surg 384: 284-293
106. Perrier ND, van Heerden JA, Goellner JR, Williams ED, Gharib H, Marchesa P, Church JM, Fazio VW, Larson DR (1998) Thyroid cancer in patients with familiar adenomatous polyposis. World J Surg 22:738–742
107. Pilotti S, Collini P, Mariani L, Placucci M, Bongarzone I, Vigneri P, Cipriani S, Falcetta F, Miceli R, Pierotti MA, Rilke F (1997) Insular carcinoma: a distinct de novo entity among follicular carcinomas of the thyroid gland. Am J Surg Pathol 21:1466–1473
108. Pisarchik AV, Ermak G, Fomicheva V, Kartel NA, Figge J (1998) The ret/PTC 1 rearrangement is a common feature of Chernobyl-associated papillary thyroid carcinomas from Belarus. Thyroid 8:133–139
109. Prasser C, Scheuba C, Prager G, Kaserer K, Flores JA, Vierhapper H, Niederle B (1999) Anaplastic (undifferentiated) thyroid carcinoma (ATC). A retrospective analysis. Langenbecks Arch Surg 384:284–293
110. Rath-Wolfson L, Koren R, Yaniv E, Sadov R, Gal R (1999) A new rapid technique for the fixation of thyroid gland surgical specimens. Pathol Oncol Res 5:70–72
111. Resnick MB, Schacter P, Finkelstein Y, Kellner Y, Cohen O (1998) Immunhistochemical analysis of p27/kip 1 expression in thyroid carcinoma. Mod Pathol 11:735–739
112. Roque L, Serpa A, Clode A, Castedo S, Soares J (1999) Significance of trisomy 7 and 12 in thyroid lesions with follicular differentiation: a cytogenetic and in situ hybridization study. Lab Invest 79:369–378
113. Rosai J, Carcangiu ML, DeLellis RA (1992) Tumors of the thyroid gland. Atlas of tumor pathology, third series, vol 5. Armed Forces Institute of Pathology, Washington, DC
114. Rosen Y, Rosenblatt P, Saltzman E (1990) Intraoperative pathologic diagnosis of thyroid neoplasms. Report on experience with 504 specimens. Cancer 66:2001–2006
115. Ruco LP, Ranalli T, Marzullo A, Bianco P, Prat M, Comoglio PM, Baroni CD (1996) Expression of Met protein in thyroid tumors. J Pathol 180:266–270
116. Rüschoff J, Prasser C, Cortez T, Höhne HM, Hohenberger W, Hofstaedter F (1993) Diagnostic value of AgNOR staining in follicular cell neoplasms of the thyroid: comparison of evaluation methods and nuclear features. Am J Surg Pathol 17:1281–1288
117. Ruschenburg I, Kubitz A, Schlott T, Korabiowska M, Droese M (1999) MAGE-1, GAGF,-1/-2 gene expression in FNAB of classic variant of papillary thyroid carcinoma and papillary hyperplasia in nodular goitre. Int J Mol Med 4:445–448
118. Ruter A, Dreifus J, Jones M, Nishiyama R, Lennquist S (1996) Overexpression of p53 in tall cell variants of papillary thyroid carcinoma. Surgery 120:1046–1050
119. Sakamoto A, Kasai N, Sugano H (1983) Poorly differentiated carcinoma of the thyroid. A clinicopathological entity for a high-risk group of papillary and follicular carcinomas. Cancer 52:1849–1855
120. Sasaki A, Daa T, Kashima K, Yokoyama S, Nakayma I, Noguchi S (1996) Insular component as a risk factor of thyroid carcinoma. Pathol Int 46:939–946

121. Scarpino S, Stoppacciaro A, Colarossi C, Cancellario F, Marzullo A, Marchesi M, Biffoni M, Comoglio PM, Prat M, Ruco LP (1999) Hepatocyte growth factor (HGF) stimulates tumor invasiveness in papillary carcinoma of the thyroid. J Pathol 189:570–575
122. Schaffler A, Palitzsch KD, Seiffarth C, Höhne HM, Riedhammer FJ, Hofstaedter F, Schölmerich J, Rüschoff J (1998) Coexisting thyroiditis is associated with lower tumor stage in thyroid carcinoma. Eur J Clin Invest 28:838–844
123. Schmid KW, Tötsch M, Öfner D, Böcker W, Ladurner D (1997) Minimally invasive follicular thyroid carcinoma: a clinicopathological study. Curr Top Pathol 91:37–43
124. Schröder S, Böcker W (1986) Clear-cell carcinomas of the thyroid gland. A clinicopathological study of 13 cases. Histopathology 10:75–89
125. Scopsi L, Sampitro G, Boracchi P, Del Bo R, Gullo M, Placucci M, Pilotti S (1996) Multivariate analysis of prognostic factors in sporadic medullary carcinoma of the thyroid. A retrospective study of 109 consecutive cases. Cancer 78:2173–2183
126. Shimizu M, Hirokawa M, Manabe T (1999) Tall cell variant of papillary thyroid carcinoma with foci of columnar cell component. Virchows Arch 434:173–175
127. Shuja S, Cai J, lacobuzio-Donahue C, Zacks J, Beazley RM, Kasznica JM, O'Hara CJ, Heinmann R, Murnane MJ (1999) Cathepsin B activity and protein levels in thyroid carcinoma, Graves disease, and multinodular goiters. Thyroid 9:569–577
128. Smit JW, van der Pluijm G, Vloedgraven HJ, Lowik CW, Goslings BM (1998) Role of integrins in the attachment of metastatic follicular thyroid carcinoma cell lines to bone. Thyroid 8:29–36
129. Soares P, Fonseca E, Wynford-Thomas D, Sobrinho-Simoes M (1998) Sporadic ret-rearranged papillary carcinoma of the thyroid: a subset of slow growing, less aggressive, thyroid neoplasms. J Patrol 185:71–78
130. Sobin LH, Wittekind Ch (1997) TNM. Classification malignant tumors, 5th edn. Wiley-Liss, New York
131. Soda G, Antonaci A, Bosco D, Nardoni S, Melis M (1999) Expression of bcl-2, c-erbB-2, p53, and p21 (waf1 cip1) protein in thyroid carcinomas. J Exp Clin Cancer Res 18:363–367
132. Sturgis CD, Caraway NP, Johnston DA, Sherman SI, Kidd L, Katz RL (1999) Image analysis of papillary thyroid carcinoma fine-needle aspirates: significant association between aneuploidy and death from disease. Cancer 87:155–160
133. Sugg SL, Ezzat S, Zheng L, Freeman JL, Rosen IB, Asa SL (1999) Oncogene profile of papillary thyroid carcinoma. Surgery 1251:46–52
134. Sugino K, Ito K Jr, Ozaki O, Mirnura T, Iwasaki H, Ito K (1998) Papillary microcarcinoma of the thyroid. J Endocrinol Invest 21:445–448
135. Sugitani I, Yanagisawa A, Shimizu A, Kato M, Fujimoto Y (1998) Clinicopathologic and immunohistochemical studies of papillary thyroid microcarcinoma presenting with cervical lymphadenopathy. World J Surg 22:731–737
136. Takano T, Miyauchi A, Yokozawa T, Matsuzuka F, Maeda I, Kuma K, Amino N (1999) Preoperative diagnosis of thyroid papillary and anaplastic carcinoma by real-time quantitative reverse transcription-polymerase chain reaction of oncofetal fibronectin messenger RNA. Cancer Res 59:4542–4545
137. Tallini G, Santoro M, Helie M, Carlomagno F, Salvatore G, Chiapetta G, Carcangiu ML, Fusco A (1998) RET/PTC oncogene activation defines a subset of papillary thyroid carcinomas lacking evidence of progression to poorly differentiated or undifferentiated tumor phenotypes. Clin Cancer Res 4:287–294
138. Tallini G, Garcia-Rostan G, Herrero A, Zelterman D, Viale G, Bosari S, Carcangiu ML (1999) Downregulation of p27K1P1 and Ki67/Mibl labeling index support the classification of thyroid carcinoma into prognostically relevant categories. Am J Surg Pathol 23:678–685
139. Tallini G, Hsueh A, Liu S, Garcia-Rostan G, Speicher MR, Ward DC (1999) Frequent chromosomal DNA unbalance in thyroid oncocytic (Hürthle cell) neoplasms detected by comparative genomic hybridization. Lab Invest 79:547–555

140. Tonacchera M, Vitti P, Agretti P, Ceccarini G, Perri A, Cavaliere R, Mazzi B, Naccarato AG, Viacava P, Micoli P, Pinchera A, Chiovato L (1999) Functioning and nonfunctioning thyroid adenomas involve different molecular pathogenetic mechanisms. J Clin Endocrinol Metab 84:4155–4158
141. Toti P, Tanganelli P, Schurfeld K, Stumpo M, Barbagli L, Vatti R, Luzi P (1999) Scarring in papillary carcinoma of the thyroid: report of two new cases with exuberant nodular fasciitis-He stroma. Histopathology 35:418–422
142. Tronko MD, Bogdanova TI, Komissarenko IV, Epstein OV, Oliynyk V, Kovalenko A, Likhtarev IA, Kairo I, Peters SB, LiVolsi VA (1999) Thyroid carcinoma in children and adolescents in Ukraine after the Chernobyl nuclear accident: statistical data and clinicomorphologic characteristics. Cancer 86:149–156
143. Tscholl-Ducommun J, Hedinger CE (1982) Papillary thyroid carcinomas. Morphology and prognosis. Virchows Arch 396:19–39
144. Tseleni S, Kavantzas N, Yova D, Alexandratu E, Karydakis V, Gogas J, Davaris P (1997) Findings of computerized nuclear morphometry of papillary thyroid carcinoma in correlation with known prognostic factors. J Exp Clin Cancer Res 16:401–406
145. Tseleni-Balafouta S, Kavantzas N, Alevizaki M, Paraskevakou H, Davaris P (1998) Neuroendocrine differentiation in follicle-cell thyroid carcinoma: correlation to prognostic factors in papillary carcinoma. J Exp Clin Cancer Res 17:533–537
146. Tworek JA, Giordano TJ, Michael CW (1998) Comparison of intraoperative cytology with frozen sections in the diagnosis of thyroid lesions. Am J Cancer Pathol 110:456–461
147. Vickery AL, Carcangiu ML, Johannessen W, Sobrinho-Simoes M (1985) Papillary carcinoma. Semin Diagn Pathol 2:90–100
148. Voutilainen PE, Multanen M, Haapiainen RK, Leppanierni AK, Sivula AH (1999) Anaplastic thyroid carcinoma survival. World J Surg 23:975–978
149. Waldmann V, Rabes HM (1997) Absence of G(s)alpha gene mutations in childhood thyroid tumors alter Chernobyl in contrast to sporadic adult thyroid neoplasia. Cancer Res 57:2358–2361
150. Walgenbach S, Sternheirn E, Bittinger F, Gorges R, Andreas J, Junginger T (1998) Prognostic value of E-cadherin in papillary thyroid carcinoma. Chirurg 69:186–190
151. Wang S, Wuu J, Savas L, Patwardhan N, Khan A (1998) The role of cell cycle regulators proteins, cyclin D1, cyclin E, and p27 in thyroid carcinogenesis. Hum Pathol 29:1304–1309
152. Wilkens L, Benten D, Tchinda J, Brabant G, Pötter E, Dralle H, v Wasielewski R (2000) Aberrations of chromosomes 5 and 8 as recurrent cytogenetic events in anaplastic carcinoma of the thyroid as detected by fluorescence in situ hybridization and comparative genomic hybridization. Virchows Arch 436:312–318
153. Winzer R, Schmutzler C, Jakobs TC, Ebert R, Rendl J, Reiners C, Jakob F, Kohrle J (1998) Reverse transcriptase-polymerase chain reaction analysis of thyrocyte-relevant genes in fine-needle aspiration biopsies of the human thyroid. Thyroid 8:981–987
154. Wong NA, Willott J, Kendall MJ, Sheffield EA (1999) Measurement of vascularity as a diagnostic and prognostic tool for well differentiated thyroid tumors' comparison of different methods of assessing vascularity. J Clin Pathol 52:593–597
155. Wynford-Thomas D (1994) Growth factors and oncogenes. In: Wheeler MH, Lazarus JH (eds) Diseases of the thyroid. Chapman and Hall, London
156. Yunta PJ, Ponce JL, Prieto M, Merino F, Sancho-Fornos S (1999) The importance of a tumor capsule in columnar cell thyroid carcinoma: a report of two cases and review of the literature. Thyroid 9:15–19
157. Zeiger MA, Smallridge RC, Clark DP, Liang CK, Carty SE, Watson CG, Udelsman R, Saji M (1999) Human telomerase reverse transcriptase (HTFRT) gene expression in FNA samples from thyroid neoplasms. Surgery 126:1195–1198

Chapter 3

Familial Differentiated Carcinoma of the Thyroid

3

M.R. Carlisle and I.R. McDougall

3.1 Introduction

In most series, thyroid cancers arising from follicular cells account for about 90% of malignant tumors of the thyroid [1–3]. The remainder are medullary cancers, which arise from parafollicular cells, lymphomas, sarcomas, and metastatic cancers. A proportion of medullary cancers are unequivocally recognized to be hereditary. These include medullary cancers occurring as part of the syndromes of multiple endocrine neoplastic syndromes MEN 2A and MEN 2B (MEN 3) and some isolated cases of medullary cancer [4]. These are discussed separately in Chap. 20. The genetics have been defined as autosomal dominant, and the cause of MEN 2A and familial medullary cancer is a mutation in the c-ret proto-oncogene [5–8].

Differentiated or nonmedullary cancers of the follicular epithelium are usually considered to be sporadic and nonfamilial. There is a growing body of evidence that some cases are familial. In my clinic about 2% of patients have a first-degree relative with similar disease. Some report an incidence of 4–5% [9, 10]. The first report was in identical twins and was published in 1955 [11]. There are now several reports of familial cases, including several from this institute [12–29]. Some investigators consider that familial thyroid cancers are more aggressive than the sporadic cases [9, 30]. This chapter will review the published reports and as far as possible analyze whether the natural history of the disease is different from the sporadic variety. The mode of inheritance and genetic susceptibility, including the relationship with Cowden's, Gardner's, and other syndromes are discussed. The molecular genetics will be reviewed. Advice about management of the patients and their families is included.

3.2 Etiology of Nonmedullary Thyroid Cancers

In most patients with differentiated thyroid cancer arising from thyroid follicular cells, there is no single causal factor which can be blamed for producing the cancer. However, there is abundant evidence that external radiation is an important cause, in particular when the patients are young at the time of exposure [31–34]. This has been shown in epidemiological studies of patients who had neck and chest radiation for benign or malignant disorders. The association has been documented for radiation to the scalp in the treatment of ringworm. These patients were exposed to doses as low as 10 rad (10 cGy) [35]. Doses of several hundred radians (100 rad = 1 Gy), prescribed to treat "status lymphaticus" and acne, caused thyroid cancer in about 5–10% of patients. Therapeutic doses of 4,000 rad (40 Gy) for Hodgkin's disease produced a 20-fold increase in thyroid cancer [36]. Currently we have identified 12 patients with thyroid cancer out of more than 1,800 patients with Hodgkin's disease who received therapeutic neck irradiation. In every report the increase in cancers was of the papillary type [26]. The data that radiation is an etiological factor, although compelling, begs the question: Why do so few patients exposed develop clinical disease? What puts some patients at risk and protects others? In evaluating familial thyroid cancers, it is important to review prior history to exclude external radiation. This brings into discussion the role of genetics. Cancers are due to a change in DNA, which results in a clone of cells having the potential to divide faster, to invade surrounding tissues, and to metastasize. This can be due to promoters of these characteristics, called "oncogenes." Alternatively there can be loss of the protective mechanisms which continually repair breaks in DNA or which suppress those characteristics of malignancy, suppressor genes. Radiation has been shown to alter both of these mechanisms.

This interplay of familial and cancerogenic factors is seen clinically. In one of the families, we reported two brothers with thyroid cancer who both had been irradiated in childhood over the neck and face, for acne [27]. One has had minimal disease, the other died from aggressive cancer that was unresponsive to all therapies. There are other similar reports [37, 38]. Were these cancers due to radiation, or familial, or both? Did the radiation cause undifferentiated disease in some but not others?

In contrast, it has generally been accepted that internal radiation from radionuclides of iodine used diagnostically or therapeutically is not associated with an increase in thyroid cancer. There are large studies showing that patients treated with radio-iodine for hyperthyroidism do not have an increase in thyroid cancers [39]. However, the dramatic increase in thyroid cancer in children

Table 3.1. Relationship of familial nonmedullary cancers with goiter and nodular goiter

Reference	Cancers (*n*)	Goiters (*n*)	Familiy members (*n*)
Burgess et al.: family 1 [15]	7	17	25
Kraimps et al.: family 1 [29]	3	4	13
Kraimps et al.: families 2, 4, and 6 combined	6	6	19
Lote et al.: family 1 [23]	7	2	42
Lote et al.: family 2	4	2	23
Osaki et al. [17]	2 (possibly 3)	2	29

exposed to radio-iodines released from the Chernobyl nuclear power plant disaster has caused this view to be reconsidered [40–44].

The incidence of differentiated thyroid cancer varies considerably among ethnic groups. The highest incidence is in populations from the Pacific rim, in particular Filipinos. In contrast, African Americans have about one-tenth the incidence of differentiated cancers. Are some ethnic groups at a higher genetic or environmental risk for cancer than others or is there an alternative explanation? One factor that appears to increase the incidence of papillary cancer is a high dietary intake of iodine. A large study of patients with papillary cancer from several ethnic backgrounds has shown some relation to dietary iodine [45]. In contrast the incidence of follicular cancer is increased in areas of iodine deficiency where nodular goiter is endemic [46, 47]. Preexisting thyroid conditions such as goiter and nodules are associated with an increased incidence of thyroid cancer. It is clear that, in some of the families with several cases of thyroid cancer, there is also a significant proportion of patients with nodules, goiter, and multinodular goiter (Table 3.1) [15]. This raises the suspicion of a growth stimulus which, in the appropriate setting, develops malignant potential. Most patients with thyroid cancer are clinically and biochemically euthyroid, therefore thyroid-stimulating hormone and thyroid-stimulating immunoglobulins are unlikely to be involved as the cause.

3.3 Could "Familial" Thyroid Cancers be a Chance Finding?

The first question to answer is whether familial cases of differentiated thyroid cancer are chance findings. Most of the published reports indicate that between 3 and 6% of patients with differentiated thyroid cancer report a first-degree relative with the same condition. Kraimps et al. [13] found that the familial incidence was 10.5% when they studied the families of 105 consecutive patients [20]. In seven families they found 15 cases. Pal et al. compared the incidence of thyroid cancer in relatives of 339 patients with differentiated thyroid cancer to that in families of 319 matched controls. They determined that there was a 10.3-fold increase (95% confidence interval 2.2–47.6) [48]. Similarly, in an analysis of 1025 patients with thyroid cancer and 5457 first-degree relatives in Norway, there was a 5.2 times increase in men and 4.9 times increase in women [49]. From a simplistic point of view, let us use data from the USA, where 19,000 new cases of thyroid cancer are diagnosed annually from a population of 250,000,000 people. If we assume that 15,000 of the cancers are differentiated and the entire population lives to be 80 years of age, the probability that a person will be diagnosed with thyroid cancer during their lifetime is 0.48%. Charkes [34], using more sophisticated mathematics, which incorporated data from the Surveillance, Epidemiology and End Results (SEER), calculated an overall risk of 0.324%, with the risk in women of 0.459% and men of 0.189% [50]. These lifetime risks are not greatly different from our simplistic calculation. From these data, the risk of two relatives having differentiated thyroid cancer would be from 0.1–0.23% (0.324×0.324% or 0.48%×0.48%). However, the size of the family and hence number of persons at risk have to be considered. Charkes, using Poisson statistics, has calculated that the risk of two cases in one family with 12 first-degree relatives is 1.9% ± 0.2%. The probability of three or more cases is less than 0.1%. Houlston [35, 36] has estimated that a family with three members with differentiated thyroid cancer would be found by chance in 100 years but does not specify whether this would be in the UK or USA [51, 52]. Malchoff et al. [37] state that the chance of finding five members with papillary cancer to be 1 in 2 billion [53].

Ron et al. [38] have found a 5.2-fold increase in thyroid cancer in relatives of an index patient with differentiated thyroid cancer [54]. Stoffer et al. [19] have determined there is a similar (4.71-fold) increase in risk in members of 222 families with an index patient [25]. These data indicate that chance is unlikely to be the cause of finding three or more members of a family with thyroid cancer.

One factor which could actually reduce the familial association is that patients may not know their relatives have thyroid cancer. In some countries physicians are reluctant to discuss the diagnosis of cancer with patients, and thyroid surgery might not be thought to be for cancer. This understanding can be strengthened by the excellent prognosis in most patients with differentiated thyroid cancer.

3.4 Genetics and Associated Syndromes

There is a definite relationship between thyroid cancer and familial adenomatous polyposis (FAP) and Gardner's syndrome [55, 56], which is the association of FAP with soft tissue tumors, osteomas, and miscellaneous neoplasms [5, 57–62]. Houlston has estimated that less than 0.1% of differentiated thyroid cancers have this association [52]. He has determined that the same percentage have the combination of differentiated thyroid cancer and Cowden's syndrome. Patients with Cowden's syndrome have nodular goiters, multiple hamartomas, skeletal abnormalities, and a 50% risk of breast cancer [63, 64]. Thyroid cancer has been described in patients with Peutz-Jeghers syndrome [51] and ataxia-telangiectasia [65]. We have also found differentiated thyroid cancer in three patients with osteogenic sarcoma [66]. Some investigators exclude patients who have differentiated thyroid cancer and FAP, or Gardner's, or Cowden's syndrome from the classification of familial nonmedullary thyroid cancer. This is not logical, because the associated disorders are also familial and the combination could be more etiologically informative.

In most of the publications of families with first-degree relatives with differentiated thyroid cancer, there are only two patients, e.g. two sisters, two brothers, one brother and one sister, mother and child, father and child, and it is not possible to assign a specific pattern of inheritance. Several population-based studies and meta-analysis of these reports also fail to answer the mode of inheritance [54, 67–71]. There are a few reports of families in which several members are affected. Table 3.2 lists families in which three or more members have thyroid cancer. Lote et al. have described two kindreds with seven and four patients [23]. Burgess et al. have also described two families with multiple patients with papillary cancer [15]. In one family of 25 individuals, 7 patients had proven thyroid cancer and 2 others probably had cancer. Nine additional members had multinodular goiter. In the second family, identical twin brothers had papillary cancer and each had a daughter who was found to have this type of cancer. They felt that the inheritance was autosomal dominant. We have con-

Table 3.2. Families with three or more differentiated thyroid cancers

Reference	Index patient	Thyroid cancers (*n*)	Family members (*n*)	Generations studied (*n*)	Relationship
Lote et al.: pedigree 1 [23]	Woman	7	51	3	2 daughters Female cousin 2 nieces, 1 nephew
Lote et al.: pedigree 2	Woman	4	33	3	Maternal aunt 2 sons
Phade et al. [24]	12-year-old boy	3	Not discussed	Same generation	Two sisters
Stoffer et al.: family B [25]	Male	5	23	4	2 cousins Aunt Great uncle
Stoffer et al.: family D	Woman	3	27	4	Mother Uncle
Stoffer et al.: family G	29-year-old woman	4	24	5	Sister Mother Maternal uncle
Malchoff et al. [53]	26-year-old woman	5	30	4	Sister 1 daughter, 1 son 1 great-niece
Burgess et al.: kindred 1 [15]	62-year-old woman	7	25	4	4 children 2 relaives (cousin and niece) 2 additional cases
Burgess et al.: kindred 2	49-year-old man	4	12	3	Twin brother Daughters of patient and twin
Kraimps et al.: kindred 1 [29]	10-year-old boy	3	13	3	11-year-old niece 27-year-old nephew
Ozaki et al.: family 8 [17]	40-year-old man	3	29	4	27-year-old sister 37-year-old brother

sulted on one member of a family with five patients over three generations with thyroid cancer, whose genetic transmission appears to be dominant.

3.4.1 Molecular Genetics of Familial Thyroid Cancer

Although most cases of nonmedullary thyroid cancer are sporadic, there is increasing evidence of a familial form. There is considerable interest in identifying a gene or genes that cause susceptibility (see Table 3.3). There is some evidence that nonmedullary thyroid cancer is autosomal dominant with partial penetrance and is not associated with other malignancies. Specific genes responsible for susceptibility to familial nonmedullary thyroid cancer without an associated comorbidity have not yet been identified [72]. Several groups of investigators are studying the molecular genetics of familial nonmedullary cancer. If a single lesion could be identified, it would allow screening of families to identify those at risk and counsel them on management. It could possibly at some future date lead to novel gene therapies.

Bignell et al. have found a gene on chromosome 14q32 which they call *MNG 1*, because members of the family studied had multinodular goiter and familial thyroid cancer [73]. In a second family, there is a gene designated *TCO* on chromosome 19q13.2, which predisposes to multinodular goiter and cancer [74]. In an analysis of 60 small families, there is no relation to *MNG 1*, *TCO*, or *RET* [75]. McKay et al. have found that *MNG 1* and *TCO* are not causal in their Tasmanian family [76]. McKay et al. in a multinational collaboration have shown a susceptibility locus on 2q21 [77].

The gene for the TSH receptor is on chromosome 14q but it has been shown to be distinct from *MNG 1* and has not been implicated in the cause of thyroid cancer [78]. Mutations of the TSH receptor gene can produce hyperfunctioning nodules, but these are almost never malignant. Mutations of this gene have also caused a hyperthyroidism in newborn. Bevan et al. have attempted to find mutations in 22 families with nonmedullary thyroid cancer [10]. They have found no evidence for MNG1, fPTC, PTEN, TSHR or TRK and their work supports the hypothesis that this condition is not homogeneous.

Rearranged forms of the RET proto-oncogene have been identified as the susceptibility genes for development of sporadic forms of papillary thyroid cancer. The RET proto-oncogene is located on chromosome 10q11.2 and encodes a transmembrane receptor of the tyrosine kinase family. *RET/PTC1*, *RET/PTC/2*, and *RET/PTC3* are chimeric oncogenes formed from the rearrangement of the RET proto-oncogene. They have been identified as one genetic event leading to the development of sporadic cases of nonmedullary thyroid cancer [79, 80]. Rearrangement of the RET proto-oncogene has also been identified in children who developed papillary cancer after exposure to radioactive iodine released during the Chernobyl reactor accident [81, 82]. In the majority of these cases, induction of papillary thyroid cancer was a consequence of *RET/PTC1* rearrangements [83]. In other cases, rearrangement of the *NTRK1* gene located on chromosome 1q22 was found to be the responsible gene. TRK family receptor genes are also known to participate in development of medullary thyroid cancer [64].

Papillary thyroid cancer is known to overexpress c-met located on 7q31. In contrast, inactivation of this gene has been shown to be significant in the development of follicular as well as anaplastic thyroid cancer. Loss of heterozygosity on chromosomes 10q, 3p, and 17p appears to be more common in follicular cancer than papillary cancer. In fact, it has been shown that papillary cancer has exceedingly low rates of loss of allelic heterozygosity [84–86].

Cowden's syndrome is an autosomal dominant disorder characterized by increased risk of thyroid cancer in combination with development of hamartomas and increased risk of development of breast tumors. The loss of a tumor suppressor gene has been found to be responsible for susceptibility to this syndrome. Deletion mapping by examination of loss of heterozygosity of polymorphic markers was employed to ascertain the fine structure of a region of chromosome 10 [87]. Using this technique, the tumor suppressor gene whose deletion is responsible for Cowden's syndrome was identified as the *PTEN* tumor suppressor gene located on 10q23.3 [88, 89]. *PTEN* encodes for a phosphatase important in the phosphatidylinositol 3-kinase signal conduction pathway. Inactivation of *PTEN* tumor suppressor gene has also been implicated in several cases of sporadic follicular thyroid tumors [90].

Familial adenomatous polyposis is an inherited autosomal dominant tumor syndrome characterized by colonic polyps with eventual malignant transformation. It is caused by germ-line mutations of the *APC* gene, which has been

Table 3.3. Genes reported to be associated with familial nonmedullary thyroid cancer

Entity	Gene	Chromosome
Nonmedullary cancer, familial	*MNG1*, *TCO*, *RET*, *TRK*, *MET*, *TSHR*, *APC*, *PTEN* have been excluded	?
Papillary cancer, sporadic	*RET/PTC1*, *RET/PTC2*, *RET/PTC3*	10q
Papillary cancer, Chernobyl	*RET/PTC1* (common) *NTRK1* rearrangement (rare)	10q 1q22
Follicular cancer, sporadic		
Familial multinodular goiter	*MNG1*	14q32
Nonmedullary thyroid cancer associated with multinodular goiter	*TCO*	19q13.2
Familial adenomatous polyposis & Gardner's syndrome	*APC*	5q21
Cowden's syndrome	*PTEN*	10q23
Thyrotropin receptor	*TSHR*	
Familial medullary thyroid cancer (men)	*RET*	10q11.2

mapped to chromosome 5q21. Malchoff et al. have studied 18 family members with both familial polyposis coli and papillary cancer [53]. They conclude that the two conditions are not caused by the same genetic abnormality. The association between nonmedullary thyroid cancer and this familial tumor syndrome is well known. Investigators have used linkage analysis, employing polymorphic markers located close to the *APC* gene, to determine whether familial papillary thyroid cancer is related to loss of the *APC* gene. It has been concluded that familial papillary thyroid cancer is genetically distinct from familial adenomatous polyposis. Gardner's syndrome is similar to familial adenomatous polyposis coli in inheritance pattern, association with papillary thyroid cancer, development of adenomas in the colon, and risk of carcinoma. Gardner's syndrome differs from polyposis coli in the addition of adenomatous polyps located in the small intestine and presence of extraintestinal lesions such as osteomas, skin fibromas, and epidermal cysts. In investigations evaluating the genetic linkage of papillary thyroid cancer, patients with Gardner's syndrome have been grouped together with patients with familial adenomatous polyposis coli; no separate investigations have been published to date [91–93].

MTS-1 encodes the tumor suppressor gene p16 and MTS-2 encodes the tumor suppressor gene p15. Structural changes in these genes have been associated with various cancers. Several investigators have concluded that deletion of MTS-1 and MTS-2 are not associated with development of thyroid cancers. However, base-pair exchange at these sites was found to contribute to development of tumor. Loss of p16 has been associated with transformation from well-differentiated thyroid cancer to anaplastic cancer [94, 95].

3.4.2
Natural History of Familial Thyroid Cancer

There is evidence that the ratio of men to women with familial thyroid cancer is nearer to unity than in sporadic cases where the ratio is about 1:3 [9]. There is conflicting data on whether familial differentiated thyroid cancer is more often multifocal, more advanced and aggressive, and has a worse prognosis than the sporadic variety [9, 28, 69, 96]. An alternative explanation is that the patients are younger, and it is accepted that, in young patients with papillary cancer, the lesions are larger, they are more likely to be multifocal, and more frequently associated with lymph node and pulmonary metastases. The younger age of patients with familial cancer could be due to increased interest in the relatives of an index case.

Recurrences of familial thyroid cancer are thought to be more common and the mortality greater. Takami et al. found that 82% had cervical metastases [30], which is an average of 65 nodes containing metastases in 61 patients subjected to modified neck dissection. Six had pulmonary metastases at presentation, 31% had a recurrence, and 5 patients died from their disease. Lote et al. found a statistically significant increased incidence in lymph node metastases compared with nonfamilial controls [23]. The average age of the patients was 37.6 years which, although similar to most series in the USA, was younger than the 52.8 years of their controls. Grossman et al. treated 14 patients, 13 of whom had multifocal disease, 57% had cervical node metastases, and 50% recurred [27]. The mean age was 40 years, and the male to female ratio 1:1.3. Uchino et al. reported on 154 families with two or more thyroid cancers from a denominator of 6,458 patients [9]. There was a higher incidence of multifocality (42% vs 30%), recurrence (16.3% vs 9.6%), and disease-free survival in the familial cases. The survival was the same in familial versus sporadic cases. It is hard to argue with data from such large numbers of patients.

Stoffer et al. found that 18 of 22 patients had multifocal disease, 5 (23%) had cervical nodal metastases, and 1 had a pulmonary metastasis [25]. They found the average age of the patients, 37.8 years, was not different from their sporadic cases. We described five pairs of sibs and have now treated 19 patients who have a first-degree relative. In general the prognosis and natural history appears similar to sporadic nonmedullary thyroid cancer. One of the male sibs developed a skeletal metastasis and died, but he had been exposed to radiation, and the familial designation as the sole cause of his cancer is questionable. The remainder of the patients who have been treated and followed at Stanford have had a good outcome.

3.5 Clinical Implications of Familial Nonmedullary Thyroid Cancer

3.5.1 Primary Treatment

The fundamentals of treatment should be no different from those for sporadic cancers. When the diagnosis is made, total or near total thyroidectomy should be undertaken. In many patients whole-body scan with ^{131}I should be conducted after surgery and abnormal uptake treated with ^{131}I. The details of these treatments are described elsewhere in this book. Because of concern that familial cancers can be more aggressive, lesser surgical procedures are not recommended. Serum thyroglobulin (Tg) measurement has the same importance in follow-up of familial thyroid cancer.

3.5.2 Screening of Families

With increasing acceptance that there are familial cases of thyroid cancer, physicians should take a careful family history before concluding a cancer is sporadic. When two patients in a family are identified with thyroid cancer, this knowledge should be disseminated through the family and, when each member next consults their physician, a careful examination of the thyroid should be conducted. Since most of the families reported have only two affected members, this is sufficient. Because the prognosis in differentiated thyroid cancer is good, the need for aggressive screening of families does not have the importance it does for medullary cancer. At the time of writing, there is no genetic or biochemical test which is of value. Any member with a nodule should have this examined by fine-needle aspiration (FNA) and all patients with suspicious and microfollicular lesions referred for thyroidectomy. When there are three or more family members with cancer, clinical screening should be more actively undertaken. In the rare families with several affected individuals in whom the cancers appear to be more aggressive, it would be reasonable to obtain ultrasound examinations and obtain an ultrasound-guided FNA of nodules more than 1 cm in diameter.

References

1. Schlumberger M, Baudin E, Travagli JP (1998) Papillary and follicular cancers of the thyroid. Presse Med 27:1479–1481
2. Sizemore GM. In: Becker KL (ed) Principles and practice of endocrinology and metabolism, 2nd edn. Lippincott, Philadelphia, pp 1555–1564
3. Wells SJ (1994) New approaches to the patient with medullary carcinoma of the thyroid gland. Thyroid Today XVII:1–9
4. Ledger G, Khosla S, Lindor NM, Thibideau SN, Gharib H (1995) Genetic testing in the diagnosis and management of multiple endocrine neoplasia type II. Ann Intern Med 122:118–124
5. Bell B, Mazzaferri EL (1993) Familial adenomatous polyposis (Gardner's syndrome) and thyroid carcinoma. A case report and review of the literature. Dig Dis Sci 38:185–190
6. Bartsch DK et al. (2000) A RET double mutation in the germline of a kindred with FMTC. Exp Clin Endocrinol Diabetes 108:128–132
7. Belli S et al. (2003) Study of RET protooncogene in multiple endocrine neoplasm 2A and in familial medullary thyroid carcinoma. Clinical pathological findings in asymptomatic carriers. Medicina (B Aires) 63:41–45
8. Marsh DJ, Mulligan LM, Eng C (1997) RET proto-oncogene mutations in multiple endocrine neoplasia type 2 and medullary thyroid carcinoma. Horm Res 47:168–178
9. Uchino S et al. (2002) Familial nonmedullary thyroid carcinoma characterized by multifocality and a high recurrence rate in a large study population. World J Surg 26:897–902
10. Bevan S et al. (2001) A comprehensive analysis of MNG1, TCO1, fPTC, PTEN, TSHR, and TRKA in familial nonmedullary thyroid cancer: confirmation of linkage to TCO1. J Clin Endocrinol Metab 86:3701–3704
11. Robinson D, Orr TG (1955) Carcinoma of the thyroid and other diseases of the thyroid in identical twins. Arch Surg 70:923
12. Nemec J et al. (1975) Familial occurrence of differentiated (nonmedullary) thyroid cancer. Oncology 32:151–157
13. Fischer DK et al. (1989) Papillary carcinoma of the thyroid: additional evidence in support of a familial component. Cancer Invest 7:323–325
14. Austoni M (1988) Thyroid papillary carcinoma in identical twins. Lancet 1:1115
15. Burgess J, Duffield A, Wilkinson SJ, Ware R, Greenaway TM, Percival J, Hoffman L (1997) Two families with an autosomal dominant inheritance pattern for papillary carcinoma of the thyroid. J Clin Endocrinol Metab 82:345–348
16. Christensen S, Ljungberg O (1983) Familial occurrence of papillary thyroid carcinoma. Br J Surg 70:908–909
17. Ozaki O et al. (1988) Familial occurrence of differentiated, nonmedullary thyroid carcinoma. World J Surg 12:565–571

18. Goldbar D, Easton DF, CannonAlbright LA, Skolnick MH (1994) A systematic population-based assessment of cancer risk in first-degree relatives of cancer probands. J Natl Cancer Inst 86:200–209
19. Gorson D (1992) Familial papillary carcinoma of the thyroid. Thyroid 2:131–132
20. Kraimps,JL, Canzian F, Jost C et al. (1999) Mapping of a gene predisposing to familial thyroid tumors with cell oxyphilia to chromosome 19 and exclusion of *JUN B* as a candidate gene. Surgery 126:1188–1194
21. Grossman R, Tu S-H, Duh Q-Y, Siperstein AE, Novosolov F, Clark OH (1995) Familial nonmedullary thyroid cancer. Arch Surg 130:892–899
22. Hrafnkelsson J et al. (2001) Familial nonmedullary thyroid cancer in Iceland. J Med Genet 38:189–191
23. Lote K, Andersen K, Nordal E, Brennhovd IO (1980) Familial occurrence of papillary thyroid carcinoma. Cancer 46:1291–1297
24. Phade V, Lawrence WR, Max MH (1981) Familial papillary carcinoma of the thyroid. Arch Surg 116:836–837
25. Stoffer S, Dyke DL van, Bach JV, Szpunar W, Weiss L (1986) Familial papillary carcinoma of the thyroid. Am J Med Genet 25:775–782
26. Szanto J, Gundy C, Toth K, Kasler M (1990) Coincidental papillary carcinoma of the thyroid in two sisters. Oncology 47:92–94
27. Grossman RF et al. (1995) Familial nonmedullary thyroid cancer. An emerging entity that warrants aggressive treatment. Arch Surg 130:892–897; discussion 898–899
28. Lupoli G et al. (1999) Familial papillary thyroid microcarcinoma: a new clinical entity. Lancet 353:637–639
29. Kraimps JL, Bouin-Pineau M-H, Amati P, Mothes D, Boneau D, Marechaud R, Barbier J (1997) Familial papillary carcinoma of the thyroid. Surgery 121:715–718
30. Takami H, Ozaki O, Ito K (1996) Familial nonmedullary thyroid cancer: an emerging entity that warrants aggressive treatment. Arch Surg 131:676
31. De Groot L, Paloyan E (1973) Thyroid carcinoma and radiation: a Chicago endemic. JAMA 225:487–491
32. Favus M, Schneider AB, Stachura ME et al. (1976) Thyroid cancer occurring as a late consequence of head-and-neck irradiation: evaluation of 1056 patients. N Engl J Med 294:1019–1025
33. Maxon HR (1985) Radiation-induced thyroid disease. Med Clin North Am 69:1049–1061
34. Ron E et al. (1995) Thyroid cancer after exposure to external radiation: a pooled analysis of seven studies. Radiat Res 141:259–277
35. Ron E (2003) Cancer risks from medical radiation. Health Phys 85:47–59
36. Hancock SL, Cox R.S, McDougall I.R (1991) Thyroid diseases after treatment of Hodgkin's disease. N Engl J Med 325:599–605
37. Fisher C, Edmonds CJ (1980) Papillary carcinoma of the thyroid in two brothers after chest fluoroscopy in childhood. Br Med J 281:1600–1601
38. Samaan N (1989) Papillary carcinoma of the thyroid: heredity or radiation induced? Cancer Invest 7:399–400
39. Ron E et al. (1998) Cancer mortality following treatment for adult hyperthyroidism. Cooperative Thyrotoxicosis Therapy Follow-up Study Group. JAMA 280:347–355
40. Kazakov VS, Demidchik EP, Astakhova LN (1992) Thyroid cancer after Chernobyl. Nature 359:21
41. Williams D (2001) Lessons from Chernobyl. BMJ 323:643–644
42. Williams ED (2003) Chernobyl, 15 years later, correlation of clinical, epidemiological and molecular outcomes. Ann Endocrinol (Paris) 64:72
43. Zelicoff AP, Pezzullo JC (2002) Thyroid cancer 15 years after Chernobyl. Lancet 359:1946–1947; author reply 1947
44. Zafra Anta MA et al. (2002) Health effects of the Chernobyl disaster. Fifteen years afterwards. An Esp Pediatr 56:324–333

45. Horn-Ross P, Morris JS, Lee M, West DW, Whittemore AS, McDougall IR, Nowels K, Stewart SL, Spate VL, Shiau AC, Krone M (2001) Iodine and thyroid cancer risk among women in a multiethnic population: The Bay Area Thyroid Cancer Study. Cancer Epidemiol Biomarkers Prev 10:979–985
46. Williams E, Doniach I, BjarnasonO, Michie W (1977) Thyroid cancer in an iodine rich area: a histopathological study. Cancer 39:215–222
47. Williams ED (1995) Mechanisms and pathogenesis of thyroid cancer in animals and man. Mutat Res 333:123–129
48. Pal T et al. (2001) Increased risk for nonmedullary thyroid cancer in the first-degree relatives of prevalent cases of nonmedullary thyroid cancer: a hospital-based study. J Clin Endocrinol Metab 86:5307–5312
49. Frich L, Glattre E, Akslen LA (2001) Familial occurrence of nonmedullary thyroid cancer: a population-based study of 5,673 first-degree relatives of thyroid cancer patients from Norway. Cancer Epidemiol Biomarkers Prev 10:113–117
50. Charkes ND (1998) On the prevalence of familial nonmedullary thyroid cancer. Thyroid 8:857–858
51. Houlston R, Stratton MR (1995) Genetics of nonmedullary thyroid cancer. Q J Med 88:685–693
52. Houlston R (1998) Genetic predisposition to nonmedullary thyroid cancer. Nucl Med Commun 19:911–913
53. Malchoff CD, Malchoff DM (1999) Familial nonmedullary thyroid carcinoma. Semin Surg Oncol 16:16–18
54. Ron E, Kleinerman RA, Boice JD Jr et al. (1987) A population based case-control study of thyroid cancer. JNCI 79:1–12
55. Gardner E (1951) A genetic and clinical study of intestinal polyposis, a predisposing factor for carcinoma of the colon and rectum. Am J Hum Genet 3:167–176
56. Gardner E, Richards RC (1953) Multiple cutaneous and subcutaneous lesions occurring simultaneously with hereditary polyposis and osteomatosis. Am J Hum Genet 5:139–148
57. Camiel M, Mule JE, Alexander LL, Benninghoff DL (1968) Association of thyroid carcinoma with Gardner's syndrome in siblings. N Engl J Med 278:1056–1058
58. Harach H, Williams GT, Williams ED (1994) Familial adenomatous polyposis associated thyroid carcinoma; a distinct type of follicular cell neoplasm. Histopathology 25:549–561
59. Piffer S (1988) Gardner's syndrome and thyroid cancer – a case report and review of the literature. Acta Oncol 27:413–415
60. Lee F, McKinnon MD (1981) Papillary thyroid carcinoma associated with polyposis coli. Am J Gastroenterol 76:138–140
61. Plail R, Bussey HJR, Glazer R, Thomson JPS (1987) Adenomatous polyposis: an association with carcinoma of the thyroid. Br J Surg 74:377–380
62. Reed M, Quayle AR, Harris SC, Talbot CH (1990) The association between thyroid neoplasia and intestinal polyps. Ann R Coll Surg Engl 72:257–359
63. Chen Y, Ott DJ, Wu WC, Gelfand DW (1987) Cowden's disease: a case report and literature review. Gastrointest Radiol 12:325–329
64. Michaels R, Shakir KA (1993) Association of multinodular goiter with breast cancer: Cowden's disease. J Endocrinol Invest 16:909–911
65. Ohta S, Katsura T, Shimada M, Shima A, Chishiro H, Matsubara H (1996) Ataxia-telangiectasia with papillary carcinoma of the thyroid. Am J Ped Hem Oncol 8:255–268
66. Verneris M, McDougall IR, Becton D, Link MP (2001) Thyroid carcinoma after successful treatment of osteosarcoma: a report of 3 patients. J Pediatric Hem Oncol 23:312–315
67. Galanti MR et al. (1997) Parental cancer and risk of papillary and follicular thyroid carcinoma. Br J Cancer 75:451–456
68. Fagin JA (1997) Familial nonmedullary thyroid carcinoma – the case for genetic susceptibility. J Clin Endocrinol Metab 82:342–344

69. Loh KC (1997) Familial nonmedullary thyroid carcinoma: a meta-review of case series. Thyroid 7:107–113
70. Ron E et al. (1991) Familial nonmedullary thyroid cancer. Oncology 48:309–311
71. Flannigan G, Clifford RP, Winslet M, Lawrence DAS, Fiddian RV (1983) Simultaneous presentation of papillary carcinoma of the thyroid in a father and son. Br J Surg 70:181–182
72. Canzian F, Stark M, Corvi R, Lesueur F (1998) High and low penetrance genes predisposing to thyroid cancer (abstract). Thyroid 8:1211
73. Bignell GR et al. (1997) Familial nontoxic multinodular thyroid goiter locus maps to chromosome 14q but does not account for familial nonmedullary thyroid cancer. Am J Hum Genet 61:1123–1130
74. Canzian F et al. (1998) A gene predisposing to familial thyroid tumors with cell oxyphilia maps to chromosome 19p13.2. Am J Hum Genet 63:1743–1748
75. Lesueur F et al. (1999) Genetic heterogeneity in familial nonmedullary thyroid carcinoma: exclusion of linkage to RET, MNG1, and TCO in 56 families. NMTC Consortium. J Clin Endocrinol Metab 84:2157–2162
76. McKay J, Williamson J, Lesueur F, Stark M, Duffield A, Canzian F, Romeo G, Hoffman L (1999) At least three genes account for familial papillary thyroid carcinoma: TCO and MNG1 excluded as susceptibility loci from a large Tasmanian family. Eur J Endocrinol 141:122–125
77. McKay JD et al. (2001) Localization of a susceptibility gene for familial nonmedullary thyroid carcinoma to chromosome 2q21. Am J Hum Genet 69:440–446
78. Cetani F, Tonacchera M, Pinchera A, Barsacchi R, Basolo G, Miccoli PM, Pacini F (1999) Genetic analysis of the TSH receptor gene in differentiated human thyroid carcinomas. J Endocrinol Invest 22:273–278
79. Curtis L, Wyllie AH, Shaw JJ et al. (1994) Evidence against the involvement of APC mutation in papillary thyroid carcinoma. Eur J Cancer 30A:984–989
80. Bongarzone I et al. (1996) Age-related activation of the tyrosine kinase receptor protooncogenes *RET* and *NTRK1* in papillary thyroid carcinoma. J Clin Endocrinol Metab 81:2006–2009
81. Bongarzone I et al. (1997) Comparison of the breakpoint regions of *ELE1* and *RET* genes involved in the generation of *RET/PTC3* oncogene in sporadic and in radiation-associated papillary thyroid carcinomas. Genomics 42:252–259
82. Beimfohr C et al. (1999) NTRK1 re-arrangement in papillary thyroid carcinomas of children after the Chernobyl reactor accident. Int J Cancer 80:842–847
83. Jhiang S, Sagartz JE, Tong Q, Parker-Thornburg J, Capen CC, Cho JY, Xing S, Ledent C (1996) Targeted expression of the *RET/PTC1* oncogene induces papillary thyroid carcinomas. Endocrinology 137:375–378
84. Valent ADG, Bernheim A (1997) Mapping of the tyrosine kinase receptors trkA (*NTRK1*), trkB (*NTRK2*) and trkC (*NTRK3*) to human chromosomes 1q22, 9q22, and 15q25 by fluorescence in situ hybridization. Eur J Hum Genet 5:102–104
85. Trovato M, Fraggetta F, Viillari D, Batolo D, Mackey K, Trimarchi F, Benvenga S (1999) Loss of heterozygosity of the long arm of chromosome 7 in follicular and anaplastic thyroid cancer, but not in papillary thyroid cancer. J Clin Endocrinol Metab 84:3235–3240
86. Zhang J, Nelson M, McIver B Hay I, Goellner JR, Grant CS, Eberhardt NL, Smith DI (1998) Differential loss of heterozygosity at 7q31.2 in follicular and papillary thyroid tumors. Oncogene 17:789–793
87. Yeh J, Marsh DJ, Zedenius J, Dwight T, Delbridge L, Robinson BG, Eng C (1999) Fine-structure deletion mapping of 10q22–24 identifies regions of loss of heterozygosity and suggests that sporadic follicular thyroid adenomas and follicular thyroid carcinomas develop along distinct neoplastic pathways. Genes Chromosomes Cancer 26:322–328
88. Dahia PL et al. (1997) Somatic deletions and mutations in the Cowden disease gene, *PTEN*, in sporadic thyroid tumors. Cancer Res 57:4710–4713

89. Marsh D, Kum JB, Lunetta KL, Bennett MJ, Gorlin RJ, Ahmed SF, Bodurtha J, Crowe C, Curtis MA, Dasouki M, Dunn T, Feit H, Geraghty MT, Graham JM Jr, Hodgson SV, Hunter A, Korf BR, Manchester D, Miesfeldt S, Murday VA, Nathanson KL, Parisi M, Pober B, Romano C, Eng C (1999) *PTEN* mutation spectrum and genotype-phenotype correlations in Bannayan-Rileyt-Ruvalcaba syndrome suggest a single entity with Cowden syndrome. Hum Mol Genet 8:1461–1472
90. Halachmi N, HS, Evron E, Cairns P, Okami K, Saji M, Westra WH, Zeiger MA, Jen J, Sidransky D (1998) Somatic mutations of the *PTEN* tumor suppressor gene in sporadic follicular thyroid tumors. Genes Chromosomes Cancer 23:239–243
91. Gardner RJ, KD, Edkins E, Walpole IR, Macrae FA, Nasioulas S, Scott WJ (1997) The clinical correlates of a 3'truncating mutation in the adenomatous polyposis coli gene. Gastroenterology 113:326–331
92. Hizawa K, Iida M, Aoyagi K, Yao T, Fujishima M (1997) Thyroid neoplasia in familial adenomatous polyposis/Gardner's syndrome. J Gastroenterology 32:196–199
93. Perrier N, Heerden JA van, Goellner JR, Williams ED, Gharib H, Marchesa P, Church JM, Fazio VW, Larson DR (1998) Thyroid cancer in patients with familial adenomatous polyposis. World J Surg 22:738–742
94. Goretzki PE, GV, Dozenrath C, Witte J, Roeher HD (1996) A frequent mutation/polymorphism in tumor suppressor gene *INK4B* (*MTS-2*) in papillary and medullary thyroid cancer. Surgery 120:1081–1088
95. Schulte K, Staudt s, Niederracher D, Finken-Eigen M, Kohrer K, Goretzki PE, Roher HD (1998) Rare loss of heterozygosity of the *MTS1* and *MTS* 2 tumor suppressor genes in differentiated human thyroid cancer. Horm Metab Res 30:549–554
96. Kwok C, McDougall IR (1995) Familial differentiated carcinoma of the thyroid: report of 5 families. Thyroid 5:395–397

Chapter 4

The Diagnosis of Thyroid Cancer 4

C. Reiners

4.1 Prevalence/Risk Assessment

The prevalence of thyroid nodules depends on iodine supply. In North America, the incidence of thyroid nodules detected by palpation is estimated to be 0.1% per year, with a prevalence of between 4% and 7% in the general population. Thyroid nodules are more common in women, with advancing age, in areas of iodine deficiency, and after exposure to external radiation [30].

According to a recent meta-analysis [35], the prevalence of thyroid nodules diagnosed by ultrasonography ranges between 20% and 70%, whereas the prevalence of abnormal findings detected by thyroid scintigraphy ranges between 30% and 40%. The relatively large variability of the prevalence of thyroid nodules detected by ultrasonography is due at least partially to the different equipment used. In the most recent studies applying 7.5–10 MHz ultrasound scanners, a prevalence of 40–70% has been revealed. By autopsy, thyroid nodules in patients with clinically normal thyroids are found in 30–50%. The risk of malignancy in asymptomatic nodules found in non-irradiated glands ranges between 0.4% and 13% (mean ± SD: 3.9±4.1%). The risk is higher in females (females:males=1.75:1) [35].

According to a study performed in Italy, thyroid nodules in children and adolescents below age of 20 years were malignant in 10% of cases, whereas the rate of malignancy with 5% was considerably lower in adults [1]. The most important risk factor for thyroid cancer is exposure to ionizing irradiation. In patients with thyroid nodules who have been irradiated during childhood or adolescence, the prevalence of thyroid cancer ranges between 30% and 50% [14].

4.2 Findings/Symptoms

Thyroid cancer frequently does not present with clinical symptoms. In a study of 835 patients who had been operated on for nodular goiter [37], 31% also had thyroid cancer (tumors with a diameter of less than 10 mm, which were clinically occult in 46% of those patients).

A study of 1.116 patients with thyroid cancer from an iodine-deficient area [29] showed that the leading symptom of thyroid cancer was an intra-thyroidal solitary nodule in 40% of the patients. Cervical lymph node enlargement as an initial symptom has been found more frequently in males (21%) than in females (10%). In patients younger than 40 years of age lymph node enlargements were three times more frequent than in patients older than 50 years. In patients aged 60 years and above, higher tumor stages (T3 and T4) have been found more frequently (42%) than in patients younger than 40 years (25%). Clinical symptoms such as hoarseness due to paresis of the laryngeal nerve were very rare, at 0.6%, and distant metastases were also found infrequently (0.8%) as initial sign of thyroid cancer. During childhood 2.6% of the patients had been irradiated for different benign diseases. Scintigraphically cold nodules were detected in 55% of the patients.

The question of the prevalence of thyroid cancer in patients with hyperthyroidism and scintigraphically hot nodules has been frequently discussed. A study performed on the same patient material [19] showed that in only 2.6% of the patients being operated on for thyrotoxicosis occult thyroid cancers were prevalent (2% of the patients with Graves' disease and 4% of the patients with functional autonomy).

The clinical signs and symptoms of thyroid cancer have very recently been evaluated in a German Patient Care Evaluation Study of thyroid cancer (PCES) and compared to a PCES Study from the USA [17]. In 4% of the German patients previous exposure to radioiodine was found; the frequency of radiation exposure in USA patients, at 4.5%, was comparable. A considerable difference could be documented concerning the prevalence of goiter: in 81% of the German patients thyroid enlargement was found, against only 45% of USA patients. A nodule could be palpated in 77% of the German and 75% of the USA patients. Dysphagia, neck pain, hoarseness and stridor could be documented in 26%, 8%, 5% and 11% of German patients as compared to 12%, 6%; 8% and 4% of the USA patients, respectively. An enlargement of neck lymph nodes was much more frequent in patients from the USA than in those from Germany (27% vs 7%).

4.3 Ultrasonography

Ultrasonography is the modality most often used for thyroid imaging. It is relatively cheap, easily accessible, rapidly performed and has the advantage of no exposure to ionizing radiation. It allows determination of the volume of the thyroid and the size of nodules, the echo structure (diffuse, uni- or multinodular), echogenicity (iso-, hyper- or hypo-echogenic) and the evaluation of adjacent neck structures. Today ultrasound scanners with high-frequency transducers (7.5–10 MHz) are recommended. They allow even very small (2–3 mm) thyroid lesions to be imaged [15].

The typical sign of malignancy is – in more than 90% of cases – a hypoechogenic solid lesion. In contrast, malignancy is very rarely found in iso- or hyper-echogenic lesions [36].

Several studies have been designed in order to evaluate whether additional criteria determinable by high-frequency ultrasound – such as the appearance of the margins (halo-sign), cystic degeneration or calcification – can be used in the differentiation of benign from malignant thyroid nodules. The general finding

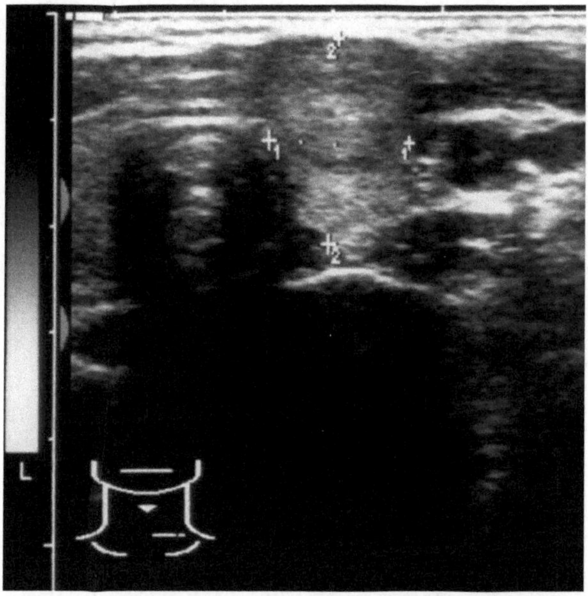

Fig. 4.1. Conventional 2D-sonography (transverse section) of a papillary thyroid cancer with irregular contours and deformation of the thyroid capsule

has been that there is no ultrasound pattern, alone or in combination with other techniques, that may be considered specific for thyroid cancer [15, 25]. The only reliable indicators of malignancy were invasive growth into surrounding structures (Fig. 4.1), metastases to cervical lymph nodes or both [15]. In contrast, thyroid cancer may be excluded in iso- or hyper-echogenic nodules with a probability of more than 90%. In the future, three-dimensional ultrasound may help to delineate thyroid nodules more precisely (Fig. 4.2).

For more than 10 years, the speed and direction of blood flow in thyroid lesions have been investigated by the color-Doppler and – more recently – the power-Doppler mode. The perfusion pattern may be delineated more clearly by means of ultrasound contrast media. However, no study has shown a specific pattern for malignancy [15, 18]. In a recent study by Rago et al. [25], intra-nodular blood flow was found to be increased in 67% of malignant and 50% of benign thyroid nodules (Fig. 4.3). However, Hegedues and Karstrup argue that at least 60–70% of cold solitary nodules can be classified as benign colloid nodules with a minimal risk of overlooking malignancy (<1%) on the basis of conventional sonography and ultrasound-guided fine-needle biopsy [15].

4.4 Scintigraphy

Scintigraphy is not a rival method to ultrasound, but complements the morphological information of sonography with the functional scintigraphic image, which shows the regional metabolic activity of the thyroid gland. Today Tc-

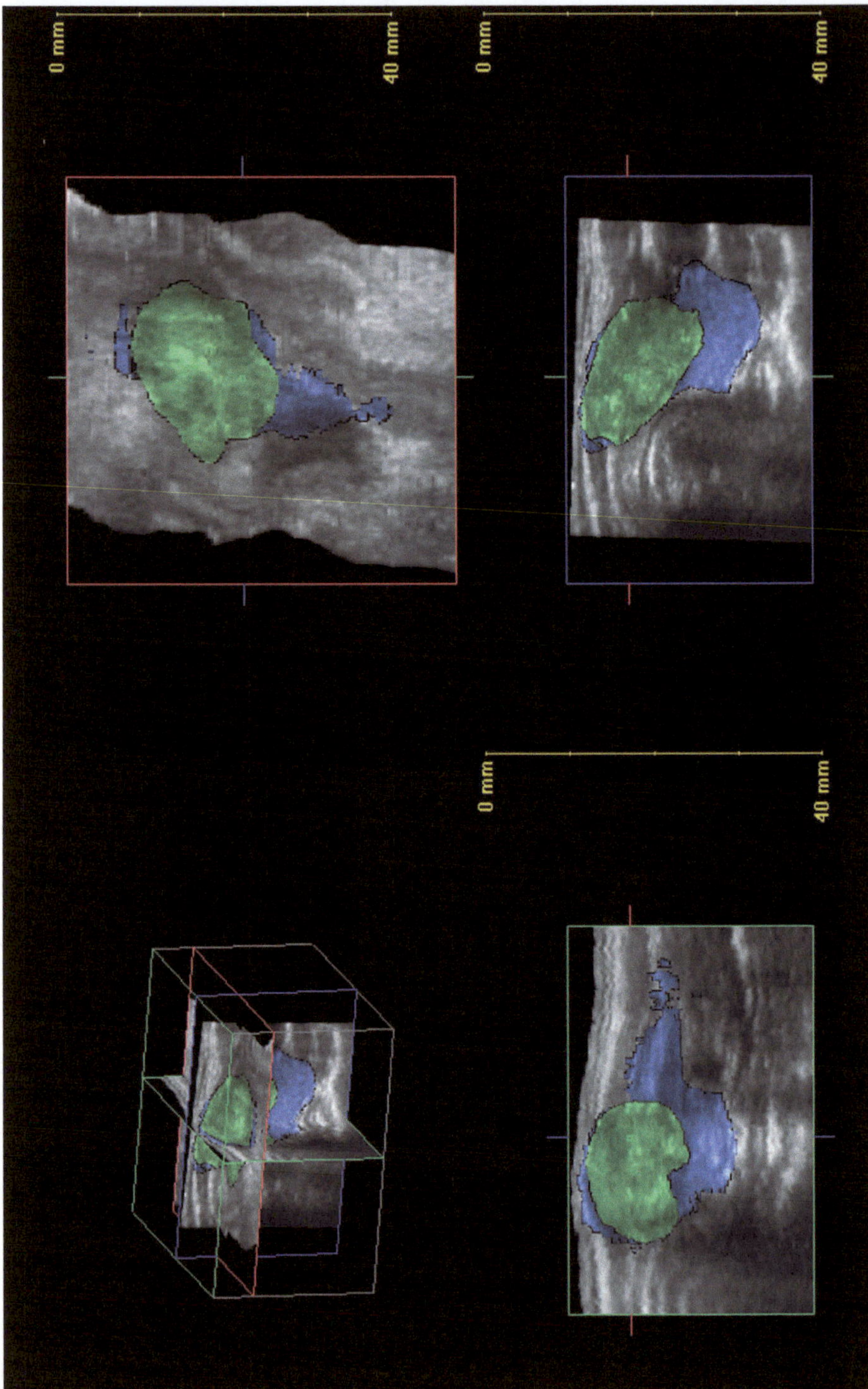
0 mm
40 mm
0 mm
40 mm
0 mm
40 mm

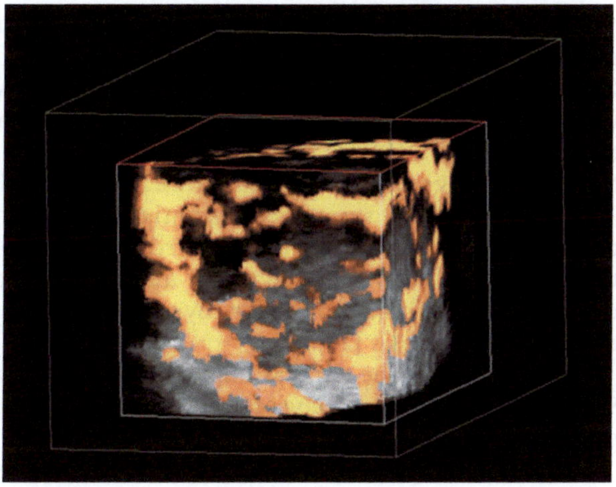

Fig. 4.3. 3D-display of color-Doppler ultrasound of a benign follicular adenoma: nonspecifically increased intra-nodular blood flow

99m-pertechnetate is used routinely for thyroid scintigraphy. For specific indications (e.g., recurrences or metastases of differentiated thyroid cancer after surgery) ^{131}I-NaI is the radiopharmaceutical of choice. For imaging the thyroid, a gamma-camera with a high-resolution collimator is necessary [10].

The typical scintigraphic sign of malignancy is a cold nodule (Fig. 4.3). Börner et al. published as early as 1965 a detailed study of scintigraphic investigations in 2,237 thyroid patients [3]. It was shown that the frequency of cold nodules increased from 21% in patients aged 15–16 years up to 44% in patients over the age of 65 years. In patients younger than 35 years, malignancy was rare in case of hypo-functionality. In contrast, thyroid cancer was histologically verified in 11% of cold nodules of patients aged 45–65 years and 25% in patients above the age of 65 years.

For follow-up of differentiated thyroid cancer, different scintigraphic procedures with a number of more or less specific radiopharmaceuticals may be used [7, 32]. The most relevant procedure is whole body scanning with diagnostic or therapeutic activities of ^{131}I NaI, frequently showing regional or distant metastases that have not been detected by other imaging procedures. The role of whole-body scintigraphy with Tl-201 chloride and Tc-99m-MIBI or -tetrofosmin in the follow-up of patients with differentiated thyroid cancer after surgery and/or radioiodine therapy is well established (especially in tumors taking up no radioiodine) [21, 23, 31]. Most recently, positron emission tomography (PET) with F-18-FDG has shown to be a promising imaging procedure especially in patients with negative radioiodine scans [12].

With respect to primary diagnosis of thyroid cancer, Tl-201, Tc-99m-MIBI and F-18-FDG have been proposed as imaging agents to determine the sus-

Fig. 4.2. 3D-ultrasound slices of a patient with papillary thyroid cancer in the left thyroid lobe: 3D-cube (*upper left*), longitudinal slice (*upper right*), horizontal slice (*lower left*) and transversal slice (*lower right*)

pected malignancy of thyroid nodules [2, 20, 32]. Kresnick et al. [20] conclude that MIBI accumulation and retention is not specific for thyroid malignancy. In combination with all other findings, a positive MIBI scan would appear to indicate an adenoma rather than a malignant tumor. This statement can be extended to the attempts to qualify malignancy of a thyroid nodule pre-operatively by scintigraphy with Tl-201 or PET with F-18-FDG.

In the past, X-ray fluorescence scintigraphy [27], which allows measurement of the stable iodine content of the thyroid and thyroidal nodules has been used to differentiate between benign and malignant lesions. However, a low iodine content, described as typical for thyroid cancer, has proved to be not specific enough for diagnosis [24].

To summarize, the clinical impact of routine thyroid scintigraphy with Tc-99m-pertechnetate has to be seen in combination with the results of ultrasonography (Table 4.1).

In patients (especially of young age) with a rapidly growing nodule, however, fine-needle aspiration biopsy (FNA) is indicated in any case and histological verification is frequently necessary.

4.5 Fine-Needle Aspiration Biopsy

According to the PCES Study [17] ultrasonography is performed in Germany before surgery in 78%, scintigraphy in 77% and FNA in 27% of patients with thyroid nodules. The corresponding figures in the USA are 39%, 40% and 43% respectively [17]. This comparison shows that FNA seems to have higher diagnostic impact in the United States. However, due to the high prevalence of goiter in Germany (81% vs 45% in the USA), the use of FNA in Germany is mostly restricted to differential diagnosis of the clinically most suspicious solitary thyroid nodules.

Table 4.1. Indications for fine-needle aspiration biopsy (FNA) of the thyroid with respect to the results of sonography and scintigraphy [28]

Sonography	Scintigraphy	Presumptive diagnosis	FNA
Iso-echogenic/hyper-echogenic	Hot	Autonomy	Relative indication
	Cold	Regressive nodule	Relative indication
Hypo-echogenic/complex	Hot	Autonomy	Relative indication
		Follicular adenoma	Relative indication
	Cold	Malignoma	**Absolute indication**
		Thyroiditis	**Absolute indication**
		Hemorrhage	**Absolute indication**
Echo-free	Cold	Cyst	Relative indication

Particularly in regions with endemic iodine deficiency, patients have to be selected for FNA. As shown in Table 4.1 sonography and scintigraphy can efficiently be used for selection. FNA is mandatory in patients with hypo-echogenic and scintigraphically cold nodules. Today disposable cannulas (no. 17 or no. 16; gauge 25–23, respectively) are used. By using such small cannulas, side effects such as hemorrhage (1 per 1000) or infections (1 per 4000) are rare [8]. Today ultrasound is usually used to guide the puncture needle during biopsy. A comparison of nine studies published since 1994, each including more than 100 cases, shows that the diagnostic accuracy can be improved by ultrasound guidance. The median sensitivity and specificity increased after introduction of ultrasound guidance from 89% and 69%, respectively, to 97% and 83% (Table 4.2).

Table 4.2. Diagnostic validity of fine needle aspiration biopsy (FNA) of the thyroid: Data from the literature

Author, year	Method	n	Insufficient material (%)	Sensitivity (%)	Specificity (%)	Accuracy (%)	PV+ (%)	PV– (%)
Cochand-Priollet [8]	US guided	132	4	79	84	83	54	95
Takashima [34]	Palpation guided	34	19	88	90	88	95	75
	US guided	99	4	96	91	94	96	91
Carpi [6]								
<1 mm	US guided	39	3	97	34	67	–	–
1–1.9 mm	US guided	52	0	90	52	66	–	–
2–3 mm	US guided	32	0	94	70	77	–	–
>3 mm	US guided	35	9	88	76	80	–	–
García-Mayor [11]	Palpation guided	403	16	94	61	72	54	95
Hatada [13]	Palpation guided	94	30	45	51	48	–	–
	US guided	72	17	62	74	68	–	–
Danese [9]	Palpation guided	522	9	92	69	73	37	98
	US guided	535	4	97	71	76	44	99
Carmeci [5]	Palpation guided	370	16	89	69	–	–	–
	US guided	127	7	100	100	–	–	–
Cáp [4]	Palpation guided (25% US guided)	516	8	90	79	81	51	97
Mikosch [22]	US guided	718	5	88	79	80	34	98

PV+/PV–: Positive/negative predictive value; US: ultrasound

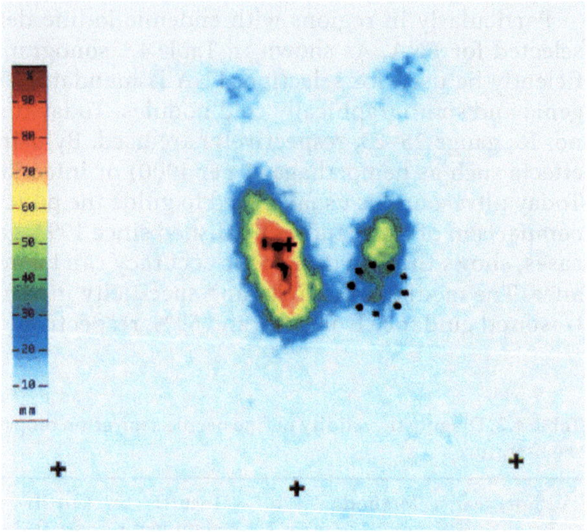

Fig. 4.4. Thyroid scan with Tc-99m-pertechnetate of a patient with papillary thyroid cancer showing a cold nodule in the lower quadrant of the left lobe

In addition, the median frequency of biopsies with insufficient material could be reduced by a factor of approximately 2 from 18% to 7% (Table 4.2). However, to date no generally acknowledged criteria for definition of an adequate biopsy smear have been approved. Usually, 5–6 groups of 10 well-preserved follicular cells each have been suggested [33].

Today the traditional classification of cytopathological smears of the thyroid according to Papanicolaou is obsolete. According to recent recommendations from the American Papanicolaou Society for Cytopathology [33] the classification should consider benign (non-neoplastic lesions), suspicious (follicular or oncocytic lesions of high cellularity) and malignant findings.

Usually the diagnosis of papillary thyroid cancer (Fig. 4.5) is not difficult, since cell-rich formations of thyroid cells organized in monolayered sheets and forming papillary clusters showing psammoma bodies, enlarged nuclei with "ground-glass" appearance containing chromatin and large and irregular nucleoli, nuclear grooves and cytoplasmic inclusions are considered to be typical [33]. However, in cases of cell-rich smears with a monomorphic or rarely pleomorphic population of epithelial cells, frequently grouped in micro-follicular clusters, distinction of a well-differentiated follicular thyroid cancer from a benign follicular adenoma is not possible (Fig. 4.5). The frequency of such findings, often judged as "follicular neoplasia", ranges between 5% and 20% [4, 8, 9, 11, 22]. In cases of "follicular neoplasia" the histological verification of the suspicious cytological finding is mandatory.

A study from Spain has shown that, since the introduction of palpation-guided FNA, the frequency of patients requiring prophylactic "surgery" has decreased from 90% to 47% and the frequency of malignancy in the surgical specimens has increased from 15% to 33% [11]. Recently, Carmeci et al. [5] from Stanford University, California, USA showed that ultrasound guidance of FNA

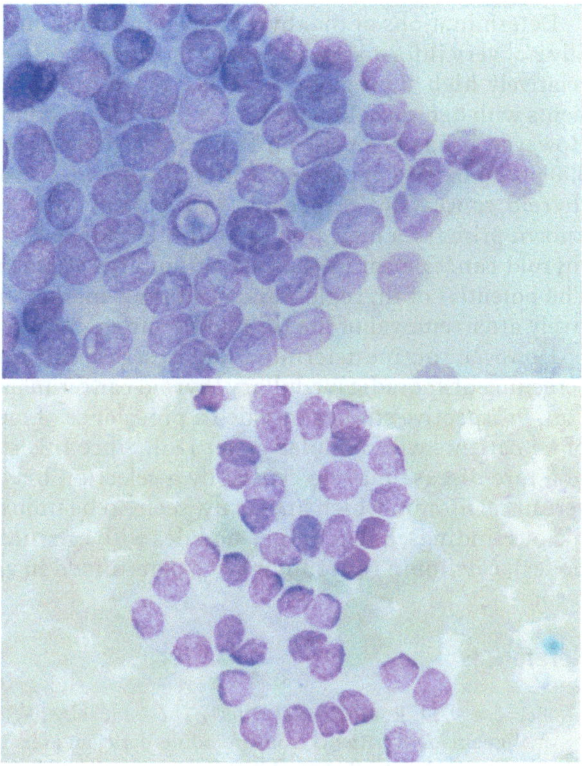

Fig. 4.5. Cytology smears of fine needle aspiration biopsies (May-Grünwald-Giemsa staining) of papillary thyroid carcinoma (*left*) and follicular neoplasia later histologically verified as benign follicular adenoma (*right*) (with permission of Prof. Dr. R. Schäffer, Institute of Pathology, University of Gießen, Germany)

leads to a considerable improvement compared to palpation-guided FNA: the cancer yield at surgery increased from 40% to 59%.

To summarize, ultrasound-guided FNA is highly recommended for differential diagnosis of especially solitary solid thyroid nodules of poor echogenicity showing decreased uptake on the scan.

4.6 Additional Diagnostic Procedures

In patients with large or multi-nodular goiters, an X-ray of the neck is useful to disclose deviation of the trachea or restriction of its lumen. For a detailed study of mediastinal involvement, CT or MRI is preferable. Particularly in cases of large invasive thyroid cancers with involvement of the sternum, MRI is highly recommended before surgery. However, CT and MRT do not allow benign and malignant thyroid lesions to be differentiated. It has to be taken into account that use of iodine-containing contrast media for CT is contraindicated in cases of suspected thyroid malignancies, as diagnostic or therapeutic applications of radioiodine may be hampered for several weeks.

Determinations of the thyroid-specific tumor marker thyroglobulin are usually not very informative in cases of suspected malignancy preoperatively, since relatively high thyroglobulin levels, up to 500 ng/ml, may be observed in patients with benign cold nodules (i.e., follicular adenoma or oncocytic adenoma). However, it has been shown that serum thyroglobulin preoperatively exceeds 500 ng/ml in 72% of patients with follicular and 56% of patients with oncocytic thyroid cancer [16]. Especially in a patient with metastases of cancer of unknown primary a high thyroglobulin level may be indicative for differentiated thyroid cancer even in the case of no large abnormalities in thyroid imaging. The potential of thyroglobulin as a tumor marker, however, is used most effectively after removal of the thyroid by surgery and radioiodine therapy.

However, routine determinations of serum calcitonin have been advocated for screening of sporadic medullary thyroid cancer in patients with thyroid nodules [26]. Prospective studies revealed a prevalence of medullary cancer in 0.6–1.3% of all patients with nodular goiter [26]. Since this surprisingly high prevalence of a rare disease may be caused by a selection bias, routine determinations of serum calcitonin, which are costly, seem to be unjustified. In patients with suspicious findings, however (i.e., nodules with calcifications, enlarged neck lymph nodes), calcitonin in serum may be determined in addition to FNA.

References

1. Belfiore A, La-Rosa GL et al. (1987) The frequency of cold thyroid nodules and thyroid malignancies in patients from an iodine-deficient area. Cancer 60:3096–3102
2. Bloom AD, Adler LP et al. (1993) Determination of malignancy of thyroid nodules with positron emission tomography. Surgery 114:728–735
3. Börner W, Lautsch M et al. (1965) Die diagnostische Bedeutung des "kalten Knotens" im Schilddrüsenszintigramm. Med Welt 17:892–897
4. Cáp J, Ryska A et al. (1999) Sensitivity and specificity of the fine needle aspiration biopsy of the thyroid: Clinical point of view. Clin Endocrinol 51:509-515
5. Carmeci C, Brooke Jeffrey R et al. (1998) Ultrasound-guided fine-needle aspiration biopsy of thyroid masses. Thyroid 8:283–289
6. Carpi E, Ferrari E et al. (1996) Needle aspiration techniques in preoperative selection of patients with thyroid nodules: A long-term study. J Clin Oncol 14:1704–1712
7. Cavalieri RR (1996) Nuclear imaging in the management of thyroid carcinoma. Thyroid 6:485–492
8. Cochand-Priollet B, Guillausseau PJ et al. (1994) The diagnostic value of fine-needle aspiration biopsy under ultrasonography in non-functional thyroid nodules: A prospective study comparing cytologic and histologic findings. Amer J Med 97:152–157
9. Danese D, Sciaccitano S et al. (1998) Diagnostic accuracy of conventional versus sonography-guided fine-needle aspiration biopsy of thyroid nodules. Thyroid 8:15–21
10. Dietlein M, Dressler J et al. (1999) Leitlinien zur Schilddrüsendiagnostik. Nuklearmedizin 38:215–218
11. García-Mayor RV, Pérez-Mendez LF et al. (1997) Fine-needle aspiration biopsy of thyroid nodules: Impact on clinical practice. J Endocrinol Invest 20:482–487
12. Grünwald F, Kaelicke T et al. (1999) Fluorine-fluorodeoxyglucose positron emission tomography in thyroid cancer: Results of a multicenter study. Eur J Nucl Med 26:1547–1552
13. Hatada T, Okada K et al. (1998) Evaluation of ultrasound-guided fine-needle aspiration biopsy for thyroid nodules. Amer J Surg 175:133–136

14. Hatipoglu BA, Gierlowski T et al. (2000) Fine-needle aspiration of thyroid nodules in radiation exposed patients. Thyroid 10:63–69
15. Hegedues L, Karstrup (1998) Ultrasonography in the evaluation of cold thyroid nodules. Eur J Endocrinol 138:30–31
16. Hocevar M, Auersperg M et al. (1998) Role of thyroglobulin in the pre-operative evaluation of follicular thyroid tumours. Eur J Surg Oncol 24:553-557
17. Hölzer S, Fremgen AM et al. (2000) Evaluation of the implications of clinical practice guidelines for patient care. Amer J Med Qual (in press)
18. Klemenz B, Wieler H, Kaiser HP (1997) Value of color-coded Doppler sonography in the differential diagnosis of thyroid nodules. Nuklearmedizin 36:245–249
19. Krause U, Olbricht T et al. (1991) Häufigkeit von Schilddrüsenkarzinomen bei Hyperthyreose. Dtsch Med Wschr 116:201–206
20. Kresnick E, Gallowitsch HJ et al. (1997) Technetium-99m-MIBI-scintigraphy of thyroid nodules in an endemic goitre area. J Nucl Med 38:62–65
21. Lind P, Gallowitsch HJ et al. (1997) Technetium-99m-Tetrofosmin-whole body scintigraphy in the follow-up of differentiated thyroid carcinoma. J Nucl Med 38:348–352
22. Mikosch P, Gallowitsch HJ et al. (2000) Value of ultrasound-guided fine-needle aspiration biopsy of thyroid nodules in an endemic goitre area. Eur J Nucl Med 27:62-69
23. Oyen WJG, Verhagen C et al. (2000) Follow-up regimen of differentiated thyroid carcinoma in thyroidectomized patients after thyroid hormone withdrawal. J Nucl Med 41:643–646
24. Patton JA, Hollifield JW et al. (1976) Differentiation between malignant and benign solitary thyroid nodules by fluorescent thyroid scanning. J Nucl Med 17:17–21
25. Rago T, Vitti P et al. (1998) Role of conventional ultrasonography and colourflow-Doppler-sonography in predicting malignancy in "cold" thyroid nodules. Eur J Endocrinol 138:41–46
26. Raue F (1998) Routine calcitonin determination in thyroid nodules–an effective approach? Exp Clin Endocrinol Diabetes 106:289-291
27. Reiners Chr, Hänscheid H et al. (1997) X-ray fluorescence analysis (XFA) of thyroidal iodine contact (TIC) with an improved measuring system. Exp Clin Endocrinol Diabetes 106:531–533
28. Reiners Chr, Becker W et al. (1986) Schilddrüsendiagnostik: Nutzen von Sonographie, Szintigraphie und Punktionszytologie für die Praxis. Intern Welt 10:294–304
29. Reinwein D, Benker G et al. (1989) Erstsymptome bei Schilddrüsenmalignomen: Einfluss von Alter und Geschlecht in einem Iodmangelgebiet. Dtsch Med Wschr 114:775–782
30. Rojewski MT, Gharib H (1985) Nodular thyroid disease. Evaluation and management. N Engl J Med 313:428–436
31. Rubello D, Mazzarotto R et al. (2000) The role of Technetium-99m-Metoxyisobutylisonitril scintigraphy in the planning of therapy and follow-up of patients with differentiated thyroid carcinoma after surgery. Eur J Nucl Med 27:431–440
32. Sisson JW (1997) Selection of the optimal scanning agent for thyroid cancer. Thyroid 7:295–302
33. Suen K (1996) Guidelines of the Papanicolaou Society of Cytopathology for the examination of fine-needle aspiration specimens from thyroid nodules. Mod Pathol 9:710-715
34. Takashima S, Fukuda H, Kobayashi T (1994) Thyroid nodules: clinical effect of ultrasound-guided fine-needle aspiration biopsy. J Clin Ultrasound 22:535–542
35. Tan GH, Gharib H (1997) Thyroid incidentalomas: management approaches to non-palpable nodules discovered incidentally on thyroid imaging. An Intern Med 126:226–231
36. Wiedemann W, Reiners Chr (1982) Die Differentialdiagnose des echoarmen Knotens der Schilddrüse. Dtsch Med Wschr 51:1972–1975
37. Yamashita H, Noduchi S et al. (1997) Thyroid cancer associated with adenomatous goitre: An analysis of the incidence and clinical factors. Jap J Surg 27:495–499

Chapter 5

The Current Surgical Approach to Non-Medullary Thyroid Cancer

5

O. Gimm and H. Dralle

5.1 Introduction

About 150 years ago, thyroid surgery was performed only in life-threatening situations. The main reason for this restrictive approach was the high mortality of up to 40%, the cause of death being usually either uncontrollable bleeding or infection. Against this background, Theodor E. Kocher and Theodor Billroth set out to improve surgery on the thyroid gland and reported their results. The "Kocher incision," a transverse, slightly curved incision about 2 cm above the sternoclavicular joints, is well known to all thyroid surgeons.

Other complications were then identified, in particular hoarseness. It was soon found that preservation of the recurrent laryngeal nerve was important in order to prevent this complication. The pathophysiology of hypoparathyroidism and tetany were not understood at that time. Kocher had a very precise operating technique. He also worked in a relatively bloodless field. These are probably the reasons why he had only a few problems with postoperative tetany. In addition, his technique enabled him to decrease the mortality from 14% in 1884 to 2.4% in 1889 and 0.18% in 1898. By 1874, Kocher had noticed symptoms of hypothyroidism in patients who successfully underwent removal of the thyroid gland. The patients became very tired, showed decreased initiative, and became cretinoid. Even though Kocher misinterpreted these findings as a result of tracheal injury, he made the correct decision in trying to avoid removal of the whole thyroid gland. After the condition of myxedema had been described, transplantation and injection of extracts of thyroid tissue were tried, and in 1892 oral therapy was introduced.

With this knowledge about the physiology, pathology, and surgery on the thyroid gland, for which Kocher received the Nobel Prize in 1909, surgery was extended to treat malignant disorders of the thyroid. Since then, surgery has been the treatment of choice for thyroid cancer. However, new therapeutic tools are required for effective treatment of thyroid cancer extending beyond the thyroid gland. Since the efficiency of the available tools (e.g., radioiodine) is limited and new tools are yet to be found, thyroid surgery will continue to play an important role in the therapy of thyroid cancer in the twenty-first century.

5.2 Prognostic Factors

Therapeutic strategies and the extent of surgery depend on factors that influence the prognosis of thyroid cancer. A variety of factors (e.g., histological type and subtype, tumor grade, tumor stage, capsular and vascular invasion, age, and sex) have been analyzed, but the data are not uniform in all studies. Histological type, size of the primary tumor, extrathyroidal tumor extension, and distant metastases are generally reported to correlate with outcome [5, 7, 20]. In contrast, while lymph node metastases have been repeatedly shown to correlate with tumor recurrence [22, 26], their significance on survival has only been reported in some studies [15].

Three histologically defined thyroid cancers derived from follicular thyroid cells comprise more than 95% of all nonmedullary thyroid malignancies (see Chaps. 1 and 2): papillary, follicular, and undifferentiated thyroid carcinoma.

Papillary thyroid carcinoma (PTC) is the most common form of thyroid cancer (up to 80%) in iodine-sufficient regions. PTCs are generally slow-growing. Despite the fact that they have a tendency to be multifocal and tend to metastasize early via the lymph nodes (about 50% at the time of diagnosis), the prognosis is considered to be good, with 10-year survival rates of 80–95% [23].

Follicular thyroid carcinoma (FTC) is more common in iodine-deficient regions but is rarely more frequent than PTC. FTC is much less often multifocal but metastasizes hematogenously rather than lymphogenously [39, 43]. Patients with FTC have 10-year survival rates of 70–95% [1, 23]. Malignant thyroid tumors that histologically show mainly the features of FTCs but also show papillary structures are classified as PTCs (see Chap. 2).

FTC and PTC have also been classified as differentiated thyroid carcinomas (DTC). Undifferentiated thyroid carcinoma (UTC) is one of the most aggressive human malignancies. Almost all patients present with a thyroid mass, which rapidly enlarges within a few weeks or months. Most patients die within a year after diagnosis due to distant metastases (often occult at the time of diagnosis) if local tumor control can be achieved [7, 24]. Clinical observation and molecular findings support the hypothesis that UTC can develop from FTC [51]. It is also well known that PTC can dedifferentiate in such a manner that it behaves like UTC [35]. The development of UTC has also been seen in patients with longstanding goiter. Whether UTCs derive directly from „normal“ follicular thyroid cells, however, is not known.

Hürthle cells (also known as oxyphilic cells or oncocytic cells) are most often found in follicular thyroid adenoma and carcinoma, but they have also been described in papillary and medullary thyroid carcinoma. They are not specific for malignant thyroid diseases. However, if they are observed in a thyroid carcinoma, they are believed to be associated with a poorer prognosis [30]. One reason might be that these tumors are less likely to take up radioiodine.

Also of particular interest are tumors with insular growth pattern. Insular growth pattern may be seen in nonneoplastic thyroid lesions [49] but is most often seen in papillary and, less often, follicular thyroid carcinoma. Insular thyroid carcinoma has been described in both adults and adolescents. Even though the presence of insular growth does not unequivocally qualify a given tumor as a poorly differentiated thyroid carcinoma, a low overall survival rate has been reported in comparison with well-differentiated thyroid carcinoma [40]. In some studies, insular thyroid carcinoma is more often associated with extrathyroidal tumor extension and metastatic spread. Interestingly, despite a lower degree of differentiation, insular thyroid carcinoma may still be capable of taking up radioiodine, which may be used as a therapeutic option if surgery is not feasible [27].

Sarcomas, lymphomas, and other rare cancers comprise about 5% of all non-medullary thyroid malignancies. Their prognosis is generally worse than DTC but often better that UTC. Because of their rareness, therapeutic recommendations are generally based on experiences analyzing small numbers of patients [2].

A variety of prognostic scoring systems (e.g., AGES, AMES, DAMES, MACIS, age-related pTNM, EORTC prognostic index [5, 19, 20, 25, 36, 46]) have been developed. Unfortunately, none of them are widely used, making comparison of studies extremely difficult if not impossible.

5.3 Surgical Treatment

5.3.1 Technique

A precise surgical technique and bloodless operation should be aimed for to provide the best treatment possible in terms of tumor removal, morbidity, and long-term outcome. Magnifying glasses, bipolar coagulation forceps, and neuromonitoring of the recurrent laryngeal nerve have proven helpful. They facilitate the identification, preparation, and preservation of important structures (e.g., parathyroid glands, recurrent laryngeal nerve) [10].

5.3.2 Primary Therapy

5.3.2.1 Thyroid gland

5.3.2.1.1 Differentiated thyroid carcinoma

The extent of thyroid gland resection has been an issue of controversy. The arguments in favor of total thyroidectomy are:

1. Thyroid cancer is often multifocal. This is particularly true for PTC [9].
2. Small intraglandular tumor remnants may dedifferentiate further and/or be the source of metastatic disease [32].

3. The rate of local recurrences is increased after less than total thyroidectomy [26].
4. In the hands of an experienced endocrine surgeon, minimal or no long-term complications can be expected [6].
5. Reoperation due to tumor remnant is associated with a higher morbidity [21, 50].
6. Thyroglobulin can be used as a marker for persistent/recurrent tumor during follow-up [3, 12].
7. Application of radioiodine application is feasible for diagnostic and/or therapeutic purposes [42].

Factors in support of less than total thyroidectomy are:

1. The rate of clinically significant recurrent thyroid cancer within the thyroid remnant is lower than the reported incidence of microscopic tumor within the thyroid remnant [17].
2. Differentiated thyroid carcinoma dedifferentiates in only a minority of patients [8].
3. Most studies have failed to demonstrate a statistically significant difference in survival rates between total thyroidectomy and less than total thyroidectomy [17].
4. In nonspecialized centers, the morbidity after less than total thyroidectomy is lower than after total thyroidectomy [45].
5. If necessary, ablation of small thyroid remnants can be achieved by application of radioiodine [28].
6. Scoring systems enable the identification of low-risk patients with a long-term disease-free and survival rate of over 90% [5, 19].

The recommendations regarding surgical extent in the presence of small, unifocal, and intrathyroidal (pT1a) PTC tumors (hemithyroidectomy or subtotal thyroidectomy) and extrathyroidal (pT4) DTC tumors (total thyroidectomy including lymphadenectomy of the cervicocentral and, if necessary, cervicolateral compartment) are uniform in Europe and the USA. However, the extent of surgery in all other stages of DTC is controversial. Epidemiological data indicate the existence of a regional and intercontinental difference with regard to tumor biology [48]. While studies from the USA have not been able to show an advantage of total thyroidectomy and cervicocentral lymphadenectomy over less extensive procedures in pT2/3-DTC [29, 41], studies from Europe have demonstrated improved survival rates when lymphadenectomy is performed in addition to total thyroidectomy [15]. Since it has been shown that morbidity correlates with surgeons‘ experience [45], these extended procedures should only be performed in specialized centers. In this regard, the conduction of prospective long-term studies would be desirable; although the feasibility is questionable.

5.3.2.1.2
Undifferentiated thyroid carcinoma

UTC occurs typically in older patients (>60 years), however, it has also been reported to occur in patients younger than 50 years.

If possible, complete surgical resection of the tumor is indicated. However, these tumors tend to grow in a rapid and invasive fashion so that complete surgical removal is often not possible. Debulking of the tumor is often all that can be achieved. In addition, adjuvant or neoadjuvant radiochemotherapy is often applied to facilitate local tumor control [33, 37]. Radioactive iodine therapy has no role in the management of UTC (see Chap. 6).

5.3.2.1.3 Rare types of thyroid cancer

Lymphomas are susceptible to radiochemotherapy, and long-term survival rates of more than 50% have been reported in patients with local disease [44, 47]. Whether total thyroidectomy can further improve patient‘s outcome has not yet been proved. Other rare types of thyroid cancer (e.g., sarcoma, carcinosarcoma, squamous cell carcinoma) are very aggressive and may behave like UTC.

5.3.2.2 Extrathyroidal tumor extension

If thyroid carcinoma extends beyond the thyroid capsule (pT4-tumor; not to be mistaken with infiltration of the tumor capsule) the tumor can infiltrate the trachea and/or the esophagus. The infiltration of these structures by DTC is a rare but surgically challenging situation. Massive hemorrhage and airway obstruction due to uncontrolled local tumor are found to be the cause of death in almost 30% of patients who die from thyroid cancer [24]. Hence, most experienced surgeons recommend the removal of as much tumor mass as possible, while preserving function; however, the exact surgical method to best approach this situation is controversial.

If tumor mass adheres to tracheal and/or laryngeal cartilage, a mere shaving procedure might be sufficient. Should tracheal and/or laryngeal cartilage be transmurally invaded, more radical procedures such as circumferential tracheal resection or total laryngectomy may be required [11, 13]. Involvement of the esophagus may require esophagectomy with interposition of free colon, stomach, or, preferably, small intestine autografts. If distant metastases are present, stent implantation is an alternative therapeutic option to prevent airway obstruction and hemorrhage.

It also should be considered that preservation of the laryngeal nerve might be worthwhile in order to maintain its function if infiltrated by differentiated thyroid carcinoma. It has been shown that this strategy neither increases the incidence of local recurrences nor affects survival [34].

Tracheal and/or esophageal invasion is more often found in patients with UTC than patients with DTC. The aggressiveness of this tumor and the likelihood that these patients will die within 1 year do not justify surgical procedures with a high morbidity rate and the patients would require long-term hospitalization.

5.3.2.3
Lymph nodes

At the time of diagnosis, lymph node metastases are a common (35–50%) finding in patients with PTC. Micrometastases are even found in up to 60–90%. The prognostic significance of these micrometastases is difficult to predict. In adults, about 15% of micrometastases are believed to become clinically significant [7]. In contrast, micrometastases in children may become clinically significant in more then 50% [18]. Only a few studies have shown a significant influence on survival [15]. It is, however, generally accepted that lymph node metastases correlate with tumor recurrence [18, 22, 31]. No scoring system clearly enables high-risk patients to be distinguished from low-risk patients. It has been shown that lymphadenectomy, in addition to thyroidectomy, does not increase the morbidity as compared to thyroidectomy alone. In contrast, the increased morbidity after reoperation is very well described [21, 50]. Therefore, in patients with PTC, a cervicocentral lymphadenectomy is justified. Of note, the ipsilateral (regarding the site of the primary tumor) cervicolateral compartment (C2 or C3) contains lymph node metastases almost as frequently as the cervicocentral compartment (C1) [16]. Lymph node metastases can even be found in the cervicolateral compartment without lymph nodes in the cervicocentral compartment [16]. However, routine dissection of the ipsilateral cervicolateral compartment is not recommended, since no survival benefit has been shown and surgery at the time lateral lymph node metastases are found is not associated with an increased morbidity.

In contrast, patients with FTC rarely (10–20%) present with lymph node metastases. It seems that they are less common in Europe [10] and more common in the USA [23, 28]. In a study published by the National Cancer Institute, lymph node metastases in FTC correlates with a decreased survival rate [14]. Whether dissection of the lymph node is able to improve survival has not yet been demonstrated. Distant metastases are more often found in patients with FTC. They may be adequately treated with radioiodine (see Chap. 6), but only if radioiodine uptake is sufficient. One prerequisite is the absence of other thyroid tissue that takes up radioiodine. In addition to total thyroidectomy, dissection of involved lymph node compartments is thus recommended [10].

Because of the tendency of UTC to grow very large, cervical adenopathy may be difficult to appreciate. Whether removal of the lymph nodes influences survival in any way is not known. It is generally recommended that lymph nodes within the cervicocentral compartment be removed, accompanied by those in the cervicolateral compartments if complications are suspected [37].

5.3.2.4
Distant metastases

Distant metastases of nonmedullary thyroid malignancies are most often reported to be present in lung and bone but may also be found in brain, liver, and even heart [24]. They are found in more than 75% of patients who die from thyroid carcinoma, and lung metastases themselves account for almost 50% of tumor-related deaths [24]. Whenever technically feasible, the treatment of choice for distant metastases is surgical resection. In the case of isolated metastases, the surgical removal may be curative and, hence, a more aggressive approach may be justified. If surgery is only indicated to alleviate symptoms, a more restricted approach should be followed. A combination therapy consisting of surgery, radioiodine, and/or external radiation may be beneficial [4].

5.3.3 Completion Thyroidectomy

About 5% of thyroid nodules are believed to be malignant [38]. Pre- and intraoperative diagnostic techniques do not always allow a clear decision whether a nodule is benign or malignant. Thus, histopathological analysis may reveal the diagnosis „thyroid cancer" postoperatively. Usually, the extent of thyroid gland resection in these cases is less than total thyroidectomy. The indications for not performing a completion thyroidectomy equal those that justify performing less than total thyroidectomy (see above). In other words, if the definitive histopathological diagnosis is thyroid cancer a completion thyroidectomy is indicated if one of the following applies:

1. Tumor remnant is proved.
2. Histology shows tumor multifocality or multifocal disease is very likely (e.g., history of external radiation).
3. Primary tumor is larger than 1 cm in diameter (>pT1), at least in pT4.
4. The presence of lymph node (N1) and/or distant metastases (M1).

5.3.4 Recurrent Disease

Patients with thyroid cancer have to be followed up for the rest of their lives. Tumor can recur even more than 20 year after primary operation. Recurrent thyroid cancer occurs most frequently in the cervical lymph nodes. Even though the complication rate of surgical therapy in patients with recurrent thyroid cancer is higher than the complication rate at primary therapy, surgery is treatment of choice if feasible.

References

1. Akslen LA, Haldorsen T, Thoresen SO, Glattre E (1991) Survival and causes of death in thyroid cancer: a population-based study of 2,479 cases from Norway. Cancer Res 51:1234–1241
2. Al-Sobhi SS, Novosolov F, Sabanci U, Epstein HD, Greenspan FS, Clark OH (1997) Management of thyroid carcinosarcoma. Surgery 122:548–552

3. Bohm J, Kosma VM, Eskelinen M, Hollmen S, Niskanen M, Tulla H, Alhava E, Niskanen L (1999) Non-suppressed thyrotropin and elevated thyroglobulin are independent predictors of recurrence in differentiated thyroid carcinoma. Eur J Endocrinol 141:460–467
4. Brierley JD, Tsang RW (1996) External radiation therapy in the treatment of thyroid malignancy. Endocrinol Metab Clin North Am 25:141–157
5. Cady B, Rossi R (1988) An expanded view of risk-group definition in differentiated thyroid carcinoma. Surgery 104:947–953
6. Clark OH (1982) Total thyroidectomy: the treatment of choice for patients with differentiated thyroid cancer. Ann Surg 196:361–370
7. Clark OH (1996) Predictors of thyroid tumor aggressiveness (see comments). West J Med 165:131–138
8. Cohn KH, Backdahl M, Forsslund G, Auer G, Zetterberg A, Lundell G, Granberg PO, Lowhagen T, Willems JS, Cady B (1984) Biologic considerations and operative strategy in papillary thyroid carcinoma: arguments against the routine performance of total thyroidectomy. Surgery 96:957–971
9. DeGroot LJ, Kaplan EL, McCormick M, Straus FH (1990) Natural history, treatment, and course of papillary thyroid carcinoma. J Clin Endocrinol Metab 71:414–424
10. Dralle H, Gimm O (1996) Lymph node excision in thyroid carcinoma. Chirurg 67:788–806
11. Dralle H, Scheumann GF, Meyer HJ, Laubert A, Pichlmayr R (1992) Cervical interventions on the airway and esophagus in infiltrating thyroid cancer. Chirurg 63:282–290
12. Duren M, Siperstein AE, Shen W, Duh QY, Morita E, Clark OH (1999) Value of stimulated serum thyroglobulin levels for detecting persistent or recurrent differentiated thyroid cancer in high- and low-risk patients. Surgery 126:13–19
13. Gillenwater AM, Goepfert H (1999) Surgical management of laryngotracheal and esophageal involvement by locally advanced thyroid cancer. Semin Surg Oncol 16:19–29
14. Gilliland FD, Hunt WC, Morris DM, Key CR (1997) Prognostic factors for thyroid carcinoma. A population-based study of 15,698 cases from the Surveillance, Epidemiology and End Results (SEER) program 1973–1991. Cancer 79:564–573
15. Gimm O, Dralle H (1997) Surgical strategies in papillary thyroid carcinoma. Curr Top Pathol 91:51–64
16. Gimm O, Rath FW, Dralle H (1998) Pattern of lymph node metastases in papillary thyroid carcinoma. Br J Surg 85:252–254
17. Grant CS, Hay ID, Gough IR, Bergstralh EJ, Goellner JR, McConahey WM (1988) Local recurrence in papillary thyroid carcinoma: is extent of surgical resection important? Surgery 104:954–962
18. Harness JK, Thompson NW, McLeod MK, Pasieka JL, Fukuuchi A (1992) Differentiated thyroid carcinoma in children and adolescents. World J Surg 16:547–553; discussion 553–544
19. Hay ID, Bergstralh EJ, Goellner JR, Ebersold JR, Grant CS (1993) Predicting outcome in papillary thyroid carcinoma: development of a reliable prognostic scoring system in a cohort of 1,779 patients surgically treated at one institution during 1940 through 1989. Surgery 114:1050–1057; discussion 1057–1058
20. Hay ID, Grant CS, Taylor WF, McConahey WM (1987) Ipsilateral lobectomy versus bilateral lobar resection in papillary thyroid carcinoma: a retrospective analysis of surgical outcome using a novel prognostic scoring system. Surgery 102:1088–1095
21. Herranz-Gonzalez J, Gavilan J, Matinez-Vidal J, Gavilan C (1991) Complications following thyroid surgery. Arch Otolaryngol Head Neck Surg 117:516–518
22. Hughes CJ, Shaha AR, Shah JP, Loree TR (1996) Impact of lymph node metastasis in differentiated carcinoma of the thyroid: a matched-pair analysis. Head Neck 18:127–132
23. Hundahl SA, Fleming ID, Fremgen AM, Menck HR (1998) A National Cancer Data Base report on 53,856 cases of thyroid carcinoma treated in the US, 1985–1995 (see comments). Cancer 83:2638–2648

24. Kitamura Y, Shimizu K, Nagahama M, Sugino K, Ozaki O, Mimura T, Ito K, Tanaka S (1999) Immediate causes of death in thyroid carcinoma: clinicopathological analysis of 161 fatal cases. J Clin Endocrinol Metab 84:4043–4049
25. Kukkonen ST, Haapiainen RK, Franssila KO, Sivula AH (1990) Papillary thyroid carcinoma: the new, age-related TNM classification system in a retrospective analysis of 199 patients. World J Surg 14:837–841; discussion 841–832
26. Loh KC, Greenspan FS, Gee L, Miller TR, Yeo PP (1997) Pathological tumor-node-metastasis (pTNM) staging for papillary and follicular thyroid carcinomas: a retrospective analysis of 700 patients. J Clin Endocrinol Metab 82:3553–3562
27. Marchesi M, Biffoni M, Biancari F, Nobili-Benedetti R, D'Andrea V, De Antoni E, Campana FP (1998) Insular carcinoma of the thyroid. A report of 8 cases. Chir Ital 50:73–75
28. Mazzaferri EL, Jhiang SM (1994) Long-term impact of initial surgical and medical therapy on papillary and follicular thyroid cancer (see comments; published erratum appears in Am J Med 1995, 98:215). Am J Med 97:418–428
29. McConahey WM, Hay ID, Woolner LB, Heerden JA van, Taylor WF (1986) Papillary thyroid cancer treated at the Mayo Clinic, 1946 through 1970: initial manifestations, pathologic findings, therapy, and outcome. Mayo Clin Proc 61:978–996
30. McLeod MK, Thompson NW (1990) Hurthle cell neoplasms of the thyroid. Otolaryngol Clin North Am 23:441–452
31. Moley JF, Wells SA (1999) Compartment-mediated dissection for papillary thyroid cancer. Langenbecks Arch Surg 384:9–15
32. Nakamura T, Yana I, Kobayashi T, Shin E, Karakawa K, Fujita S, Miya A, Mori T, Nishisho I, Takai S (1992) p53 gene mutations associated with anaplastic transformation of human thyroid carcinomas. Jpn J Cancer Res 83:1293–1298
33. Nilsson O, Lindeberg J, Zedenius J, Ekman E, Tennvall J, Blomgren H, Grimelius L, Lundell G, Wallin G (1998) Anaplastic giant cell carcinoma of the thyroid gland: treatment and survival over a 25-year period. World J Surg 22:725–730
34. Nishida T, Nakao K, Hamaji M, Kamiike W, Kurozumi K, Matsuda H (1997) Preservation of recurrent laryngeal nerve invaded by differentiated thyroid cancer. Ann Surg 226:85–91
35. Ozaki O, Ito K, Mimura T, Sugino K (1999) Anaplastic transformation of papillary thyroid carcinoma in recurrent disease in regional lymph nodes: a histologic and immunohistochemical study. J Surg Oncol 70:45–48
36. Pasieka JL, Zedenius J, Auer G, Grimelius L, Hoog A, Lundell G, Wallin G, Backdahl M (1992) Addition of nuclear DNA content to the AMES risk-group classification for papillary thyroid cancer. Surgery 112:1154–1159; discussion 1159–1160
37. Passler C, Scheuba C, Prager G, Kaserer K, Flores JA, Vierhapper H, Niederle B (1999) Anaplastic (undifferentiated) thyroid carcinoma (ATC). A retrospective analysis. Langenbecks Arch Surg 384:284–293
38. Piromalli D, Martelli G, del Prato I, Collini P, Pilotti S (1992) The role of fine needle aspiration in the diagnosis of thyroid nodules: analysis of 795 consecutive cases. J Surg Oncol 50:247–250
39. Rao RS, Parikh HK, Deshmane VH, Parikh DM, Shrikhande SS, Havaldar R (1996) Prognostic factors in follicular carcinoma of the thyroid: a study of 198 cases (see comments). Head Neck 18:118–124; discussion 124–116
40. Rodriguez JM, Parrilla P, Moreno A, Sola J, Pinero A, Ortiz S, Soria T (1998) Insular carcinoma: an infrequent subtype of thyroid cancer. J Am Coll Surg 187:503–508
41. Rossi RL, Cady B, Silverman ML, Wool MS, Horner TA (1986) Current results of conservative surgery for differentiated thyroid carcinoma. World J Surg 10:612–622
42. Samaan NA, Schultz PN, Hickey RC, Goepfert H, Haynie TP, Johnston DA, Ordonez NG (1992) The results of various modalities of treatment of well differentiated thyroid carcinomas: a retrospective review of 1,599 patients. J Clin Endocrinol Metab 75:714–720
43. Segal K, Arad A, Lubin E, Shpitzer T, Hadar T, Feinmesser R (1994) Follicular carcinoma of the thyroid. Head Neck 16:533–538

44. Skarsgard ED, Connors JM, Robins RE (1991) A current analysis of primary lymphoma of the thyroid. Arch Surg 126: 1199–1203; discussion 1203–1194
45. Sosa JA, Bowman HM, Tielsch JM, Powe NR, Gordon TA, Udelsman R (1998) The importance of surgeon experience for clinical and economic outcomes from thyroidectomy. Ann Surg 228:320–330
46. Tennvall J, Biorklund A, Moller T, Ranstam J, Akerman M (1986) Is the EORTC prognostic index of thyroid cancer valid in differentiated thyroid carcinoma? Retrospective multivariate analysis of differentiated thyroid carcinoma with long follow-up. Cancer 57:1405–1414
47. Tsang RW, Gospodarowicz MK, Sutcliffe SB, Sturgeon JF, Panzarella T, Patterson BJ (1993) Non-Hodgkin's lymphoma of the thyroid gland: prognostic factors and treatment outcome. The Princess Margaret Hospital Lymphoma Group. Int J Radiat Oncol Biol Phys 27:599–604
48. Wang C, Crapo LM (1997) The epidemiology of thyroid disease and implications for screening. Endocrinol Metab Clin North Am 26:189–218
49. Wenig BM, Heffess CS, Adair CF (1997) Atlas of endocrine pathology. Saunders, Philadelphia
50. Wilson DB, Staren ED, Prinz RA (1998) Thyroid reoperations: indications and risks. Am Surg 64:674–678; discussion 678–679
51. Wynford-Thomas D (1997) Origin and progression of thyroid epithelial tumours: cellular and molecular mechanisms. Horm Res 47:145–157

Part II

Differentiated Thyroid Cancer II

Chapter 6

Radioiodine Therapy for Thyroid Cancer 6

M. Dietlein, D. Moka, and H. Schicha

6.1 Introduction

Therapy with radioiodine (^{131}I) has been used for over 50 years in the treatment of patients with papillary and follicular thyroid carcinoma, both to ablate any remaining normal thyroid tissue and to treat the carcinoma. Patients treated with surgery and radioiodine have a survival rate that exceeds the rate for most other cancers. Recurrence rates are high in patients treated by surgery alone. However, no treatment protocols have been evaluated in a randomized controlled manner, nor is a prospective study likely in the near future, since the case rate is low, the presentation too variable, and the necessary observation period too long given the low mortality rate. The improvement of survival rates and decrease in rates of recurrence after radioiodine ablation has been documented by retrospective, long-term studies: Samaan et al. [72] followed 1,599 patients with well-differentiated thyroid carcinoma for up to 43 years. Treatment with radioiodine was the single most powerful prognostic indicator for a disease-free interval and increased survival. Those patients categorized as low risk also had significantly lower recurrence and death rates if they received ^{131}I. In the study by Mazzaferri and Jhiang [48], 1,355 patients with papillary and follicular cancer had a median follow-up of 15.7 years; 42% of the patients were followed for 20 years and 14% for 30 years. When patients with stage II or III tumors (WHO classification, Hedinger et al. [29]) were considered, those treated with ^{131}I had lower 30-year recurrence rates (16% compared with 38%) and cancer-specific mortality rates (3% compared with 9%) than those not treated with ^{131}I.

However, management varied widely for the recommendation of radioiodine ablation and for the ablative dose of ^{131}I. Clinical members of the American Thyroid Association were surveyed in regard to their treatment and long-term assessment of differentiated papillary thyroid carcinoma [86]. For a 39-year-old female with a well-encapsulated, 2-cm solitary carcinoma and no history of radiation (index patient), only a small majority of clinicians (61%) would recommend radioiodine administration after surgery. Solomon et al. [86] concluded the need for more formal practice guidelines for patients with thyroid cancer.

6.2 Radioiodine Ablation and Radioiodine Therapy

Radioiodine ablation and therapy is dependent upon uptake of ^{131}I in residual thyroid tissue or metastatic lesions. The beta-particles emitted by ^{131}I penetrate and destroy tissue only within 2 mm, making destruction of large deposits difficult. In addition, the uptake of iodine in malignant thyroidal tissue has been estimated to be 0.04 – 0.6% of the dose/gram of tumor tissue, considerably less than normal thyroid uptake. Therefore, the first step to treat differentiated thyroid cancer is surgery. Near-total or total thyroidectomy improves the ability of ^{131}I to ablate the remaining gland and to concentrate in regional and distant metastases. ^{131}I therapy for thyroid cancer has frequently been divided into radioiodine ablation and radioiodine therapy, the latter term being used to indicate the treatment of residual or recurrent thyroid cancer at the thyroid bed or of metastatic lesions elsewhere [90]. The possible presence of microscopic multifocal thyroid cancer that may be undetected limits the assumption of a disease-free thyroid remnant.

6.2.1 Ablation of Residual Thyroid Tissue

Routine thyroid remnant ablation is widely used and has appeal for several reasons:

1. Thyroid cancer is frequently multifocal, multicentric, and microscopic. Mazzaferri and Jhiang [48] found more than one thyroid tumor in 319 of 1,355 patients (24%). Total thyroidectomy is rarely achievable in practice. Radioiodine may destroy occult microscopic carcinoma within the thyroid remnant because the carcinoma cells receive radiation from ^{131}I taken up by adjacent normal thyroid cells.
2. Residual thyroid tissue may prevent the visualization of distant or local metastatic disease on follow-up ^{131}I scanning. ^{131}I uptake in normal thyroid tissue is far greater than the uptake in thyroid cancer. In the case of large amounts of thyroid tissue, the scan usually shows a starburst effect of high ^{131}I uptake in the remnant that makes visualizing uptake nearby impossible (Fig. 6.1).
3. Residual thyroid tissue may synthesize significant amounts of thyroid hormone, which suppresses thyroid-stimulating hormone (TSH) and further impedes diagnostic imaging. A high level of TSH stimulation (>30 mU/l) is necessary for proper scanning.
4. Follow-up care of patients with thyroid cancer has improved with the utilization of serum thyroglobulin levels. Thyroid ablation allows for greater specificity of testing for serum thyroglobulin by eliminating the endogenous production of thyroglobulin by normal or recovering tissue [54].

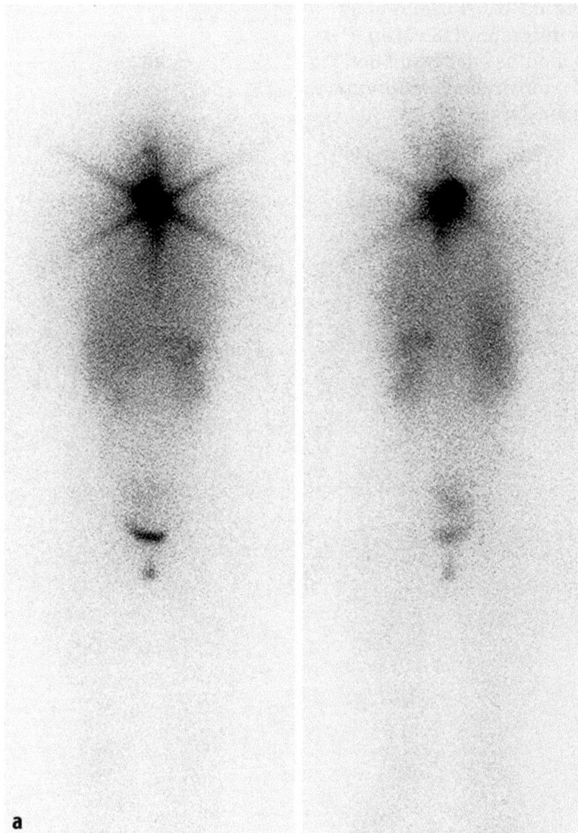

Fig. 6.1 a–d. Twenty-year-old patient with papillary thyroid cancer pT4N1M1 (pulmonary). **a** The first ^{131}I whole-body scintigraphy (1.85 GBq ^{131}I) showed a starburst effect of high uptake in the thyroid remnant. The lung metastases were not visible. **b** ^{123}I whole-body scintigraphy (185 MBq ^{123}I) 3 months later could not demonstrate the pulmonary metastases. **c** Subsequent ^{131}I whole-body scintigraphy (7.4 GBq ^{131}I) and **d** SPECT showed iodine-avid lung metastases

6.2.2
Ablative Dose

An absorbed dose of 300–500 Gy seems to be appropriate with the administered activity calculated as follows:

$$\text{Activity (MBq)} = \frac{\text{Dose (Gy)} \times \text{remnant weight (g) x 24.8}}{\text{Effective T 1/2 (days)} \times {}^{131}\text{I uptake (24 h)}}$$

With two variables that are difficult to measure (weight of thyroid remnants and effective half-life of ^{131}I), this method is neither attractive or suitable for most hospital departments. A fixed activity of ^{131}I is the easier alternative, but what should this activity be?

The answer requires a clear definition as to what constitutes a 'successful ablation.' Chopra et al. [15] showed that visual assessment of ^{131}I scans overestimated thyroid bed uptake in 22% of cases. They argued in favor of quantitation of uptake of an administered activity and recommended that anything below

Fig. 6.1 b. ^{123}I whole-body scintigraphy (185 MBq ^{123}I) 3 months later could not demonstrate the pulmonary metastases

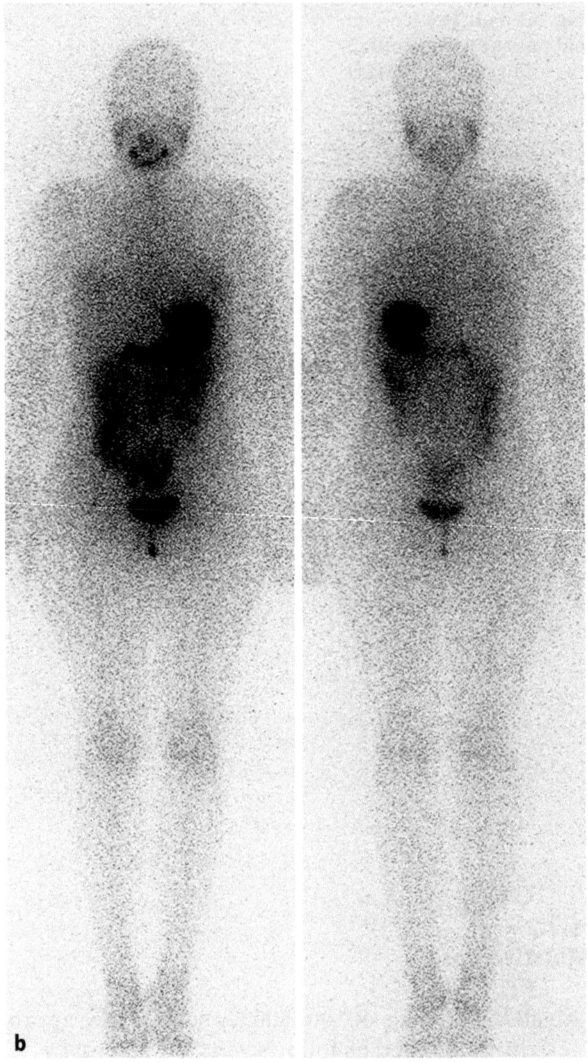

1% was indicative of successful ablation. Application of more stringent criteria for ablation, such as the absence of uptake or uptake less than twice the background, could be the reason for reports of failed ablation [2]. It is essential that the presence of uptake in the postablation scan is not a reliable predictor for future treatment and that time should be allowed for the combined effects of ^{131}I and suppressive thyroxine treatment to exert their effect [65].

Proponents of higher-dose ablations suggest that a 3.7- to 5.5-GBq ablative dose may actually be considered adjuvant radiation therapy for occult metastases not detected by ^{131}I imaging [5, 7]. Administering ^{131}I to small remnants

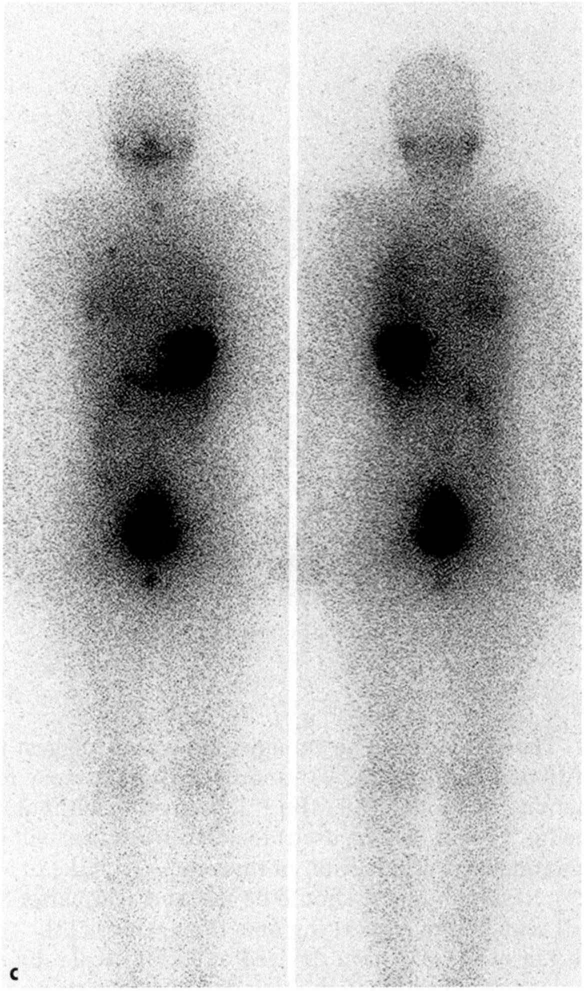

Fig. 6.1 c. Subsequent ^{131}I whole-body scintigraphy (7.4 GBq ^{131}I)

(<5% ^{131}I uptake) can have a tumoricidal rather than an ablative effect by eliminating multiple microscopic foci in 'normal' thyroid tissue that can be alarmingly abundant, thus reducing the possibility of local recurrence.

Comtois et al. [16] compared the efficacy of low (925–1110 MBq), intermediate (≥1,850 MBq) and high activities (≥3.7 GBq) of ^{131}I and observed an ablation rate of 7–83% with a low activity and 60–100% with intermediate or high activities of ^{131}I. Some of the factors that have contributed to the initial high failure rate of low-dose ablation trials can now be identified. Poor success rates were noted following high-dose diagnostic scans using 185 MBq, with higher success rates being achieved after diagnostic scans of 37–74 MBq ^{131}I, indicating a possible stunning effect. Other factors contributing to the poorer success rates were incomplete surgical excision, failure to reduce preablation iodine intake, and very stringent criteria for ablation.

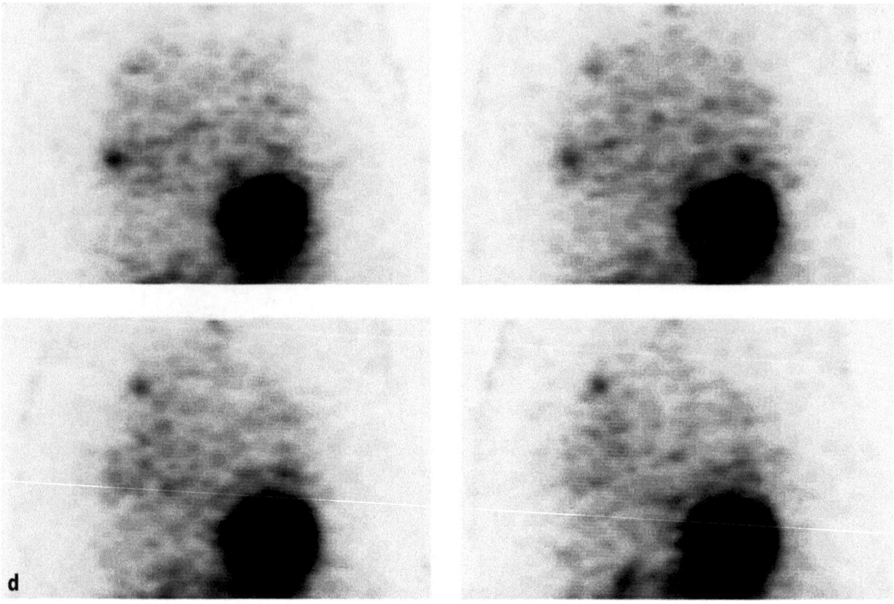

Fig. 6.1 d. SPECT showed iodine-avid lung metastases

There appears to be enough evidence to suggest that, in nonmetastatic well-differentiated thyroid carcinoma, radical surgery followed by an intermediate activity of about 1,850 MBq ^{131}I, preferably without a preceding diagnostic scan using ^{131}I (^{123}I may be used) to avoid stunning, will achieve a reasonable rate of ablation with a reduction in thyroid bed uptake of a tracer ^{131}I dose of less than 1%. Residual uptake should be checked again after 3–6 months with a low-dose ^{131}I scan before embarking on a therapy dose [2].

Lin et al. [35] have devised a 'sliding scale' by which patients with higher uptake receive higher ablation doses. A recommendation of 2–5 GBq ^{131}I for ablation of detectable residual thyroid is given by the German Society of Nuclear Medicine [19].

6.2.3 In Which Patients Is Ablation Unnecessary?

In the study by Mazzaferri and Jhiang [48], low-risk patients, defined as those with tumors smaller than 1.5 cm completely confined to the thyroid, were not found to benefit from thyroid ablation. In contrast, Samaan et al. [72] examined the use of radioactive iodine in 1,156 low-risk patients and found beneficial effects in low-risk patients, with significantly fewer recurrences and deaths. They recommended radioactive iodine therapy for all patients who have a positive scan after surgery.

Regarding the biological behavior of the papillary microcarcinomas and the frequency in autopsy studies, most authors do not generally recommend radioiodine administration for patients with solitary papillary microcarcinoma, diameter up to 1.0 cm, a subgroup of the pT1NOMO stage [18, 74, 94]. If a patient with papillary microcarcinoma wishes to undergo this therapy, radioiodine ablation can be selectively performed.

6.2.4 Radioiodine Therapy for Thyroid Cancer

For those patients with proven or assumed residual or recurrent thyroid cancer, the term 'radioiodine therapy' is usually used.

However, there are differing theories regarding the activity of ^{131}I needed for proper therapy. Of the dosimetry methods available, the most widely used and simplest is to administer a large fixed dose. Most clinics use this method regardless of the percentage uptake of ^{131}I in the remnant or metastatic lesion. Patients with distant metastases are treated with 3.7 – 11 GBq ^{131}I. There is no convincing evidence that treatment is improved by quantitative methods of measurement of retention, uptake, and effective half-times necessary for dosimetric studies [24].

A second approach is to use quantitative dosimetry methods. If the calculated dose to be delivered is less than 35 Gy, it is unlikely that the cancer will respond to ^{131}I therapy. These patients should be considered for surgery, external radiation, or medical therapy. Doses that deliver more than 85 Gy to metastatic foci are likely to be effective [45].

A third approach is to administer a dose calculated to deliver a maximum of 2 Gy to the bone marrow, keeping the whole-body retention less than 4.5 GBq at 48 h and the amount in the lungs less than 3 GBq when there is diffuse pulmonary uptake. The maximum dose is kept at 11 GBq ^{131}I [47].

6.2.5 Radioiodine Therapy with Negative Radioiodine Scan

A distinct group of patients who warrant special consideration are those with differentiated thyroid cancer with positive or rising serum thyroglobulin levels and negative radioiodine scans. Although definitions vary, a positive thyroglobulin level means a value greater than 2 ng/ml in a patient who has undergone total thyroidectomy and ^{131}I ablation. This special case of elevated serum thyroglobulin levels and absent radioactive iodine uptake poses a clinical dilemma. The following explanations should be considered:

- Diffuse metastases that are too small for detection
- Thyroid cancer that produces thyroglobulin but does not take up enough iodine for detection
- High levels of 'cold' iodine blocking the uptake of radioiodine
- Normal thyroid tissue that hinders the imaging of metastatic disease
- A falsely positive elevation of thyroglobulin level

Table 6.1. Studies reporting documented disease in thyroglobulin-positive patients with negative radioiodine scans (from Sweeney and Johnston [90])

Study	No. of patients	Elevated thyroglobulin levels	Negative diagnostic ^{131}I scan	Evidence of disease
Pacini et al. [58]	17	17/17 (15–976 ng/ml)	17/17 (185 MBq ^{131}I)	16/17 had positive post-therapy scan
Robbins [67]	10	10/10 (>10 ng/ml)	10/10 (370 MBq ^{131}I)	9/10 had positive post-therapy scan
Pineda et al. [63]	17	17/17 (8–480 ng/ml)	17/17 (55–185 MBq ^{131}I)	16/17 had positive post-therapy scan 13/16 had decreased thyroglobulin levels post ^{131}I
Ronga et al. [69]	10	10/10	10/10	7/10 had positive post-therapy scan
Schlumberger et al. [79]	25	25/25	25/25 (74–185 MBq ^{131}I)	18/25 had positive post-therapy scan
Total	79	79/79	79/79	66/79 had positive post-therapy scan

Table 6.1 lists reports of thyroglobulin-positive patients with negative diagnostic scans who had documented metastatic or persistent thyroid cancer. These results highlight the failure of small diagnostic doses of ^{131}I to visualize recurrent or metastatic disease. Therapeutic doses of ^{131}I may be warranted in thyroglobulin-positive patients with negative radioiodine diagnostic imaging. The decrease in thyroglobulin-levels after the administration of 3.7 GBq ^{131}I despite the absence of clear ^{131}I uptake [63] suggested a possible benefit of such an ^{131}I dose. Furthermore, these patients should have urinary iodine measured to ensure that the values are less than 200 µg/day per gram creatinine, thus excluding artifactual suppression of ^{131}I uptake.

6.2.6 Radioiodine Therapy in Patients on Maintenance Hemodialysis

The behavior of radioiodine in hemodialyzed patients with thyroid carcinoma was described by Daumerie et al. [17]. Over six treatments, blood activity decreased with a half-life of 3.4±0.5 h (1 SD) during hemodialysis. Taking the physical half-life of 8.06 days between dialyses and carrying out the first dialysis 24 h after radioiodine administration, the total body irradiation was 3.9 times greater in hemodialyzed patients than in nondialysis subjects. Daumerie et al. [17] recommended delivering 25% of the currently prescribed activity and performing the first dialysis session after 24 h to reduce total body irradiation.

6.3 Prognostic Factors and Therapeutic Strategies in Metastatic Thyroid Cancer

The study by Schlumberger et al. [77] highlighted the prognostic significance of the early discovery of distant metastases by the combined use of thyroglobulin-measurement and ^{131}I whole-body scanning. Of 394 patients with lung and/or bone metastases, two-thirds of the patients had ^{131}I uptake in their metastases, but only 46% achieved a complete response. Prognostic factors for complete response were: younger age, presence of ^{131}I uptake in the metastases and small extent of disease. Patients who achieved a complete response following treatment of distant metastases had a 15-year survival rate of 89%, while those who did not achieve complete response had a survival rate of only 8%.

6.3.1 Lymph Node Metastases

At the time of initial therapy, cervical or mediastinal lymph node metastases were found in 32% of 535 patients [28] and in 42% of 1355 patients [48] with papillary and follicular cancer. Radioiodine therapy reduced both the recurrence rate and death rate in these patients [7, 48]. Because ^{131}I uptake may vary from one tumor deposit to another, the complete dissection of involved lymph node areas is highly recommended. When surgery is performed, a complete dissection of the affected lymph node area is preferred to lymph node sampling.

Travagli et al. [91] described the combination of radioiodine and probe-guided surgery for the treatment of patients with functioning lymph node metastases. Fifty-four patients had already undergone total thyroidectomy (51 patients) or lobectomy with isthmusectomy (3 patients), with lymph node dissection in 33 patients. Surgical excision of neoplastic foci might have been difficult in these patients and was facilitated by accurate localization on the preoperative ^{131}I scan and the use of an intraoperative probe. The following protocol was used at the Institute Gustave Roussy:

Day 0: Administration of 3.7 GBq ^{131}I
Day 4: Whole-body scan
Day 5: Surgery using an intraoperative probe
Day 7: Control whole-body scan

The probe made a major contribution to the operative procedure in 86% of patients (in 22% for unusual sites, in 20% for neoplastic foci embedded in sclerosis, and in 44% for easy localization of neoplastic foci). Finally, it confirmed the completeness of surgical excision. Further studies are required for a more general recommendation.

6.3.2 Pulmonary Metastases

In the study by Schlumberger et al. [79], the four independent variables that adversely affected survival were extensive metastases, older age at discovery of the metastases, absence of ^{131}I uptake, and moderately differentiated follicular cell type. Nemec et al. [55] achieved a 10-year survival rate of 80% in young patients with papillary carcinoma whose chest X-rays showed fine pulmonary metastases. The best prognosis is with lung metastases seen only on ^{131}I imaging and not by X-ray or computed tomography (Table 6.2). Schlumberger et al. [75] observed 23 patients treated with ^{131}I for diffuse pulmonary metastases detected only by ^{131}I imaging, and 87% of these patients had no lung uptake on subsequent scans and thyroglobulin became undetectable (Fig. 6.2).

In contrast, the experience of Sisson et al. [84] with patients manifesting pulmonary micronodular lung metastases demonstrated that radioiodine therapy uncommonly produced complete remissions. The authors asked whether the tumors might be too small for effective irradiation from radioiodine. Less than 40% of the beta and electron emission energy is deposited within a spherical

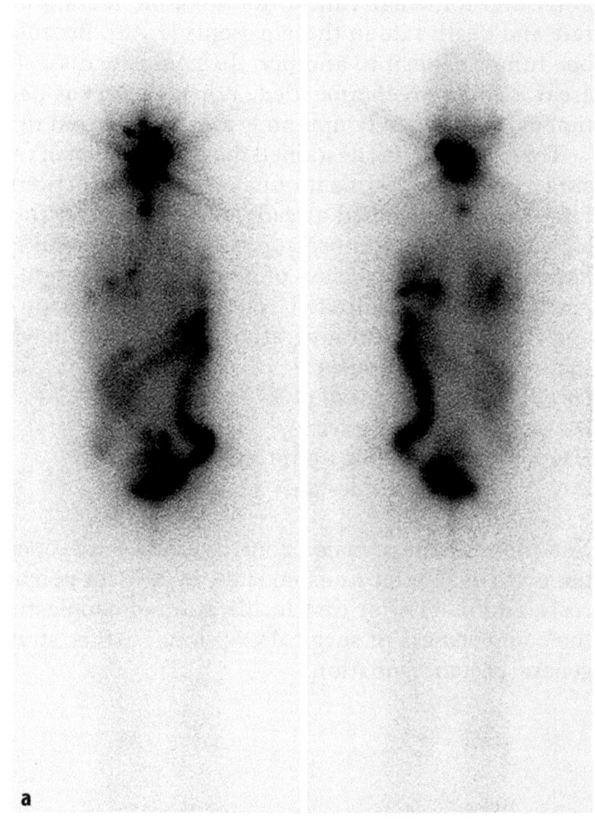

Fig. 6.2 a, b. Thirty-seven-year-old patient with papillary thyroid cancer pT2N1aM1 (pulmonary). **a** The first ^{131}I whole-body scintigraphy (3.7 GBq ^{131}I) showed lung metastases that concentrated radioiodine.

Table 6.2. Survival rates for patients with thyroid cancer with pulmonary and/or bone metastases

Study	No. of patients	1-year survival (%)	5-year survival (%)	10-year survival (%)	Remission (%)
Lung metastases					
Brown et al. [10]	20	–	63	54	–
Massin et al. [42]	58	68	44	28 (8 years)	–
Casara et al. [12]					
Normal X-rays, ^{131}I positive	42	100	100	95	–
Visible on X-rays, ^{131}I positive	54	92	59	40	–
Visible on X-rays, ^{131}I negative	38	90	18	8	–
Schlumberger et al. [79]					
Normal X-rays	73	–	–	91	83
Micronodules	64	–	–	63	53
Macronodules	77	–	–	11	14

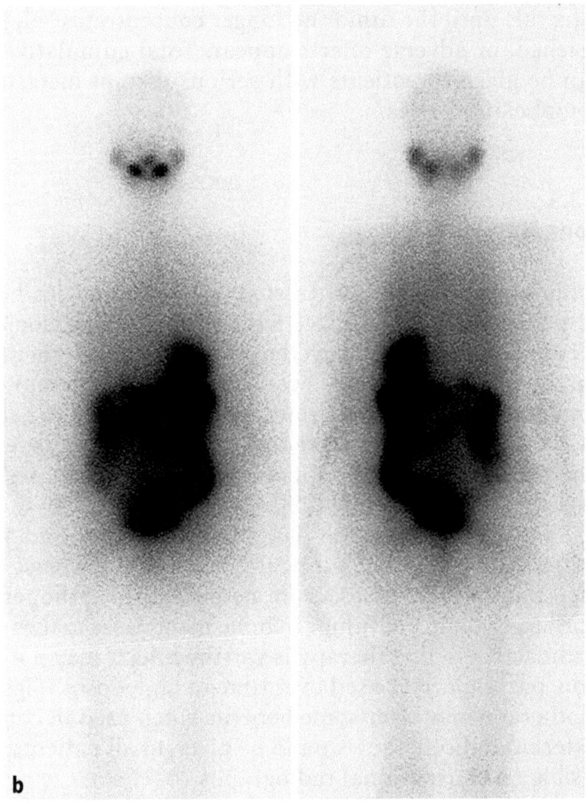

Fig. 6.2 b. The second ^{131}I whole-body scintigraphy (7.4 GBq ^{131}I) demonstrated complete remission 3 months later

Table 6.2. *Continued.*

Study	No. of patients	1-year survival (%)	5-year survival (%)	10-year survival (%)	Remission (%)
Bone metastases					
Brown et al. [10]	21	–	7	0	–
Schlumberger et al. [79]					
Single	37	–	–	total 21	22
Multiple	71	–	–		3
Lung and bone metastases					
Schlumberger et al. [79]	72	–	–	13	7

target with a diameter of 0.5 mm and much less if the target is smaller. Sisson et al. [84] did not mean that treatments with ^{131}I were not useful because the measured tumor volumes might have underestimated the total tumor volumes and the actual absorbed dose of ^{131}I might be higher than the calculated dose.

Mazzaferri [47] recommended a dose of 7.4 GBq ^{131}I when the metastases concentrate ^{131}I. Scanning and treatment with ^{131}I are repeated at 6- to 12-month intervals until the tumor no longer concentrates ^{131}I, large cumulative doses are reached, or adverse effects appear. Total cumulative doses of 37 GBq or more can be given to patients with serious distant metastases, but the frequency of complications rises.

6.3.3 Bone Metastases

Schlumberger et al. [79] treated 142 patients with bone metastases. A total of 92 patients had radioactive iodine therapy in association with external radiotherapy, 18 patients received only external radiotherapy, 45 patients underwent surgery, and 35 patients were given chemotherapy. Fourteen patients had a complete response to therapy, and each of the 14 had been treated with ^{131}I in association with external radiotherapy. No patients responded to chemotherapy. The poor prognosis of patients with bone metastases is linked to the bulkiness of the lesions (Table 6.2) [75].

Sweeney and Johnston [90], Mazzaferri [47], and Schlumberger [75] gave the recommendation that surgical resection to decrease the bulk of disease, to resect solitary metastases, or for neurologic or orthopedic palliation is important. The large volume of tumor in bone metastases makes ^{131}I therapy alone difficult. Radioactive iodine therapy is worthwhile; it may not cure but does offer palliation, particularly if used over time in high doses (Figs. 6.3 and 6.4). External radiotherapy may offer some benefits when used in conjunction with ^{131}I therapy. External radiotherapy should be given to all patients who have bone metastases visible on conventional radiographs.

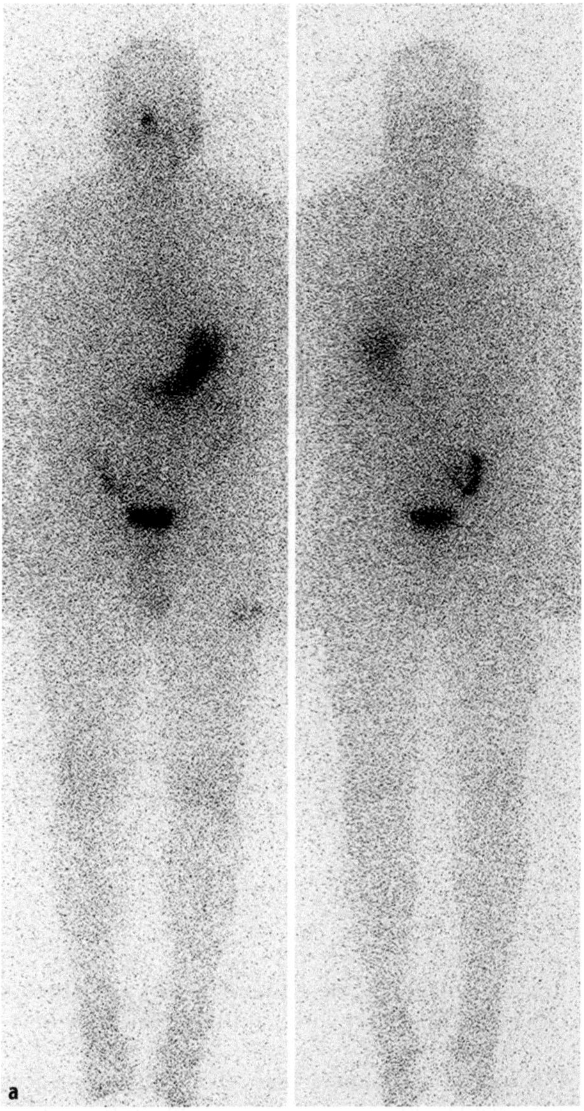

Fig. 6.3 a, b. Sixty-two-year-old patient with follicular thyroid cancer pT2N0M1 (right os ilium). The first radioiodine therapy (3.7 GBq ^{131}I) and subtotal resection of the osseous metastasis had already been performed. **a** ^{123}I whole-body scintigraphy (185 MBq ^{123}I) 3 months later, and **b** ^{131}I whole-body scintigraphy (7.4 GBq ^{131}I) demonstrated the osseous metastasis in the right pelvis and thyroid remnant on the right side. Misinterpretation as residual activity in the large bowel must be avoided. Subsequently, the patient underwent external radiation therapy

Fig. 6.3 b. ^{131}I whole-body scintigraphy (7.4 GBq ^{131}I) demonstrated the osseous metastasis in the right pelvis and thyroid remnant on the right side. Misinterpretation as residual activity in the large bowel must be avoided. Subsequently, the patient underwent external radiation therapy

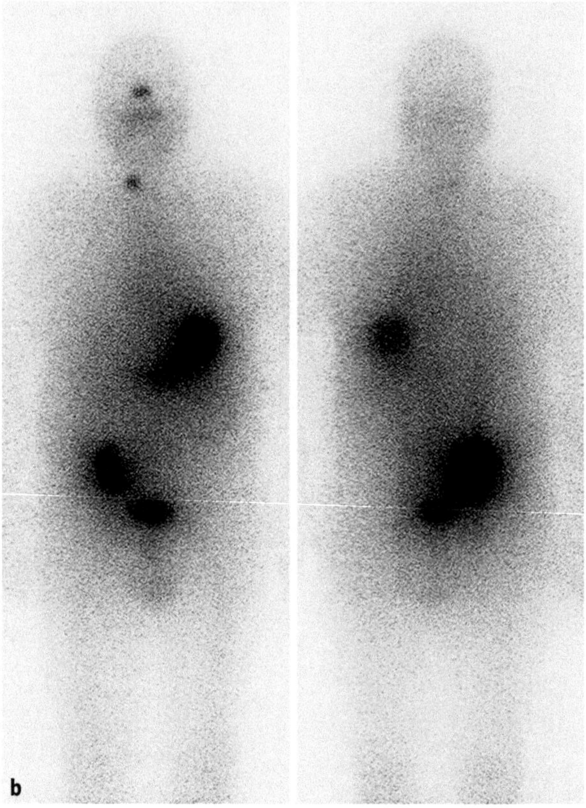

6.3.4 Brain Metastases

Brain metastases are rare in thyroid cancer and were found in 1 of 325 patients by Maheshwari et al. [40] and in 2 of 571 patients with papillary cancer by Mazzaferri and Young [50].

Chiu et al. [14] analyzed 47 cases of brain metastases from thyroid cancer seen at one institution over five decades. Brain metastases from thyroid carcinoma are a poor prognostic sign. Although selection bias and other unidentified factors inherent to retrospective analysis limit their conclusion, surgical resection of brain metastases may be associated with prolonged survival. However, no evidence of survival benefit was found from radioiodine therapy, external beam radiotherapy, or chemotherapy.

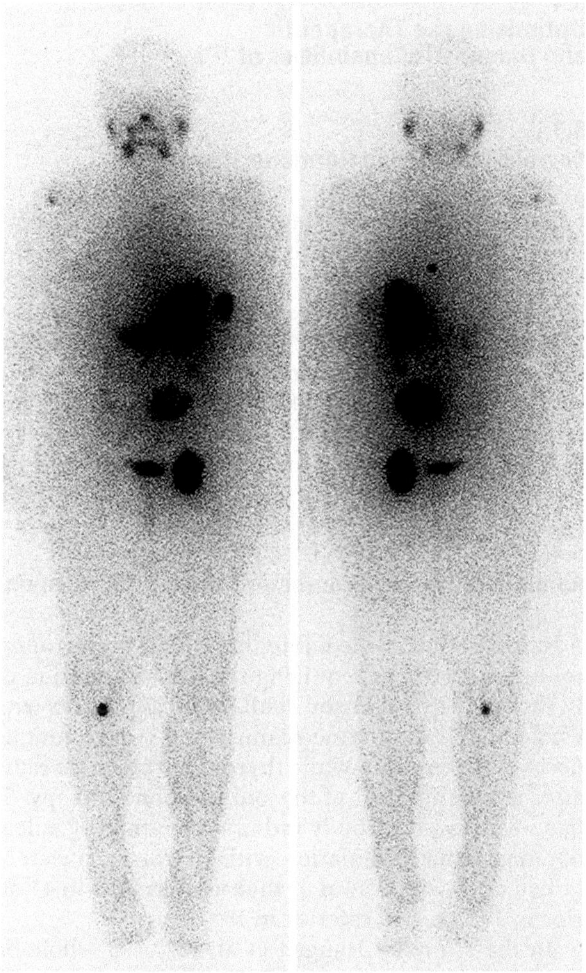

Fig. 6.4. Seventy-four-year-old patient with follicular thyroid cancer pT2N0M1 (os sacrum, left acetabulum, thoracic spine, right humerus, right tibia, left adrenal gland). ^{123}I whole-body scintigraphy demonstrated iodine avid metastasis following two radioiodine therapies (14.8 GBq ^{131}I)

6.3.5 Locally Invasive Thyroid Cancer

Locally invasive, surgically unresectable thyroid cancer is associated with a high cancer mortality and recurrence rate. Radioiodine is useful in these patients if uptake is proven. Some investigators report the use of radiosensitizers such as adriamycin, along with ^{131}I to increase the tumoricidal effect [67], but this approach has not yet been incorporated into clinical practice.

Adjuvant external radiotherapy improves the recurrence-free survival in patients older than 40 years with invasive papillary thyroid cancer pT4 and lymph node involvement [21]. Further details are included in Chap. 7.

6.4 Optimizing the Therapeutic and Diagnostic Capabilities of ^{131}I

6.4.1 Thyroid-Stimulating Hormone Stimulation

Following total or near-total thyroidectomy, TSH elevation reaches a maximum in 3–5 weeks. However, in patients with a large thyroid remnant, elevation of TSH may occur slowly or minimally. In the follow-up care, patients are maintained on suppressive doses of thyroid hormone. Before whole-body imaging or ^{131}I therapy, levothyroxine replacement must be discontinued for approximately 4–5 weeks. Short-term administration of triiodothyronine (40–60 μg) alleviates some of the symptoms of prolonged hypothyroidism and must be stopped 2 weeks before radioiodine administration. There is no significant evidence that rapid tumor growth is stimulated by a brief rise in TSH concentration [47].

6.4.2 Administration of Recombinant Human Thyrotropin

Administration of recombinant human thyrotropin (Thyrogen) stimulates thyroid tissue without requiring the discontinuation of thyroid hormone therapy. In the study by Ladenson et al. [34], 127 patients with thyroid cancer underwent whole-body radioiodine scanning by two techniques: first after receiving two doses of thyrotropin while thyroid hormone therapy was continued, and second after the withdrawal of thyroid hormone therapy. Sixty-two of the 127 patients had positive whole-body radioiodine scans by at least one technique. The scans obtained after stimulation with thyrotropin were equivalent to the scans obtained after withdrawal of thyroid hormone in 41 of these patients (66%), superior in 3 (5%), and inferior in 18 (29%).

In the study by Haugen et al. [27], ^{131}I whole-body scans were concordant between the recombinant TSH-stimulated and thyroid hormone withdrawal phases in 195 of 220 (89%) patients. Of the discordant scans, 8 (4%) had superior scans after recombinant human TSH administration, and 17 (8%) had superior scans after thyroid hormone withdrawal.

The use of Thyrogen allows for radioiodine imaging while the patients are euthyroid on triiodothyronine and/or thyroxine. Data on ^{131}I kinetics indicate that the clearance of radioiodine is approximately 50% greater in euthyroid patients than in hypothyroid patients, who have decreased renal function. Thus, radioiodine retention is less in euthyroid patients at the time of imaging, and this factor should be considered when selecting the activity of radioiodine for use in radioiodine imaging.

Thyrotropin also stimulates the production of thyroglobulin, which may increase the usefulness of this tumor marker in patients treated with thyroid hormone who have had thyroid tissue ablated. Based on a serum Tg level of 2 ng/ml or more in the study by Haugen et al. [27], thyroid tissue or cancer was detected during thyroid hormone therapy in 22%, after recombinant human TSH stimulation in 52%, and after thyroid hormone withdrawal in 56% of patients with disease or tissue limited to the thyroid bed and in 80%, 100%, and 100% of patients, respectively, with metastatic disease.

The use of recombinant human TSH is recommended in patients who have no evidence of recurrent or metastatic thyroid cancer and whose serum thyroglobulin is undetectable during thyroid hormone suppression of TSH [49, 76]. Special indications for Thyrogen testing concern patients who are unable to mount an adequate endogenous TSH response to thyroid hormone withdrawal or in whom withdrawal is medically contraindicated due to comorbidity (e.g., severe cardiovascular or pulmonary diseases, diabetes mellitus, psychotic disorders).

Dosage and administration: Thyrogen 0.9 mg intramuscularly may be administered every 24 h in two doses. For radioiodine imaging, radioiodine administration should be given 24 h following the final Thyrogen injection. Scanning should be performed 48 h after radioiodine administration. For serum thyroglobulin testing, the serum sample should be obtained 72 h after the final injection of Thyrogen.

Recombinant human TSH is also allowed as a preparation for radioiodine thyroid-remnant ablation under thyroid hormone replacement. Robbins et al. [68] retrospectively have reviewed the rate of complete remnant ablation in patients having radioiodine ablation after hormone withdrawal (n = 42 patients, ^{131}I ablation activity 4.77 ± 2.74 GBq) compared with those having radioiodine ablation after recombinant human TSH (n = 45 patients, ^{131}I ablation activity 4.07 ± 2.41 GBq). A successful ablation was defined as no visible radioiodine uptake on the follow-up diagnostic scans, performed with 185 MBq ^{131}I. Robbins et al. [68] have found that 84% of those prepared by recombinant human TSH and 81% of those prepared by hormone withdrawal have complete resolution of visible thyroid bed uptake after radioiodine ablation. The likelihood of a complete ablation appears to be similar for these two methods of preparation. Pacini et al. [59] have used, for postsurgical ablation of thyroid remnants, a 1.1-GBq (30 mCi) standard dose of ^{131}I and prospectively compared three treatment arms: in the first arm, patients (n = 50) were treated while hypothyroid; in the second arm, patients (n = 42) were treated while hypothyroid and stimulated in addition with rh TSH; in the third arm, patients (n = 70) were treated while euthyroid on thyroid hormone therapy and stimulated with rh TSH. The outcome of thyroid ablation was assessed by conventional ^{131}I scan performed in the hypothyroid state 6–10 months after ablation. The rate of successful ablation was similar in the hypothyroid and hypothyroid + rh TSH groups (84% and 78.5%, respectively). A significantly lower rate of ablation (54%) was achieved in the euthyroid + rh TSH group. The mean radiation dose delivered during the 1st h of treatment was significantly lower in the euthyroid + rh TSH group (10.7 ± 12.6 Gy/h) compared with the hypothyroid + rh TSH group (48.5 ± 43 Gy/h) and the hypothyroid group (27.1 ± 42.5 Gy/h). The study of Pacini et al. [59] indicates that by using stimulation with rh TSH, a 1.1-GBq (30 mCi) standard dose of radioiodine is not sufficient for a satisfactory thyroid ablation rate. Possible reasons for this failure rate may be the low 24-h radioiodine uptake, the low initial dose rate delivered to the residues, and the accelerated iodine clearance observed in euthyroid patients. Possible alternatives for obtaining a satisfactory rate of thyroid ablation with rh TSH may consist of increasing the dose of radioiodine or using different protocols of rh TSH administration, producing more prolonged stimulation of the thyroid cells.

The clinical use of recombinant human TSH in patients with advanced metastases of thyroid cancer has been described by several centers [6,30,32,36,39,53,62]. The observation studies provide preliminary evidence that rh TSH safely aids radioiodine treatment of advanced differentiated thyroid cancer. The use of rh TSH may reduce the effective half-life of ^{131}I, mainly due to a reduced renal iodine clearance in the hypothyroid state [53]. The therapeutic consequences of this changed bioavailability of ^{131}I is an open point of discussion. As prospectively controlled clinical trials have not been carried out, Thyrogen is not yet recommended as the therapeutic standard for the purpose of radioiodine therapy of metastatic thyroid cancer. Rh TSH is suitable in advanced recurrent or metastatic thyroid cancer patient who may be intolerant to TSH stimulation by levothyroxine withdrawal or who suffer from severe comorbidity.

6.4.3 Low-Iodine Diet

The total body iodine pool should be as low as possible. A low daily intake of iodine (approximately 50 μg) can increase the ^{131}I uptake and can double the thyroid dose in Gy per each 3.7 GBq of ^{131}I administered [41, 43]. A daily iodine intake of 50 μg can be achieved by restricting the use of iodized salt, dairy products, eggs, and seafood (Table 6.3). It appears to be practical to limit the time patients spend on the diet to approximately 2 weeks prior to therapy. Iodine excretion in the urine should be measured in doubtful cases.

Table 6.3. Instructions for low-iodine diet

Avoid the following foods for 1–2 weeks
Iodized salt, sea salt
Milk or other dairy products (e.g., cheese, chocolate, ice cream, yogurt)
Eggs
Seafood (e.g., fish, kelp)
Foods that contain the additives carrageenan, algin, alginate, agar-agar
Cured and corned foods (e.g., ham, lox, corned beef, sauerkraut)
Breads made with iodate dough conditioners
Foods and medications containing red food dyes (found in cereals, candies, and vitamins)
Soy products (e.g., soy sauce, soy milk)
Additional guidelines
Avoid restaurant foods and 'fast' food
Foods that contain small amounts of milk or eggs may be used
Consult doctor before discontinuing any red-colored medication

Exogenous stimulation using recombinant human TSH (rh TSH) enables the continuous substitution of levothyroxine, which contains 65.4% of its molecular weight in iodine. Thus, a substantial source of iodine intake is maintained during exogenous stimulation. Although this amount of stable iodine is comparable with the iodine intake in regions of normal iodine supply, it may reduce the accumulation of radioiodine in thyroid carcinoma tissue [37]. Park and Hennessey [61] compared a 7-day and a 14-day low-iodine diet for outpatient preparation for radioiodine rh TSH scanning in patients taking levothyroxine. Measuring urine iodine to creatinine ratios (I/Cr), the 2 weeks of preparation resulted in 71% of patients having a urinary iodine-to-creatinine ratio in the adequate range (<100 μg I/g Cr) versus 41% after 1 week. The authors [61] suggest that rh TSH protocols for monitoring residual thyroid tissue or recurrent thyroid carcinoma may have an improved efficacy if patients are prepared with a low-iodine diet. This study also supports the necessity of a 2-week diet preparation for adequate reduction in total body iodine.

6.4.4 Optimal Diagnostic Scan Dose

The studies of Jeevanram et al. [31] and Park et al. [60] suggested that a 'non-cancericidal' dose of ^{131}I may impair the ability of thyroid tumors to concentrate subsequent therapeutic doses, a phenomenon later termed 'stunning.' The optimum dose of ^{131}I for diagnostic scanning allows visualization of the thyroid remnant and all local and distant metastases without causing a sublethal radiation stunning of the thyroid tissue.

Arnstein et al. [3] performed a series of phantom studies to evaluate the ^{131}I dose that would be sufficient to detect metastatic deposits. Detectability depends on lesion volume and depth, the radioiodine uptake, background activity, and imaging equipment. With assumptions made for these variables, they found that 10- and 30-μl lesions (lesion volumes assumed to represent treatable tumor) with uptakes of 0.05% or more of ^{131}I/g of tissue would only be detected by a 74-MBq diagnostic dose if the lesion was at the surface and in the absence of background activity. Investigating this troubling hypothesis even further, they concluded that some potentially treatable lesions probably cannot be detected even with a diagnostic dose of 1.1 GBq ^{131}I.

Park et al. [60] published retrospective data comparing pretherapy and post-therapy scans done with ^{123}I and ^{131}I. Twenty-six patients were included in the ^{131}I diagnostic scan group (receiving 110–370 MBq ^{131}I) and 14 patients underwent ^{123}I diagnostic scanning. Subsequently, ^{131}I therapy was given to all of these patients. Uptake was compared by visual inspection on a posttherapy scan performed approximately 48 h after the large dose of ^{131}I was given. The uptake of the therapeutic dose was found to be impaired (defined as a qualitative visual decrease in lesion) in 20 of 26 patients in the ^{131}I diagnostic dose group and in none of the 14 patients previously scanned with ^{123}I. It was suggested that ^{123}I may be a better diagnostic agent for use before ^{131}I therapy.

McDougall [51] compared 147 scintiscans, completed 48–72 h after 74 MBq ^{131}I, with scintiscans done on average 7.8 days after therapeutic doses of ^{131}I. The therapeutic doses ranged from 1,100 to 7,400 MBq ^{131}I. The posttreatment scans showed less uptake in one region in 2 of the 147 patients (1.4%), and showed more lesions in 12 patients (8%). McDougall [51] concluded that 74 MBq ^{131}I seldom interferes with subsequent therapy and does not cause stunning.

Based on the important goals of optimal imaging of treatable lesions and subsequent maximum therapeutic dosing, doses of 100–400 MBq ^{131}I should be used for diagnostic scanning, with the higher range preferred when therapeutic dosing is not likely (e.g., for scans used in yearly posttherapy follow-up). Prompt therapeutic dosing following diagnostic scanning is important. The radiation effect of the diagnostic dose on thyroid uptake and function takes place over time, and prompt therapeutic dosing will allow little time for the physiological effects of early radiation damage. Practically, this means that ^{131}I therapy should be administered within 1 day after diagnostic scanning. Low-dose scans may be adequate for therapeutic decision-making but are not sensitive enough for imaging to determine the extent of disease.

6.4.5 Redifferentiation Therapy and Future Therapeutic Options

Retinoic acid [8, 22, 23, 82, 83] or chemotherapy [53, 67] should be considered in patients with radioiodine-negative metastases for tumor redifferentiation in preparation for radioiodine therapy. A decrease in thyroglobulin level and an increase in radioiodine uptake has been found in up to one-third of the study groups of Grünwald et al. [23], Börner et al. [8], and Simon et al. [83]. But the results from other clinical observations are inconsistent [22], and the general use of isotretinoin in all patients with otherwise untreatable thyroid cancer cannot be recommended [18]. Haugen et al. [26] have investigated the mRNA expression of the six retinoic acid receptor and retinoid X-receptor isoforms (RARα, -β, -γ and RXRα, -β, -γ) in human thyroid cell lines. The RARβ and RXRγ isoforms seem to predict response to retinoid therapy in thyroid cancer cell lines. These experimental data offer a future perspective on a more selective use of retinoid therapy in patients in whom retinoid therapy may be beneficial. For widely metastatic disease, high-dose adriamycin therapy provides a 30–40% partial response of disease, but long-term cures are rare. Octreotide and tamoxifen therapies are currently being studied as future therapeutic possibilities, but these agents are still experimental [25]. Further details are included in Chap 10.

6.4.6 Lithium

This drug enhances tumor ^{131}I retention by reducing release of iodine from normal thyroid and tumor tissue [64]. In a dosage of 400–800 mg daily (10 mg/kg) for 7 days, lithium increases ^{131}I uptake in metastatic lesions while only slightly increasing ^{131}I uptake in normal tissue. Serum lithium concentrations should be measured frequently and maintained between 0.8 and 1.2 mmol/l. Radiation of tumors in which the biological half-life of iodine is short can be enhanced by lithium without increasing radiation to other organs. Mazzaferri [47] recommended using lithium in this setting generally, but larger groups of patients were not studied. Thus, the clinical benefit was not clearly documented in the radioiodine therapy for thyroid cancer.

6.4.7 Further Optimization of ^{131}I Imaging

Decreasing background activity may be important for visualizing small metastases, and delaying the imaging beyond 72 h is necessary. Constipation should be treated with cathartics. The efficiency of a system for imaging ^{131}I is dependent on the collimator and the thickness of the crystal. A gamma camera equipped with a high-energy collimator and a thick crystal is most important:

- Whole-body images should be acquired for a minimum of 30 min and/or should contain a minimum of 140,000 counts.
- Scanning times for single (spot) images of body regions should be 10–15 min or less if the minimum number of counts is reached sooner (e.g., 60,000 counts for a camera with a large field of view, 35,000 counts for a small field of view).

The diagnostic ^{131}I scan is most sensitive and specific for treatable metastases. Although the specificity of ^{131}I imaging is approximately 99%, false-positive scans may result from body secretions, pathological transudates and inflammation, non-specific mediastinal uptake, or tumors of nonthyroidal origin. Misleading scans can be caused by physiological secretion of ^{131}I from the nasopharynx, salivary and sweat glands, and stomach, from genitourinary excretion or spilling, and from skin contamination with sputum. Pathological pulmonary transudates and inflammation due to cyst and lung lesions caused by fungal and other inflammatory disease may produce false-positive scans.

Given a therapeutic ^{131}I dose, an additional posttreatment scan should always be performed. About 25% of these post-treatment scans show lesions not detected by the diagnostic scan done before therapy, which may or may not be clinically important. Posttreatment ^{131}I scans are especially likely to yield the most information when diagnostic scans are negative and serum thyroglobulin concentrations are elevated.

6.4.8 Diuretic-Enhanced ^{131}I Clearance

Because renal excretion of ^{131}I may be reduced in patients with hypothyroidism, diuretic-enhanced ^{131}I renal clearance offers a potential method for decreasing whole-body radiation burden. In the study by Seabold et al. [81], the enhanced clearance appeared primarily due to the effect of furosemide and not to a water diuresis. Oral hydration alone did not substantially alter the mean posttreatment ^{131}I clearance from the mean pretreatment clearance in the patients who did not receive diuretics.

6.5 Side Effects of ^{131}I Therapy

6.5.1 Radiation Thyroiditis

Radiation thyroiditis occurs in about 20% of patients, most often in patients with large thyroid remnants given doses of ^{131}I that deliver about 500 Gy. It usually appears 2–4 days after ^{131}I administration and is characterized by neck and ear pain, painful swallowing, and thyroid swelling and tenderness. Patients with mild pain can be treated with salicylate or diclofenac, but those with severe pain or swelling should receive corticosteroid therapy; for example, prednisone 30 mg daily for several days.

6.5.2 Painless Neck Edema

Painless neck edema within 48 h after ^{131}I administration is a much less common problem than radiation thyroiditis. It responds to corticosteroid therapy.

6.5.3 Sialadenitis

Pain, tenderness, and dysfunction of the salivary glands is a well-recognized early complication of ^{131}I therapy. Acute and chronic sialadenitis occurred in 12% of patients in the prospective study by Allweiss et al. [1]. Symptoms included dry mouth, bitter taste, recurrent salivary tenderness, and swelling. Onset of symptoms occurred at a median of 6 days after therapy and lasted a median of 2 years.

Radiation sialadenitis appears to occur secondary to direct radiation injury to the glands. Salivary glands concentrate iodide, resulting in high iodide concentration in saliva 30–40 times higher than in plasma. Salivary gland scintigraphy with pertechnetate has been used to quantify the damage done to the salivary glands by ^{131}I therapy. A dose-dependent reduction in salivary function was found due to ^{131}I therapy (cumulative doses less than 10 GBq). It was estimated that complete loss of salivary gland secretion may occur after a cumulative dose of 18.5 GBq ^{131}I [87].

Radiation exposure can be reduced one-fifth to one-tenth by the use of salivary flow-increasing foods such as lemons. Sufficient fluid intake is also important. Patients are encouraged to drink enough to stimulate urination at least hourly when awake over the 24 h following radiation dosage. Transient salivary gland pain can be treated with anti-inflammatory agents, but patients with more persistent pain are referred to ear, nose, and throat specialists for a full evaluation.

Parenchymal damage in salivary glands can significantly be reduced by amifostine, an organic thiophosphate, thus preventing patients from xerostomia. In 25 control patients [9], the parenchymal function of parotid and submandibular glands was significantly reduced by 40% at 3 months after the administration of 3 GBq or 6 GBq ^{131}I. Nine control patients developed grade I and two grade II xerostomia. In 25 amifostine-treated patients, parenchymal function of salivary glands was not significantly altered and xerostomia did not occur in any of these patients. On the other hand, the effect of amifostine (radiation protector) on the tumor uptake is not clearly documented. The experiences from other centers should be published. Thus, generally accepted guidelines regarding the use of amifostine have not been implemented so far. An increased incidence of salivary gland tumors in patients previously treated with radioiodine has been observed by Dottorini et al. [19].

6.5.4 Taste Dysfunction

Varma et al. [93] report a 48% incidence of taste dysfunction, described as loss of taste with or without taste distortion (phantom, metallic, or chemical taste). Onset was usually after 24–168 h, transient in a majority but persisting for 4 weeks to 1 year in 37% of the patients. This potential side-effect should be mentioned to patients.

6.5.5 Gastrointestinal Symptoms

Nausea is an early side-effect of ^{131}I therapy and is thought to be caused by radioiodine uptake in the stomach wall. In a report by van Nostrand et al. [56], gastrointestinal complaints were noted in 67%. These patients experienced mild nausea without vomiting as early as 2 h following therapy and usually within 36 h. The symptom lasted 1 h to 2 days and was well-controlled with antiemetics in most cases. The prophylactic use of metoclopramide can be recommended.

6.5.6
Testicular Function and Male Fertility

Because thyroid cancer strikes at all ages and long-term survival is excellent, the effect of ^{131}I therapy on fertility is an important consideration. Young men may develop permanent testicular damage with a reduction in sperm count that is roughly proportional to the ^{131}I dose administered. According to gamma-dose measurement by thermoluminescent dosimeters and MIRD calculation of beta contribution from blood, the absorbed radiation dose to the testes is 30–43 mGy/GBq ^{131}I for thyroid cancer [13]. The detrimental effect of ^{131}I on spermatogenesis appears to be, in a majority of cases, reversible in the long term. Reports of infertility from ^{131}I treatment with complete and permanent aspermia are rare despite the frequency of transient impairment of testicular germinal cell function [90].

Sarkar et al. [73] interviewed 33 patients (13 males and 20 females) with respect to their reproductive histories and the health of their children. All patients had undergone ^{131}I therapy when they were younger than 21 years of age and had received a mean total dose of 7.25 GBq. The average follow-up period was 18.7 years. The incidence of infertility (12%) was not significantly different from that in the general population.

Exposure of the testes can be diminished somewhat by good hydration and frequent urination during the first 24 to 48 h following therapy. Long-term storage of semen has been suggested for patients in whom high-dose cumulative therapy is anticipated [57].

6.5.7
Ovarian Function and Female Fertility

There are only a few reports on the possible damage to the gonads of females treated with ^{131}I [11, 38]. Dottorini et al. [19] found no significant difference in fertility rate, birth rate, and prematurity between 627 women treated with ^{131}I and 189 untreated women.

6.5.8
Pregnancy Outcome

Schlumberger et al. [78] obtained data on 2,113 pregnancies by interviewing female patients treated for thyroid carcinoma. The incidence of miscarriages was 11% before any treatment for thyroid cancer; this number increased slightly after surgery for thyroid cancer, both before (20%) and after (20%) ^{131}I, but did not vary with the cumulative ^{131}I dose. Miscarriages were more frequent (40%) in the 10 women who were treated with ^{131}I during the year preceding conception. Incidences of stillbirth, preterm birth, low birth weight, congenital malformation, and death during the 1st year of life were not significantly different before and after ^{131}I therapy. The incidence of thyroid disease and nonthyroidal malignancy was similar in children born either before or after their mothers were exposed to ^{131}I.

Therefore, it is recommended that conception be postponed for 1 year after treatment with ^{131}I . There is no evidence that pregnancy affects tumor growth in women receiving adequate thyroxine therapy [75]. In women of childbearing age, pregnancy must be ruled out before radioiodine therapy by using a pregnancy test (beta-human chorionic gonadotrophin).

6.5.9 Bone Marrow Suppression

Temporary bone marrow suppression is seen in patients treated with ^{131}I [80]. Bone marrow depression is usually maximal at 1 month to 6 weeks after therapy. However, the baseline leukocyte count may be decreased even 1 year after high-dose therapy. Patients with skeletal or extensive metastases or those who have received external radiation or chemotherapeutic agents may be more susceptible to this side-effect.

Menzel et al. [52] treated 26 patients suffering from advanced differentiated thyroid cancer with repeated activities of 11.1 GBq. Use of repetitive highactivity, with a maximum of 44.4 GBq ^{131}I applied during 1 year and a maximum of 99.9 GBq accumulated activity resulted in a significant increase in hematotoxicity. Thirty-eight percent of patients had mild hematotoxic side effects (WHO I), 8% evinced moderate hematotoxicity (WHO II), and one patient developed severe leucopenia and thrombopenia (WHO III). None of these patients revealed clinical symptoms during the mean follow-up period of 4 years.

The separation and transplantation of autologous hematopoietic stem cells appear to be in an experimental stage. The feasibility of separation should be discussed before a large cumulative dose of ^{131}I has been administered. The long-term benefit for patients in whom the administration of large ^{131}I doses is expected needs to be evaluated by future studies.

6.5.10 Leukemia

Acute myeloid leukemia, the type associated with ^{131}I therapy, may occur within 10 years after treatment in patients given ^{131}I every few months and in whom the total blood doses per administration are more than 2 Gy or when cumulative doses are greater than approximately 37 GBq ^{131}I [66]. The absolute risk of life lost because of recurrent thyroid carcinoma exceeds that from leukemia by 4-fold to 40-fold, depending on the age at which the patient is treated [95].

Treatment regimes that include individual ^{131}I doses of as much as 7.4 GBq at intervals of greater than 6 months, with 12 months preferred, and that do not exceed 30 GBq per total patient dose probably do not significantly increase the risk for leukemia [4].

6.5.11
Solid Tumors

There is a low incidence of bladder cancers following repeated high-dose radioiodine therapies [20]. Attention to adequate hydration for urine dilution and emptying the bladder hourly during waking hours over the first 2 days following administration will reduce the bladder wall exposure to radiation and, perhaps, decrease the frequency of bladder cancer.

The risk of second primary malignancies was evaluated in a Swedish, Italian, and French cohort of papillary and follicular thyroid cancer patients. The study concerned 6,481 thyroid cancer patients, diagnosed during the period 1934–1995, at a mean age of 44 years [70]. In all, 17% were treated with external radiotherapy and 62% received radioiodine therapy. In total, 576 patients were diagnosed with a second primary malignancy. The mean interval of time between thyroid cancer diagnosis and second primary cancer was 15 years (range: 2–55 years). Compared with the general population of each of the three countries, an overall significantly increased risk of second primary malignancy of 27% (95% confidence interval: 15–40%) was seen in the European cohort. An increased risk of both solid tumors and leukemias was found with increasing cumulative activity of ^{131}I administered, with an excess absolute risk of 14.4 solid tumors and 0.8 leukemias/GBq of ^{131}I and 10^5 person-years of follow-up. A relationship was found between ^{131}I administration and occurrence of bone and soft tissue, colorectal, and salivary gland cancers. No interaction was evidenced between external radiotherapy and ^{131}I administration for the risk of secondary primary malignancy. The excess relative risk for solid tumors did not vary widely with time after exposure to ^{131}I: among the 3,211 patients followed for at least 10 years after thyroid cancer treatment, the excess relative risk of a second primary malignancy more than 10 years after the last ^{131}I treatment was 6% (95% confidence interval: 1–12%) per gigabecquerel of ^{131}I administered.

Among the 344 patients aged less than 20 years at thyroid cancer diagnosis, 13 second primary malignancies occurred. Compared with the general population, the overall risk of second primary malignancies was significantly increased (standardized incidence ratio 2.5), independent of the therapy. In all, 61% of the young patients were treated by ^{131}I and no carcinogenic effect of ^{131}I was found in this subgroup (relative risk 1.1). As the dose-response relationships for ^{131}I administration were linear, it seems necessary to restrict the repeated use of radioiodine therapy to thyroid cancer patients in whom clinical benefits are expected.

6.5.12
Pulmonary Fibrosis

Pulmonary fibrosis is seen in patients with diffuse pulmonary metastases from differentiated thyroid carcinoma who have been treated with ^{131}I in doses that exceed 9.25 GBq [20]. Although rarely observed, this potential side effect must be considered in patients with disseminated pulmonary metastases.

6.5.13 Neurological Complications

Because brain metastases in thyroid cancer are rare, screening measures are not common. However, because of the dire consequences of cerebral edema, certain precautions are recommended. The head should always be included in pretherapy diagnostic scanning with ^{131}I. Furthermore, in patients with widespread metastatic disease or bulky local disease, a magnetic resonance imaging study is appropriate before ^{131}I therapy. Surgical debulking of spinal lesions may be prudent before ^{131}I is given.

Pretreatment with corticosteroid, as used in preventing cerebral edema in patients receiving external beam therapy, is suggested in patients with brain metastases who are to be treated with ^{131}I.

6.5.14 Parathyroid Dysfunction

Anatomical location of the parathyroid glands outside the thyroid bed may be protective due to the physical properties of the beta-radiation from ^{131}I. Overall, the parathyroid gland can be considered relatively radioresistant, and parathyroid glands seem clinically unaffected by high-dose ^{131}I therapy. However, the management of patients should include long-term follow-up of calcium levels due to possible operative damage.

6.5.15 Lacrimal Gland Dysfunction

The symptoms from radiation-induced ocular dryness are rather discrete, in contrast to the symptoms caused by salivary gland dysfunction. Lacrimal gland dysfunction might be permanently impaired after high-dose radioiodine therapy. Zettinig et al. [96] investigated 88 patients with a history of radioiodine therapy for thyroid carcinoma and compared them with a sex- and age-matched control group. The mean administered activity was 5.3 ± 4.7 GBq ^{131}I (range: 3.0–22.3 GBq), and 66 of the patients (75%) had a single radioiodine treatment. A total of 81 patients (92%) had at least one abnormal function test indicating impaired lacrimal gland dysfunction. Schirmer's test was decreased (<10 mm/5 min) in 47 of the 88 patients and definitely abnormal (< 5 mm/5 min) in 35 patients. A tear film breakup time of <10 s was found in 78 patients and 62 patients had a definitely abnormal breakup time of <5 s. The lacrimal lipid layer was impaired in 43 patients. The following symptoms of dry eye were recorded: xerophthalmia (16%), epiphora (11%), or epiphora and photophobia (1%). Similar results were reported by Solans et al. [85] using a standardized questionnaire ($n = 79$ patients): Xerophthalmia persisted to the 2nd year of follow-up in 17.7% of cases and was still present in the 3rd year of follow-up in 13.9% of cases. Keratoconjunctivitis sicca persisted in 11 patients (13.9%) to the 2nd year of follow-up but was only present in 6 patients (7.6%) more than 3 years after the last radioiodine application. A dependence on cumulative dose of radioiodine was significant for subjective xerophthalmia, with a linear trend to cumulative activity. The data indicate that lacrimal gland dysfunction (sicca syndrome) is relatively frequent after radioiodine therapy. In most cases this is a transient side-effect, but in some patients it may persist for a long period or appear late.

6.6 Radiation Considerations in the Treatment of Thyroid Cancer

Sodium iodide ^{131}I is available in capsule and liquid forms for oral and intravenous administration. The capsular form is associated with easier handling. Recommendations for inpatient therapy and whole-body scintigraphy with ^{131}I in Germany are outlined by the 'Strahlenschutzverordnung,' the 'Richtlinie Strahlenschutz in der Medizin' [33] and the 'Strahlenschutzkommision' [88].

References

1. Allweiss P, Braunstein GD, Kate A et al. (1984) Sialadenitis following I-131 therapy for thyroid cancer. J Nucl Med 25:755–758
2. Al-Nahhas AM (1999) Ablation in differentiated thyroid carcinoma: How much surgery? How much iodine? [Editorial] Nucl Med Commun 20:595–597
3. Arnstein NB, Carey JE, Spaulding SA et al. (1986) Determination of iodine-131 diagnostic dose for imaging metastatic thyroid cancer. J Nucl Med 27:1764–1769
4. Beierwaltes WH (1978) The treatment of thyroid carcinoma with radioactive iodine. Semin Nucl Med 8:79–94
5. Beierwaltes WH, Rabbani R, Dmuchowski C et al. (1984) An analysis of "ablation of thyroid remnants" with I-131 in 511 patients from 1947–1984: experience at University of Michigan. J Nucl Med 25:1287–1293
6. Berg G, Lindstedt G, Suurküla M et al. (2002) Radioiodine ablation and therapy in differentiated thyroid cancer under stimulation with recombinant human thyroid-stimulating hormone. J Endocrinol Invest 25:44-52
7. Biersack HJ, Helpap B, Koch U et al. (1983) Should treatment of highly differentiated thyroid carcinoma be conservative? Nuklearmedizin 20:20–23
8. Börner AR, Petrich T, Weckesser E et al. (2002) Monitoring isotretinoin therapy in thyroid cancer using ^{18}F-FDG PET. Eur J Nucl Med Mol Imaging 29:231-236
9. Bohuslavizki KH, Klutmann S, Brenner W et al. (1998) Salivary gland protection by amifostine in high-dose radioiodine treatment: result of a double-blind placebo-controlled study. J Clin Oncol 16:3542–3549
10. Brown AP, Greening WP, McCready VR et al. (1984) Radioiodine treatment of metastatic thyroid carcinoma: the Royal Marsden Hospital experience. Br J Radiol 57:323–327
11. Casara D, Rubello D, Saladini G et al. (1993) Different features of pulmonary metastases in differentiated thyroid cancer: natural history and multivariate statistical analysis of prognostic variables. J Nucl Med 34:1626–1631
12. Casara D, Rubello D, Saladini G et al. (1993) Pregnancy after high therapeutic doses of iodine-131 in differentiated thyroid cancer: potential risks and recommendations. Eur J Nucl Med 20:192–194

13. Ceccarelli C, Battisti P, Gasperi M et al. (1999) Radiation dose to the testes after ^{131}I therapy for ablation of postsurgical thyroid remnants in patients with differentiated thyroid cancer. J Nucl Med 40:1716–1721
14. Chiu AC, Delpassand ES, Sherman SI (1997) Prognosis and treatment of brain metastases in thyroid carcinoma. J Clin Endocrinol Metab 82:3637–3642
15. Chopra S, Wastie ML, Chan S et al. (1996) Assessment of completeness of thyroid ablation by estimation of neck uptake of ^{131}I on whole-body scans: comparison of quantification and visual assessment of thyroid bed uptake. Nucl Med Commun 17:687–691
16. Comtois R, Theriault C, Del Vecchio P (1993) Assessment of the efficacy of iodine-131 for thyroid ablation. J Nucl Med 34:1927–1930
17. Daumerie C, Vynckier S, Caussin J et al. (1996) Radioiodine treatment of thyroid carcinoma in patients on maintenance hemodialysis. Thyroid 6:301–304
18. Dietlein M, Dressler J, Farahati J et al. (2004) Procedure Guidelines for radioiodine therapy of differentiated thyroid cancer (version 2) (in German). Nuklearmedizin 43:115–120
19. Dottorini ME, Lomuscio G, Mazzucchelli L et al. (1995) Assessment of female fertility and carcinogenesis after I-131 therapy for differentiated thyroid carcinoma. J Nucl Med 36:21–27
20. Edmonds CJ, Smith T (1986) The long-term hazards of the treatment of thyroid cancer with radioiodine. Br J Radiol 59:45–51
21. Farahati J, Reiners C, Stuschke M et al. (1996) Differentiated thyroid cancer: impact of adjuvant external radiotherapy in patients with perithyroidal tumor infiltration (stage pT4). Cancer 77:172–180
22. Grüning T, Tiepolt C, Zöphel K, et al. (2003) Retinoic acid for redifferentiation of thyroid cancer – does it hold its promise? Eur J Endocrinol 148:395-402
23. Grünwald F, Menzel C, Bender H et al. (1998) Redifferentiation therapy-induced radioiodine uptake in thyroid cancer. J Nucl Med 39:1903–1906
24. Harbert JC (1987) Nuclear medicine therapy. Thieme, New York
25. Haugen BR (1999) Management of the patient with progressive radioiodine non-responsive disease. Semin Surg Oncol 16:34–41
26. Haugen BR, Larson LL, Pugazhenthi U, et al. (2004) Retinoic acid and retinoid receptors are differentially expressed in thyroid cancer and thyroid carcinoma cell lines and predict response to treatment with retinoids. J Clin Endocrinol Metab 89:272-280
27. Haugen BR, Pacini F, Reiners C et al. (1999) A comparison of recombinant human thyrotropin and thyroid hormone withdrawal for the detection of thyroid remnant or cancer. J Clin Endocrinol Metab 84: 3877–3885
28. Hay ID, Grant CS, van Heerden JA et al. (1992) Papillary thyroid microcarcinoma: a study of 535 cases observed in a 50-year period. Surgery 112:1139–1147
29. Hedinger C, Williams ED, Sobin LH (1989) The WHO histological classification of thyroid tumors: a commentary on the second edition. Cancer 63:908–911
30. Jarzab B, Handkiewicz-Junak D, Roskosz J, et al. (2003) Recombinant human TSH-aided radioiodine treatment of advanced differentiated thyroid carcinoma: a single-centre study of 54 patients. Eur J Nucl Med Mol Imaging 30:1077-1086
31. Jeevanram RK, Shah DH, Sharma M et al. (1986) Influence of initial large dose on subsequent uptake of therapeutic radioiodine in thyroid cancer patient. Nucl Med Biol 13:277–279
32. Keizer de B, Brans B, Hoekstra A, et al. (2003) Tumour dosimetry and response in patients with metastatic differentiated thyroid cancer using recombinant human thyrotropin before radioiodine therapy. Eur J Nucl Med Mol Imaging30:367-373
33. Kemmer W, Michalczak H (2003) Richtlinie Strahlenschutz in der Medizin 2002. Hildegard Hoffmann, Berlin
34. Ladenson PW, Braverman LE, Mazzaferri EL et al. (1997) Comparison of administration of recombinant human thyrotropin with withdrawal of thyroid hormone for radioactive iodine scanning in patients with thyroid carcinoma. N Engl J Med 337:888–896

35. Lin JD, Chaa TC, Huang MJ et al. (1998) Use of radioactive iodine for thyroid remnant ablation in well differentiated thyroid carcinoma to replace thyroid re-operation. Am J Clin Oncol 21:77–81
36. Lippi F, Capezzone M, Angelini F et al. (2001) Radioiodine treatment of metastatic differentiated thyroid cancer in patients on L-thyroxine, using recombinant human TSH. Eur J Endocrinol 144:5-11
37. Löffler M, Weckesser M, Franzius C et al. (2003) Iodine excretion during stimulation with rh TSH in differentiated thyroid carcinoma. Nuklearmedizin 42:240-243
38. Lushbaugh CC, Casarett GW (1976) The effects of gonadal radiation in clinical radiation therapy. A review. Cancer 37:1111–1120
39. Luster M, Lassmann M, Haenscheid H et al. (2000) Use of recombinant human thyrotropin before radioiodine therapy in patients with advanced differentiated thyroid carcinoma. J Clin Endocrinol Metab 85:3640-3645.
40. Maheshwari YK, Hill CS, Haynie TP et al. (1981) ^{131}I therapy in differentiated thyroid carcinoma: M.D. Anderson Hospital experience. Cancer 47:664–671
41. Maruca J, Santner S, Miller K et al. (1984) Prolonged iodine clearance with a depletion regimen for thyroid carcinoma. J Nucl Med 25:1089–1093
42. Massin JP, Savoie JC, Garnier H et al. (1984) Pulmonary metastases in differentiated thyroid carcinoma. Cancer 53:982–992
43. Maxon HR, Boehringer TA, Drilling J (1983) Low iodine diet in I-131 ablation of thyroid remnants. Clin Nucl Med 8:123–126
44. Maxon HR, Englaro EE, Thomas SR et al. (1992) Radioiodine-131 therapy for well-differentiated thyroid cancer – a quantitative radiation dosimetric approach: outcome and validation in 85 patients. J Nucl Med 33:1132–1136
45. Maxon HR, Thomas SR, Hertzberg VS et al. (1983) Relation between effective radiation dose and outcome of radioiodine therapy for thyroid cancer. N Engl J Med 309:937–941
46. Mazzaferri EL (1995) Treating high thyroglobulin with radioiodine: a magic bullet or a shot in the dark? J Clin Endocrinol Metab 80:1485–1487
47. Mazzaferri EL (1996) Radioiodine and other treatments and outcomes. In: Braverman LE, Utiger RD (eds) The thyroid. Lippincott-Raven, Philadelphia, pp 922–945
48. Mazzaferri EL, Jhiang SM (1994) Long-term impact of initial surgery and medical therapy on papillary and follicular thyroid cancer. Am J Med 97:418–428
49. Mazzaferri EL, Robbins RJ, Spencer CA et al. (2003) A consensus report of the role of serum thyroglobulin as a monitoring method for low-risk patients with papillary thyroid carcinoma. J Clin Endocrinol Metab 88:1433-1441
50. Mazzaferri EL, Young E (1981) Papillary thyroid carcinoma: a 10-year follow-up report of the impact of therapy in 576 patients. Am J Med 70:511–518
51. McDougall IR (1997) 74 MBq radioiodine ^{131}I does not prevent uptake of therapeutic doses of ^{131}I (i.e. it does not cause stunning) in differentiated thyroid cancer. Nucl Med Commun 18:505–512
52. Menzel C, Grünwald F, Schomburg A et al. (1996) "High-dose" radioiodine therapy in advanced differentiated thyroid carcinoma. J Nucl Med 37:1496–1503
53. Morris JC, Kim CK, Padilla ML et al. (1997) Conversion of non-iodine-concentrating differentiated thyroid carcinoma metastases into iodine-concentrating foci after anticancer chemotherapy. Thyroid 7:63–66
54. Moser E, Fritsch S, Braun S (1988) Thyroglobulin and 131 I uptake of remaining tissue in patients with differentiated carcinoma after thyroidectomy. Nucl Med Commun 9:262–266
55. Nemec J, Zamrazil V, Pohunkova D et al. (1979) Radioiodine treatment of pulmonary metastases of differentiated thyroid cancer. Results and prognostic factors. Nuklearmedizin 18:86–90
56. Nostrand van DV, Neutze J, Atkins F (1986) Side effects of "rational dose" iodine-131 therapy for metastatic well-differentiated thyroid carcinoma. J Nucl Med 27:1519–1527

57. Pacini F, Gasperi M, Fugazzda L et al. (1994) Testicular function in patients with differentiated thyroid carcinoma treated with radioiodine. J Nucl Med 35:1418–1422
58. Pacini F, Lippi F, Formica N et al. (1987) Therapeutic doses of iodine-131 reveal undiagnosed metastases in thyroid cancer patients with detectable serum thyroglobulin levels. J Nucl Med 28:1888–1891
59. Pacini F, Molinaro E, Castagna MG et al. (2002) Ablation of thyroid residues with 30 mCi ^{131}I: a comparison in thyroid cancer patients prepared with recombinant human TSH or thyroid hormone withdrawal. J Clin Endocrinol Metab 87:4063-4068
60. Park HM, Perkin OW, Edmondson JW et al. (1994) Influence of diagnostic radioiodines on the uptake of ablative dose of iodine-131. Thyroid 4:49–54
61. Park JT II, Hennessey JV (2004) Two-week low iodine diet is necessary for adequate outpatient preparation for radioiodine rh TSH scanning in patients taking levothyroxine. Thyroid 14:57-63
62. Pellegriti G, Scollo C, Giuffrida D et al. (2001) Usefulness of recombinant human thyrotropin in the radiometabolic treatment of selected patients with thyroid cancer. Thyroid 11:1025-1030
63. Pineda JD, Lee T, Ain K et al. (1995) Iodine-131 therapy for thyroid cancer patients with elevated thyroglobulin and negative diagnostic scan. J Clin Endocrinol Metab 80: 1488–1492
64. Pons F, Carrio I, Estorch M et al. (1987) Lithium as an adjuvant of iodine-131 uptake when treating patients with well-differentiated thyroid carcinoma. Clin Nucl Med 12:644–647
65. Ramacciotti C, Pretorius HT, Line BR et al. (1982) Ablation of non-malignant thyroid remnants with low doses of radioiodine: concise communication. J Nucl Med 23:483–489
66. Reiners C (1991) Stochastische Risiken der I-131-Therapie des Schilddrüsenkarzinoms. Nuklearmediziner 20:331–334
67. Robbins J (1991) Thyroid cancer: a lethal endocrine neoplasm. Ann Intern Med 115:133–147
68. Robbins RJ, Larson SM, Sinha N et al. (2002) A retrospective review of the effectiveness of recombinant human TSH as a preparation for radioiodine thyroid ablation. J Nucl Med 43:1482-1488
69. Ronga G, Fiorentino A, Paserio E et al. (1990) Can iodine-131 whole body scan be replaced by thyroglobulin measurement in the postsurgical follow-up of differentiated thyroid carcinoma? J Nucl Med 31:1766–1771
70. Rubino C, Vathaire F de, Dottorini ME et al. (2003) Second primary malignancies in thyroid cancer patients. Br J Cancer 89:1638-1644
71. Samaan NA, Schultz PN, Haynie TP et al. (1985) Pulmonary metastasis of differentiated thyroid carcinoma: treatment results in 101 patients. J Clin Endocrinol Metab 60:376–380
72. Samaan NA, Schultz PN, Hickey R et al. (1992) The results of various modalities of treatment of well-differentiated thyroid carcinoma: a retrospective review of 1599 patients. J Clin Endocrinol Metab 75:714–720
73. Sarkar SD, Beierwaltes WH, Gill SP et al. (1976) Subsequent fertility and birth histories of children and adolescents treated with ^{131}I for thyroid cancer. J Nucl Med 17:460–464
74. Schicha H, Dietlein M, Scheidhauer K (1999) Therapie mit offenen radioaktiven Stoffen. In: Büll U, Schicha H, Biersack HJ et al. (eds) Nuklearmedizin. Thieme, Stuttgart, pp 512–545
75. Schlumberger MJ (1998) Papillary and follicular thyroid carcinoma (review). N Engl J Med 338:297–306
76. Schlumberger M, Berg G, Cohen O et al. (2004) Follow-up of low-risk patients with differentiated thyroid carcinoma: a European perspective. Eur J Endocrinol 150:105-112
77. Schlumberger M, Challeton C, de Vathaire F et al. (1996) Radioactive iodine treatment and external radiotherapy for lung and bone metastases from thyroid carcinoma. J Nucl Med 37:598–605

78. Schlumberger M, de Vathaire F, Ceccarelli C et al. (1996) Exposure of radioactive iodine-131 for scintigraphy or therapy does not preclude pregnancy in thyroid cancer patients. J Nucl Med 37:606–612
79. Schlumberger M, Tubiana M, De Vathaire F et al. (1986) Long-term results of treatment of 283 patients with lung and bone metastases from differentiated thyroid carcinoma. J Clin Endocrinol Metab 63:960–967
80. Schober O, Günter HH, Schwarzrock R et al. (1987) Hämatologische Langzeitveränderungen bei der Radioiodtherapie des Schilddrüsenkarzinoms. I.) Periphere Blutbildveränderungen. Strahlenther Onkol 163:464–474
81. Seabold JE, Ben-Haim S, Pettit WA et al. (1993) Diuretic-enhanced I-131 clearance after ablation therapy for differentiated thyroid cancer. Radiology 187:839–842
82. Simon D, Köhrle J, Schmutzler C et al. (1996) Redifferentiation therapy of differentiated thyroid carcinoma with retinoid acid: basics and first clinical results. Exp Clin Endocrinol Diabetes 104 [Suppl 4]:13–15
83. Simon D, Körber C, Krausch M et al. (2002) Clinical impact of retinoids in redifferentiation therapy of advanced thyroid cancer: final results of a pilot study. Eur J Nucl Med Mol Imaging 29:775-782
84. Sisson JC, Jamadar DA, Kazerooni EA et al. (1998) Treatment of micronodular lung metastases of papillary thyroid cancer: are the tumors too small for effective irradiation from radioiodine? Thyroid 8:215–221
85. Solans R, Bosch J-A, Galofré P et al. (2001) Salivary and lacrimal gland dysfunction (sicca syndrome) after radioiodine therapy. J Nucl Med 42:738-743
86. Solomon BL, Wartowsky L, Burman KD (1996) Current trends in the management of well differentiated papillary thyroid carcinoma. J Clin Endocrinol Metab 81:333–339
87. Spiegel W, Reiners C, Börner W (1985) Sialadenitis following iodine-131 therapy for thyroid carcinoma [letter]. J Nucl Med 26:816
88. Strahlenschutzkommission (2004) Notwendigkeit der stationären Durchführung der Ganzkörperszintigraphie mit I-131 beim Schilddrüsenkarzinom. Empfehlung der Strahlenschutzkommission. Verabschiedet in der 190. Sitzung der Strahlenschutzkommission am 22/23. April 2004
89. Strahlenschutzverordnung 2001 (2002) Bundesanzeiger, Köln
90. Sweeney DC, Johnston GS (1995) Radioiodine therapy for thyroid cancer. Endocrinol Metabol Clin North Am 24:803–839
91. Travagli JP, Cailleux AF, Ricard M et al. (1998) Combination of radioiodine (^{131}I) and probe-guided surgery for persistent or recurrent thyroid carcinoma. J Clin Endocrinol Metab 83:2675–2680
92. Varma VM, Beierwaltes WH, Nofal MM et al. (1970) Treatment of thyroid cancer: death rates after surgery and after surgery followed by sodium iodine I-131. JAMA 214:1437–1442
93. Varma VM, Dai WL, Henkin RI (1992) Taste dysfunction in patients with thyroid cancer following treatment with I-131. J Nucl Med 33:996
94. Wittekind C, Meyer JH, Bootz F (2003) TNM Klassifikation maligner Tumoren. 6. Aufl. Springer, Berlin Heidelberg New York
95. Wong JB, Kaplan MM, Meyer KB et al. (1990) Ablative radioactive iodine therapy for apparently localized thyroid carcinoma. A decision analytic perspective. Endocrinol Metab Clin North Am 19:741–760
96. Zettinig G, Hanselmayer G, Fueger BJ et al. (2002) Long-term impairment of the lacrimal glands after radioiodine therapy: a cross-sectional study. Eur J Nucl Med Mol Imaging 29:1428–1432

^{124}I Positron Emission Tomographic Dosimetry and Positron Emission Tomography/Computed Tomography Imaging in Differentiated Thyroid Cancer

7

L.S. Freudenberg, A. Bockisch, and W. Jentzen

7.1 Introduction

Patients with well-differentiated thyroid cancer (DTC) of follicular origin usually undergo total thyroidectomy and at least one radioiodine therapy using ^{131}I. Besides the therapeutic effect, ^{131}I whole body imaging offers excellent accuracy for the detection of DTC metastases; however, it is limited only for those accumulating iodine. Additional useful diagnostic tools in the follow-up of thyroidectomized patients with DTC are thyroglobulin, ultrasonography (US), US-guided fine-needle biopsy, and [^{18}F]fluorodeoxyglucose positron emission tomography (FDG-PET) [1–6]. Recent studies show that FDG-PET leads to changes in approaches to surgical treatment plans in a significant number of patients. In detail, in cases with poor tumor differentiation, reduced or lost iodine-accumulating ability leads to false-negative ^{131}I scanning results [1–3].

In the majority of patients, however, iodine uptake in the tumor is adequate for scintigraphy and somewhat less frequent for radioiodine therapy. Although ^{131}I therapy and diagnostics are not only well established but also very successful, they suffer from two drawbacks. Due to physical restrictions of gamma cameras used for ^{131}I imaging, the special resolution is limited and there is significant septa penetration degrading the scintigram. Therefore, in the presence of the extremely high uptake of thyroid remnant, many local metastases may not be detected by the scintigraphy following the first therapy. The resulting uncertainty in staging probably requires in a certain way an overtreatment. The second drawback in conventional therapy is the unfeasible or inaccurate dosimetry. Iodine imaging is very selective and therefore the morphological correlate is often missing. In the face of the unknown depth of the lesion, attenuation correction cannot be applied and, in addition, due to the missing volume information, dosimetry is completely impossible. Therefore, the usual radioiodine therapy is performed using risk-adapted standard activities.

7.2
^{124}I Characteristics

The above-mentioned drawbacks may be mostly overcome by replacing the gamma camera by PET using ^{124}I. ^{124}I is a positron emitter with a half-life of 4.2 days, but only 23% of the transition results in positron emission. The complex decay scheme of ^{124}I includes several high-energy gamma rays, making ^{124}I imaging a challenge even for high-quality PET systems. There are single gamma quanta – in cascade with positron emission – with energies of 603 keV and 723 keV and abundance of 62% and 10%, respectively. Since the typical discriminator energy window of PET ranges from 350 to 650 keV, additional random counts resulting from gamma coincidences, scatter (versus the annihilation coincidences) will occur and result in lower image contrast. The mean positron energy is less than 1 MeV; therefore, a degradation of image resolution caused by long-range positrons does not occur.

Widespread application is hampered today by its very restricted availability. ^{124}I is preferably produced using a high-energetic cyclotron. We apply the ^{124}Te(d,2n)^{124}I reaction using a 14-MeV deuteron beam (a detailed description of the radiopharmaceutical production, preparation, and its impurities is given elsewhere [7]). A variety of PET scanners have been characterized for the use of ^{124}I, and satisfactory imaging results can be achieved in realistic settings [13, 15–19]. Thus, ^{124}I is suitable for quantitative PET imaging and has been used for dosimetry [8–14].

The requested high specificity of the tracer that makes it ideal for detecting lesions results in a lack of identifiable anatomical structures, thus making an accurate localization of foci of tracer uptake highly problematic [20, 22]. This disadvantage is overcome by correlating the PET information with available anatomical background information obtained, for instance, from a combined PET/CT.

We propose to apply 50 MBq ^{124}I for dosimetric purposes and 25 MBq if only cervical imaging is intended. After oral administration measurements after 4, 24, 48, 72, and 96 h are proposed for accurate dosimetry. We expect that a single uptake measurement (after 2 or 3 days) may replace the multiple measurements that have already been proven for benign thyroid diseases [21]. In spite of the above-mentioned randoms due to high-energy gamma rays, it could be proven that the use of the three-dimensional (3D) mode is appropriate [16–19], and acquisition times of 5-min emissions per bed position are suitable. Therefore, a whole body scan in the PET/CT requires approximately 30 min. It has to be said that if PET/CT scans are performed the application of iodinated contrast agents is strictly forbidden.

7.3
Metastases Dosimetry Using ^{124}I PET

Furhang and coworkers [23] published a reasonable procedure for dosimetry using ^{124}I PET. Our modifications have resulted in a quite complex bundle of measurements. There are two targets for dosimetry: determining the lesion

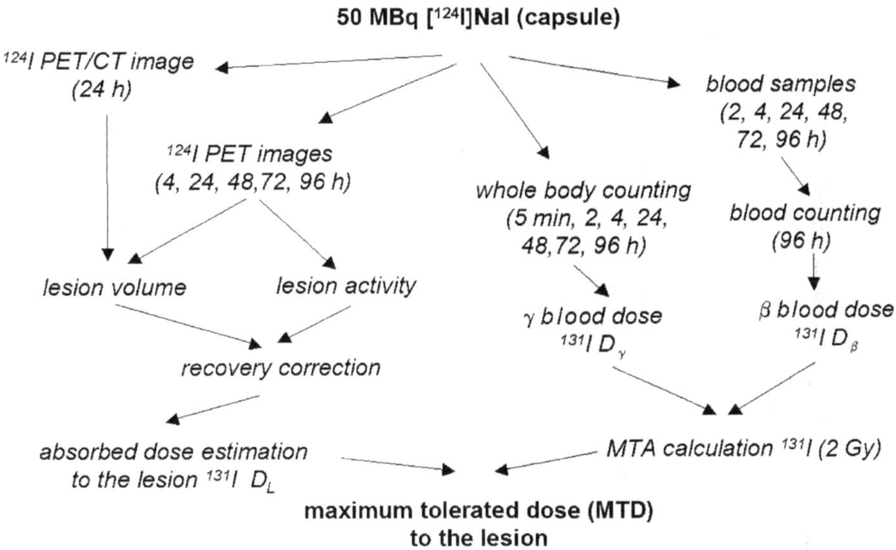

Fig. 7.1 The radioiodine dosimetry procedure for differentiated thyroid cancer (DTC) using ^{124}I (MTA maximum tolerated activity)

dose and the dose deposited in the bone marrow that is the organ at risk. Blood is taken as the surrogate marker for bone marrow toxicity. Parallel to external beam radiation, 2 Gy is used as dose constraint to the bone marrow. Thus, 2 Gy to the blood is used to calculate the maximum tolerated activity (MTA) assuming that the iodine kinetics during the ^{124}I dosimetry is similar to that of the ^{131}I under therapeutic conditions. Finally, using the calculated MTA, the maximum potential dose in each lesion is calculated. Depending on the result, the indication for radioiodine therapy is derived. Apart from small local metastases, absorbed doses well above 100 Gy are needed for cure. Absorbed doses below 30 Gy usually have only limited effect.

As illustrated in Fig. 7.1, the radioiodine dosimetry procedure consists of two parts: blood and whole-body counting as well as PET(/CT) imaging. The blood and whole-body counting monitors the respective radioiodine kinetics. The time activity curves are then used to estimate the absorbed dose to blood per unit of administered activity to the lesion.

Specifically, the patient was given an activity of about 50 MBq of ^{124}I. The blood dose is derived from measurements of daily blood samples. In addition, whole-body clearance measurements need to be carried out, e.g., employing an uncollimated gamma camera with the patient standing a large distance away (4 m). The measurements need to be taken in anterior and posterior view to account for absorption. The blood dose per unit of administered activity consists of two components, β blood and γ blood dose, and are estimated using their corresponding time-activity curves. PET imaging is performed using (single) PET and combined PET/CT. The daily whole-body measurements were carried out

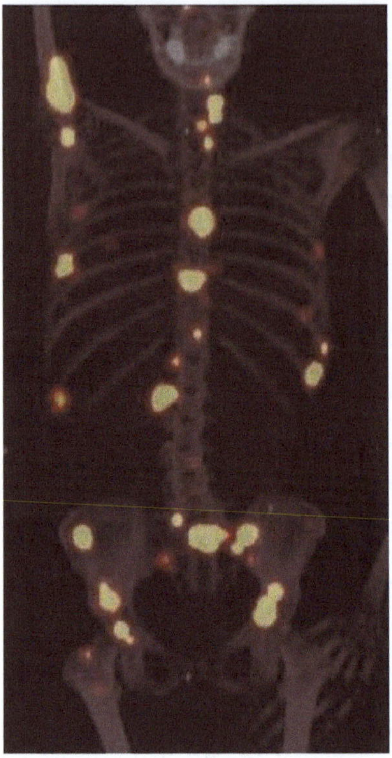

Fig. 7.2 ^{124}I PET/CT image acquired 24 h after oral administration of 45 MBq shows multiple bone metastases

with PET, and after 24 h one PET/CT image was taken. Both sets of images were used to obtain the lesion volume, either from PET images using the threshold technique [24] and/or directly from the CT images. The lesion activity corrected with the measured recovery coefficient was used to estimate the absorbed dose per unit of administered activity of each lesion.

In summary, the absorbed dose to the lesions per unit of administered activity and the MTA are used to calculate the maximum tolerated dose (MTD) to the DTC lesions that is essential in estimating the success of radioiodine therapy. A clinical example illustrates the usefulness of the ^{124}I dosimetry.

A 49-year-old woman suffered from a pathological fracture of the right humerus. The following clinical workup resulted in an advanced follicular thyroid carcinoma (pT4 pN1 M1 os). Three weeks after thyroidectomy, the patient presented with severe bone pain, and multiple bone metastases were seen in bone scintigraphy. Blood concentration of thyroglobulin was 16,800.0 ng/ml with undisturbed recovery test and negative thyroglobulin antibodies. As desired was risen to TSH 43 mU/l. Due to the extent of the disease, the patient received ^{124}I dosimetry in order to apply maximum activity.

^{124}I PET imaging showed multiple iodine-avid bone metastases (see Fig. 7.2). Lesion dosimetry yielded a dose of 30–150 Gy/GBq and a MTA of 5 GBq, thus revealing a MTD of 150–750 Gy. As this high-risk patient had a poor prognosis

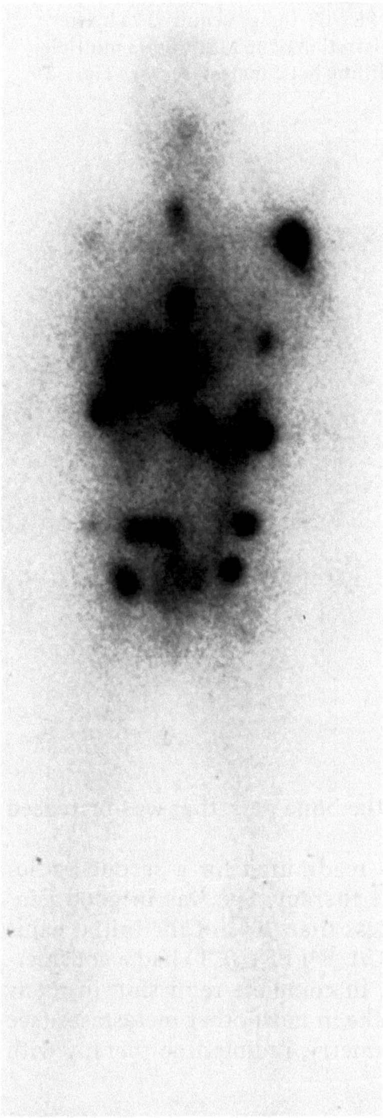

Fig. 7.3 ^{131}I whole-body scan acquired 10 days after oral administration of 10 GBq showing bone metastases

and the algorithm to qualify the MTA is conservative, the patient was treated with 10 GBq of ^{131}I with a hematological backup. Side-effects of this high-dose therapy were transient decrease in lymphocytes (from 2.1/nl to a minimum of 0.2/nl on posttherapy day 6), recurrent fever requiring antibiotic therapy and intermittent worsening of bone pain resulting in morphine therapy. The ^{131}I whole-body scan 10 days after application of 10 GBq ^{131}I demonstrated an extensive activity retention in the lesions known from the ^{124}I PET (see Fig. 7.3). At

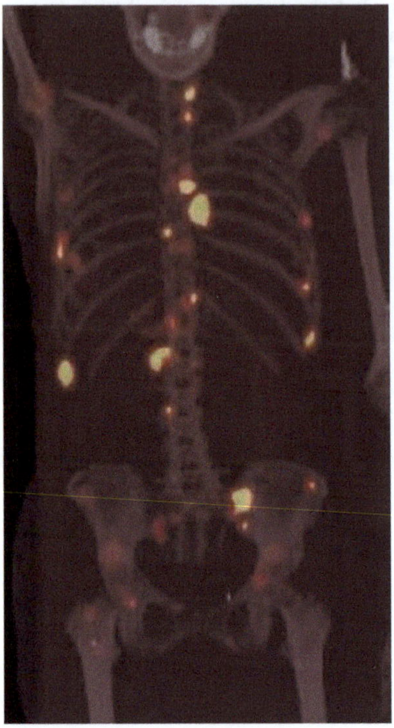

Fig. 7.4 ^{124}I PET/CT image acquired 24 h after oral administration of 48 MBq shows multiple, clearly declining bone metastases (see Fig. 7.2)

that time the patient already recovered from the bone pain that was increased as a flair phenomenon.

Four months posttherapy, the patient was readmitted for a second radioiodine dosimetry and subsequent radioiodine therapy. She was in good general health. Thyroglobulin was decreased to less than 10% of the initial value (1,240.0 ng/ml), again undisturbed, TSH 52 mU/l. ^{124}I PET(/CT) had a considerable effect on patient management, resulting in complete remission in many lesions and a dramatic decrease in iodine uptake in most other metastases (see Fig. 7.4). As a consequence of the second dosimetry, radioiodine therapy with 8 GBq ^{131}I was given.

7.4 PET/CT Imaging with ^{124}I

As of February 2005, there have been no studies examining the impact of ^{124}I PET on the management of differentiated thyroid cancer, although ^{124}I PET has been shown to be an useful imaging technique for the diagnosis and management of thyroid diseases [13]. However, interpreting PET scans with highly specific tracers such as ^{124}I is challenged by the lack of identifiable anatomical

Fig. 7.5 ^{124}I PET acquired 24 h after oral administration of 50 MBq showing pathological tracer uptake cervically or mediastinally

structures in PET images. This shortcoming of diagnostic procedures using radioactive iodine is reduced by PET/CT.

An example illustrates this finding. A 54-year-old man with a history of well-differentiated (G1) follicular thyroid carcinoma (1 cm in diameter, with penetration of the thyroid capsule, pT4 pN0 MX) developed an increased thyroglobulin blood concentration of 1.8 ng/ml; recovery test 68%; thyroid stimulating hormone 68 mU/l, fT3 2.9 ng/ml, and fT4 2.8 ng/ml. Cervical ultrasonography showed no pathological structures. Prior to further treatment, an accurate staging was desired.

Images on a combined PET/CT system were acquired (Biograph, Siemens) 24 h after oral administration of 50 MBq of ^{124}I. Projections from head to pelvis were obtained. The PET scan alone showed pathologically increased tracer uptake in two foci located cervically or mediastinally (see Fig. 7.5). An accurate anatomical localization of these foci was not completely possible as the tracer is highly specific. The CT scan alone showed no pathology. Image fusion of PET and the coregistered CT enabled to attribute the pathological tracer uptake to an area close to the aorta representing mediastinal micrometastases (see Fig. 7.6).

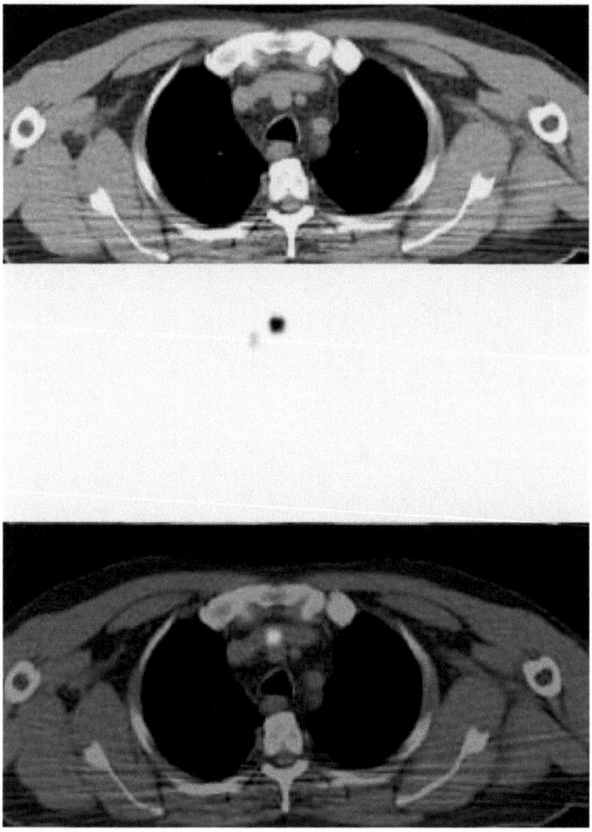

Fig. 7.6 ^{124}I PET (A), CT (B), and PET/CT (C) acquired 24 h after oral administration of 85 MBq pathological tracer uptake mediastinally, representing mediastinal micrometastases close to the aorta

This case illustrates the potential of ^{124}I PET/CT in exact anatomical localization of DTC metastases.

In a pilot study, we showed the clinical usefulness of ^{124}I PET/CT with lesion detection rates of 97% compared with high-dose ^{131}I whole-body scan with lesion detection rates of 83% [19]. PET/CT not only adds the morphological information to the ^{124}I PET, but also has the power to assess iodine-negative metastases. Due to the small patient group, the impact of ^{124}I PET/CT on patient management could not be evaluated. However, with ^{124}I PET/CT being superior to ^{131}I whole-body scan with respect to lesion detectability on a lesion-by-lesion basis, an impact on patient management appears to be likely. Several case reports support this finding [16–20, 25].

Another advantage of combined ^{124}I PET and CT are synergistic effects. Although the combined assessment of fused PET and CT images in a fusion display does not reveal additional tumor manifestations compared with PET and CT alone, the accurate topographic localization of the tumor can result in a change of staging and in therapy management [16–19, 25]. From these consid-

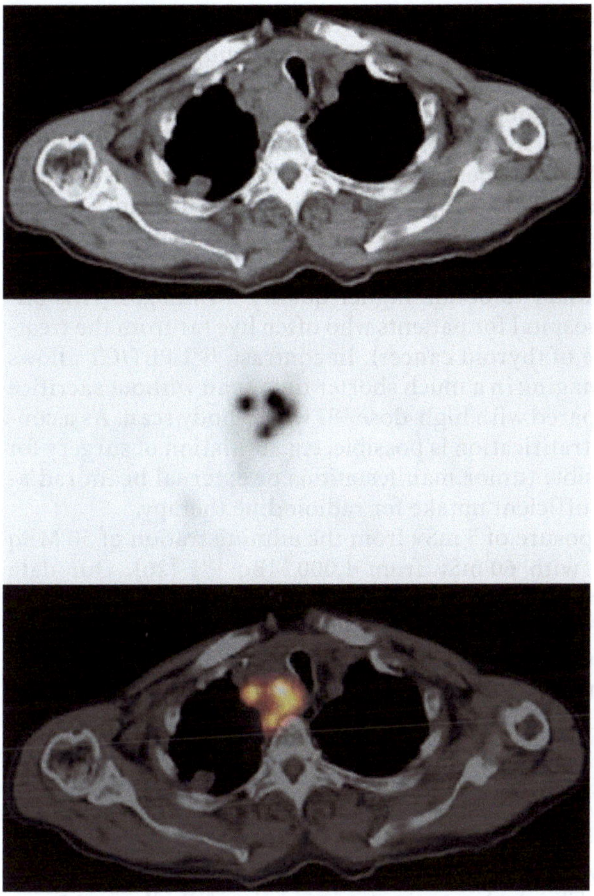

Fig. 7.7 ^{124}I PET (A), CT (B), and PET/CT (C) images acquired 24 h after oral administration of 50 MBq show pathological tracer uptake mediastinally representing four iodine-avid mediastinal metastases. Additional non-iodine-avid metastases were found in the mediastinum and lung

erations, it is clear that ^{124}I PET/CT may provide incremental diagnostic value over the individual imaging modalities.

As an example, a 46-year-old man with advanced papillary thyroid carcinoma (pT4 pN1 MX) was referred to the Department of Nuclear Medicine for radioiodine therapy. The physical examination showed a patient in good general health. On admission, the following pathological laboratory values were seen: thyroglobulin 29.0 ng/ml; recovery test 81%; thyroid-stimulating hormone 51 mU/l, fT3 2.3 ng/ml, and fT4 2.5 ng/ml. Results of cervical ultrasonography suggested a cervical metastasis. Prior to therapy, this high-risk patient received ^{124}I dosimetry to allow individual treatment planning. Images on a combined PET/CT system were acquired (Biograph, Siemens) 26 h after oral administration of 50 MBq ^{124}I. The PET scan alone showed pathologically increased tracer uptake in four mediastinal metastases (see Fig. 7.7); however, the additional CT and subsequent PET/CT showed additional, non-iodine-avid metastases (mediastinal and pulmonary). The patient was referred to the Department of Radiation Therapy for further treatment and underwent external beam radiotherapy. Hence, PET/CT allowed fast treatment stratification and therapy.

In addition, logistics and economics of the diagnostic tests have to be analyzed. PET/CT certainly adds significant costs to the diagnostic workup; nevertheless, there are savings too from shortening the workup and keeping the patient at work. ^{124}I PET/CT can be performed on a outpatient basis – another economic factor. A high-dose, whole-body scan is typically performed 3–8 days after the administration of ^{131}I. Nevertheless scanning can be difficult in terms of septal penetration at high ^{131}I activity. Sometimes a secondary scan, e.g., 4–5 days later, may be necessary to obtain higher-quality ^{131}I images. This implies a separate visit to the hospital for patients who often live far from the treatment center (low prevalence of thyroid cancer). In contrast, ^{124}I PET/CT allows us to complete diagnostic imaging in a much shorter time span without sacrifice in diagnostic accuracy compared with high-dose ^{131}I whole-body scan. As a consequence, faster treatment stratification is possible, e.g., initiation of surgery for the removal of easily accessible tumor manifestations or external beam radiation for metastases with insufficient uptake for radioiodine therapy.

Moreover, a radiation exposure of 5 mSv from the administration of 50 MBq of ^{124}I compares favorably with 60 mSv from 1,000 MBq ^{131}I [26]. Our data showed the superiority of ^{124}I PET over planar ^{131}I whole-body scan even at lower ^{124}I activities. Thus, ^{124}I PET presumably is a suitable alternative for high-dose diagnostic ^{131}I whole-body scan [27] in follow-up of DTC that is less time-consuming and more convenient for the patient.

7.5 Conclusions

^{124}I is an efficient diagnostic tool in DTC and allows not only sensitive imaging but also precise dosimetry. The dosimetry procedure using ^{124}I allows estimation of the maximum tolerated dose to the lesions with acceptable accuracy. In contrast to the conventional procedures using, for instance, gamma cameras, it allows absolute quantification. The ^{124}I dosimetry has been clinically proven to be useful. It is a promising approach in patients suffering from advanced DTC before radioiodine therapy and patients with suspected recurrence and/or metastases.

In addition to the synergistic effects of combining morphological imaging with highly specific functional imaging, ^{124}I PET/CT represents a suitable, low-dose alternative to the clinical standard of high-dose ^{131}I whole-body scan in follow-up of patients with DTC. The diagnostic and logistic advantages of ^{124}I PET dosimetry and PET/CT imaging can only be utilized clinically if ^{124}I becomes more widely available.

References

1. Frilling A, Gorges R, Tecklenborg K, Gassmann P, Bockhorn M, Clausen M, Broelsch CE (2000) Value of preoperative diagnostic modalities in patients with recurrent thyroid carcinoma. Surgery 128:1067–1074
2. Alnafisi NS, Driedger AA, Coates G, Moote DJ, Raphael SJ (2000) FDG PET of recurrent or metastatic iodine-131-negative papillary thyroid carcinoma. J Nucl Med 41:1010–1015
3. Chung JK, So Y, Lee JS, Choi CW, Lim SM, Lee DS, Hong SW, Youn YK, Lee MC, Cho BY (1999) Value of FDG PET in papillary thyroid carcinoma with negative iodine-131 whole-body scan. J Nucl Med 40:986–992
4. Grunwald F, Kalicke T, Feine U, Lietzenmayer R, Scheidhauer K, Dietlein M, Schober O, Lerch H, Brandt-Mainz K, Burchert W, Hiltermann G, Cremerius U, Biersack HJ (1999) Fluorine-18 fluorodeoxyglucose positron emission tomography in thyroid cancer: results of a multicenter study. Eur J Nucl Med 26:1547–1552
5. Hooft L, Hoekstra OS, Deville W, Lips P, Teule GJ, Boers M, van Tulder MW (2001) Diagnostic accuracy of ^{18}F-fluorodeoxyglucose positron emission tomography in the follow-up of papillary or follicular thyroid cancer. J Clin Endocrinol Metab 86:3779–3786
6. Gorges R, Eising EG, Fotescu D, Renzing-Kohler K, Frilling A, Schmid KW, Bockisch A, Dirsch O (2003) Diagnostic value of high-resolution B-mode and power-mode sonography in the follow up of thyroid cancer. Eur J Ultrasound 16:191–206
7. Knust EJ, Dutschka K, Weinreich R (2000) Preparation of ^{124}I solutions after thermodistillation of irradiated $^{124}TeO_2$ targets. Appl Radiat Isot 52:181–184
8. Frey P, Townsend D, Flattet A, de Gautard R, Widgren S, Jeavons A, Christin A, Smith A, Long A, Donath A (1986) Tomographic imaging of the human thyroid using I-124. J Clin Endocrinol Metab 63:918–927
9. Lambrecht RM, Woodhouse N, Phillips R, Wolczak D, Qureshi A, Reyes ED, Graser C, Al-Yanbawi S, Al-Rabiah A, Meyer W et al (1988) Investigational study of iodine-124 with a positron camera. Am J Physiol Imaging 3:197–200
10. Crawford DC, Flower MA, Pratt BE, Hill C, Zweit J, McCready VR, Harmer CL (1997) Thyroid volume measurement in thyrotoxic patients: comparison between ultrasonography and iodine-124 positron emission tomography. Eur J Nucl Med 24:1470–1478
11. Erdi YE, Macapinlac H, Larson SM, Erdi AK, Yeung H, Furhang EE, Humm JL (1999) Radiation dose assessment for I-131 therapy of thyroid cancer using I-124 PET imaging. Clin Pos Imag 2:41–46
12. Frey P, Townsend D, Jeavons A, Donath A (1985) In vivo imaging of the human thyroid with a positron camera using ^{124}I. Eur J Nucl Med 10:472–476
13. Pentlow KS, Graham MC, Lambrecht RM, Daghighian F, Bacharach SL, Bendriem B, Finn RD, Jordan K, Kalaigian H, Karp JS, Robeson WR, Larson SM (1996) Quantitative imaging of iodine-124 with PET. J Nucl Med 37:1557–1562
14. Eschmann SM, Reischl G, Bilger K, Kupferschlager J, Thelen MH, Dohmen BM, Besenfelder H, Bares R (2002) Evaluation of dosimetry of radioiodine therapy in benign and malignant thyroid disorders by means of iodine-124 and PET. Eur J Nucl Med 29:760–767
15. Herzog H, Tellmann L, Qaim SM, Spellberg S, Schmid A, Coenen HH (2002) PET quantitation and imaging of the non-pure positron-emitting iodine isotope ^{124}I. Appl Radiat Isot 56:673–679
16. Freudenberg LS, Antoch G, Görges R, Beyer T, Debatin JF (2002) Combined PET/CT with iodine-124 in diagnosis of mediastinal micrometastases in thyroid carcinoma. Internet J Radiol 2
17. Freudenberg LS, Antoch G, Görges R, Knust EJ, Beyer T, Brandau W, Bockisch A, Debatin JF (2002) ^{124}I-PET/CT in metastatic follicular thyroid carcinoma. Eur J Nucl Med 29:1106
18. Freudenberg LS, Antoch G, Gorges R, Knust J, Pink R, Jentzen W, Debatin JF, Brandau W, Bockisch A, Stattaus J (2003) Combined PET/CT with iodine-124 in diagnosis of spread metastatic thyroid carcinoma: a case report. Eur Radiol 13 [Suppl 4]:L19–L23

19. Freudenberg LS, Antoch G,Knust J, Müller SP, Jentzen W, Görges R, Beyer T, Pink R, Stattaus J, Bockisch A, Debatin JF, Brandau W (2004) Value of ^{124}I-PET/CT in staging of patients with differentiated thyroid cancer. Eur Radiol 14:2092–2098
20. Beyer T, Townsend DW, Brun T, Kinahan PE, Charron M, Roddy R, Jerin J, Young J, Byars L, Nutt R (2000) A combined PET/CT scanner for clinical oncology. J Nucl Med 41:1369–1379
21. Bockisch A, Jamitzky T, Derwanz R, Biersack HJ (1993) Optimized dose planning of radioiodine therapy of benign thyroidal diseases. J Nucl Med 34:1632–1638
22. Townsend DW, Cherry SR (2001) Combined anatomy and function: the path of true image fusion. Eur Radiol 11:1968–1974
23. Furhang EE, Larson SM, Buranapong P, Humm JL. Furhang EE (1999) Larson thyroid cancer dosimetry using clearance fitting. J Nucl Med 40:131–136
24. Erdi YE, Mawlawi O, Larson SM, Yeung H, Finn R, Humm JL (1997) Segmentation of lung lesion volume by adaptive positron emission tomography image thresholding. Cancer 80 [Suppl]:2505–2509
25. Görges R, Antoch G, Brandau W, Freudenberg LS, Knust EJ, Dutschka K, Müller S P, Jentzen W, Bockisch A, Stattaus J (2002) Kombinierte PET/CT mit dem Positronenstrahler ^{124}I bei metastasiertem follikulären Schilddrüsenkarzinom. Nuklearmedizin 5:N68–N71
26. International Commission on Radiological Protection (eds) (1998) ICRP publication 80. Addendum to publication 53 – radiation dose to patients from radiopharmaceuticals. Ann ICRP 28
27. Filesi M, Signore A, Ventroni G, Melacrinis FF, Ronga G (1998) Role of initial iodine-131 whole-body scan and serum thyroglobulin in differentiated thyroid carcinoma metastases. J Nucl Med 39:1542–1546

Chapter 8

External Beam Radiotherapy 8

M. Biermann, M.K. Pixberg, A. Schuck,
N. Willich, A. Heinecke, and O. Schober

8.1 Introduction

While surgery, radioiodine therapy (RIT) and TSH suppression therapy are generally accepted mainstays of therapy for differentiated thyroid carcinoma (DTC) [52, 67, 76], the role of external beam radiotherapy (RTx) remains controversial.

Unequivocal indications for RTx of thyroid neoplasms are undifferentiated/anaplastic thyroid carcinoma, thyroid lymphoma, locoregional recurrences and (pre-)symptomatic metastases when radical surgery is not possible and the tumour tissue or tumour residues after surgery have no sufficient I-131 uptake [64, 67, 75].

The case for adjuvant RTx in addition to surgery, RIT and TSH-suppressive therapy is however open to debate. With the exception of two prospective but inconclusive studies [6, 90], evidence is available only from retrospective surveys, with sometimes poorly defined inclusion criteria, inconsistent treatment regimens (different surgical procedures with or without ablative ^{131}I therapy), or inconsistent or obsolete standards of radiotherapy. In the following we present a systematic review of the available evidence on adjuvant RTx for DTC. We do not discuss RTx for medullary carcinoma, which has been reviewed elsewhere [60].

8.2 Methods

8.2.1 Literature Search

The primary search was based on our earlier reviews [66, 77]. All cited papers and all review articles known to us [11, 30, 64, 66, 67, 71, 77, 83, 86] were systematically searched for potentially relevant references. Finally, a PubMed search was performed using the medical subject heading (MeSH) term "thyroid neoplasms", with the subheading "radiotherapy" ("thyroid neoplasms/radiotherapy [MH]"), which yielded 1,697 results as of 1 June 2004. Of all potentially relevant titles, the abstract was checked when available and in most instances the full paper. Our inclusion criteria were all original research articles published since

1970 in English, German, or French on adjuvant RTx of DTC which comprised at least one arm with and without RTx, with a minimum of 10 patients each. Only the most recent article on each patient cohort was to be included in the review. Pre-1970 papers were included out of historical interest. As a shorthand notation for tumour staging, the tumour-node-metastasis (TNM) classification of 1997 [98] is used throughout this chapter wherever applicable.

8.2.2 Statistical Analysis

With the exception of two prospective studies [6, 90], all studies were retrospective and not randomised, representing evidence-based medicine (EBM) levels of evidence III–IV [92]. It was therefore not possible to perform a systematic meta-analysis based on Cochrane principles, for the funnel plot methodology is based on the assumption that all known and unknown risk factors are equally distributed across therapy groups through randomisation [18]. We have chosen a conservative approach and determined 5-year survival and 5-year freedom of recurrence for each study whenever possible, this being the longest interval of follow-up covered by the majority of studies. Significance tests are only those contained in the original papers.

8.3 Results

8.3.1 Literature Search

The 22 studies that met the above inclusion criteria are listed in Table 8.1. The following seven studies represent earlier publications on the same cohorts and are therefore not included in Table 8.1: Tubiana 1975 [95] (same cohort as [94]); Heinze 1976 [33] (same as [45]); Mazzaferri 1977 [54], Young 1980 [100], Mazzaferri 1991 [53] (same as [51]); Glanzmann 1979 [25] and 1992 [26] (same as [27]); Benker 1990 (same as [21]).

The following papers were not included in the analysis for the reasons stated: Hare 1941 [28] (231 patients with RTx; no information on treatment assignment, no control group); Jakobson 1954 [37] (144 patients with RTx; no control group); Windeyer 1954 [97] (157 patients irradiated for TC; no control group); Sheline 1966 [82] (58/147 patients with RTx, but insufficient data on control group); Smedal 1967 [88] (59 patients with RTx for DTC; no control group); Chung 1980 [16] (38 patients with RTx; no control group); Schümichen 1983 [79] (75/382 patients with DTC received RTx, but insufficient data for comparison between groups); Adamietz 1999 [1] (138/178 patients with pT4 or N1 DTC received RTx, but no data on control group); Kleinert 1989 [41] (56/89 patients with TC received RTx; insufficient data on control group); Kuijpens 1998 [42] (only 7/343 patients received RTx); Hölzer 2000 [34, 35] (142/1685 patients with

Table 8.1 Retrospective studies on external beam radiotherapy

Study	Patients (*n*)	Follow-up years	RTx	Inclusion criteria	Groups	Patients in groups (*n*)	Outcomes					Comment
							5 years		*n* years			
							Survival (%)	Freedom from recurrence (%)	n	Survival (%)	Freedom from recurrence (%)	
Pemberton 1939 [61]: 1 institution (USA) 1907–1937	774			TC	R	106	63[a]		10	54[a]		
					R+RTx	221	73[a]			60[a]		
					RTx	138	23[a]			14[a]		
Portmann 1941 [65]: 1 institution (USA) 1922–1936	200			TC	R	52	52[a]					
					R+RTx	79	57[a]					
					RTx	29						
Mabille 1961 [49]: 1 institution (France) 1919–1958	143	≥5	XR 200 kV, 40–50 Gy	TC	R	30	83[a]					Only 18 patients received ^{131}I
					R+RTx	23	83[a]					
					iR+RTx	24	38[a]					
					RTx	66	16[a]					
Simpson 1978 [84]: 1 institution (Canada) 1958–1977	137	≤20	40 Gy	DTC	R	34					50[a]	14 patients in RTx group received ^{131}I
					R+I	19					84[a]	
					R+RTx	49					95[a]	

Table 8.1 *Continued*

Study	Patients (*n*)	Follow-up years	RTx	Inclusion criteria	Groups	Patients in groups (*n*)	Outcomes					Comment
							5 years		*n* years			
							Survival (%)	Freedom from recurrence (%)	n	Survival (%)	Freedom from recurrence (%)	
Leisner 1982 [45]: 2 institutions (Germany) 1960–1980	621		^{60}Co uh	TC	–							2 university hospitals in Munich; 1 used RTx, 1 did not
			XR, 60 Gy	DTC pT4	TT+I	67	68*		8	38*	10.5[a]	
					TT+I+RTx	167	88*			75*	10.7[a]	
Tubiana 1985 [94]: 1 institution (France) 1943–1976	539		RM, 200 kV <50 Gy; ^{60}Co, MVe+ph 50–60 Gy	TC	TT	275	94	81	15	81	64	10% local recurrences with RTx >50 Gy vs 15% with <50 Gy
					TT+I	61	93	67		75	44	
					TT+RTx±I	66	81	70		62	53	
					R2+RTx	97	78	58		57	39	
					RTx	23	60	55		14	7	
Wu 1987 [99]: 1 institution (China) 1958–1979	405		ov XR, 4–20 MVe 40–70 Gy	TC	cR	238	92		15	62		No ^{131}I
					cR+RTx	59	78			54		
					iR	57	33*			17		
					iR+RTx	51	71*			43		
Rossi 1988 [69]: 1931–1980	97	5–27	XR 200 kV, 35 Gy, 2–4 MV	TC R2	"Low risk"							
					iR	17	76[a]					
					iR+RTx	21	95[a]					
			48–60 Gy, TB, CL, UM		"High risk"							
					iR	12	50[a]*					$p<0.001$
					iR+RTx	31	10[a]*					

Table 8.1 *Continued*

Study	Patients (*n*)	Follow-up years	RTx	Inclusion criteria	Groups	Patients in groups (*n*)	Outcomes					Comment
							5 years		*n* years			
							Survival (%)	Freedom from recurrence (%)	n	Survival (%)	Freedom from recurrence (%)	
Simpson 1988 [85]: 13 institutions (Canada)	1,578	4–24	35–50 Gy TB/CL/ML (variable)	DTC	R	821	96[b]	81[a]	20	89[b]		
					R+RTx	144	94[b]	85[a]		87[b]		
					R+I	170	93[b]	86[a]		88[b]		
					R+I+RTx	88	96[b]	84[a]		88[b]		
				PTC R1	R1	38	97[b]	26*	20	36[b]*		Any radiotherapy better than none
					R1+RTx	52	97[b]	90*		97[b]		
					R1+I	39	93[b]	82*		82[b]		
					R1+I+RTx	43	100[b]	86*		89[b]		
Müller-Gärtner 1991 [55]: 1 institution (Germany) 1960–1987	149	5, median; 7, mean		FTC	TT+I	70	88[a]	82[a]				
					TT+I+RTx	79	87[a]	83[a]				
Samaan 1992 [70]: 1 institution (USA) 1948-1989	1,599	11 median	R+I(a)	DTC	447				11 median	98[a]*	90[a]*	
			R+I(r)		289					90[a]*	76[a]*	
			R+RTx		113					77[a]*	63[a]*	

Table 8.1 *Continued*

Study	Patients (*n*)	Follow-up years	RTx	Inclusion criteria	Groups	Patients in groups (*n*)	Outcomes					Comment
							5 years		*n* years			
							Survival (%)	Freedom from recurrence (%)	n	Survival (%)	Freedom from recurrence (%)	
Glanzmann 1992 [27]: 1 institution (Switzerland) 1960–1988	339		40–70 Gy ^{60}Co 4–6 MV el.+ph; TB, CL, UM	DTC	uR	2			>15		50[a]	
					uR+RTx	18					100[a]	
					TT+I	4					100[a]	
					TT+I+RTx	50					100[a]	
Phlips 1993 [62]: 1 institution (Belgium) 1974–1989	94	6 median	55 Gy ^{60}Co 18 MV LA; TB, CL, UM	DTC	R+I	56	94		6 median		75[a]	Worse survival in RTX group despite better local control
					R+I+RTx	38	84				97[a]	
Esik 1994 [20]: 1 institution (Hungary) 1961–1991	114		oV >40 Gy, ^{60}Co >45 Gy; else „iRTx“	TC	PTC+iRTx	10	90[b]	38[b]	20	40[b]*	38[b]*	Better survival and local control for PTC; better local control for FTC
					PTC+RTx	48	100[b]	98[b]		100*	82[b]*	
					FTC+iRTx	13	83	68[b]		72[b]	47[b]*	
					FTC+RTx	43	96[b]	97[b]		82[b]	97[b]*	
Mazzaferri 1994 [51]: >3 institutions 1950–1993	1,355		–	DTC	R–LT_4	151	–	–	30	88*	60*	RTx patients had more advanced disease
					R	760				94*	70*	
					R+I	388				97*	85*	
					R+RTx	56				68*	37*	

Table 8.1 *Continued*

Study	Patients (*n*)	Follow-up years	RTx	Inclusion criteria	Groups	Patients in groups (*n*)	Outcomes					Comment
							5 years		*n* years			
							Survival (%)	Freedom from recurrence (%)	n	Survival (%)	Freedom from recurrence (%)	
O'Connel 1994 [58]: 1 institution (England) 1969–1991	113		^{60}Co 5 MV ph, 60 Gy; TB, CL, UM	DTC	R+RTx	74	65[b]		10	46[b]		
					R+I-RTx	39	49[b]			23[b]		
Farahati 1996 [21]: 1 institution (Germany) 1997–1992	169	6 0	50–60 Gy MVe+ph; TB+CL ±UM	DTC pT4	TT+I	70	94[a]	77[a]	10	91[a]	70[a]	
				M0	TT+I+RTx	99	100[a]	93[a]		100[a]	93[a]	
				PTC pT4	TT+I	20	85[a]	54[b]		75[a]	90[b]*	5 died without RTx, 0 with RTx (n.s.).
				N1 ≥ age 40	TT+I+RTx	21	100[a]	90[b]		100[a]	45[b]*	
Tsang 1998 [93]: 1 institution (Canada) 1986–1996	382	11 median	40–65 Gy; 88% ≥40 Gy 65% el. TB 19% TB, CL, UM	DTC	R±I	197	95[b]	90[b]	10		89[a]	
					R+RTx±I	185	94[b]	86[b]			86[a]	
				PTC R1	R1±I	65	93[b]	86[b]		93*	78*	^{131}I but not RTx reduces recurrence in TB
					R1+RTx±I	90	100[b]	98[b]		100*	93*	

Table 8.1 *Continued*

Study	Patients (*n*)	Follow-up years	RTx	Inclusion criteria	Groups	Patients in groups (*n*)	Outcomes					Comment
							5 years		*n* years			
							Survival (%)	Freedom from recurrence (%)	n	Survival (%)	Freedom from recurrence (%)	
Sautter-Bihl 2001 [73]: 2 institutions (Germany) 1970–1987	441		50–60 Gy ^{60}Co, ph. 6–18 MV; TB, CL, UM	DTC	TT±I	218	96[b]		10	91		10-year survival n.s. (*p* = 0.06)
					TT+RTx±I	223	93[b]			93		
				DTC pT4	TT±I	14	57[b]		10	46		
					TT+RTx±I	60	87[b]			87		
Chow 2002 [14]: 1 institution (Hong Kong) 1960–1997	758		5 MV ph. & 13 MVe 60 Gy; TB,CL	PTC	R+I	567			10	99	89	
					R+I+RTx	20				100	100	
					R1+I	43				100	95	
					R1+I+RTx	4				100	75	
					R2+I	55		40[b]		58	24*	
					R2+I+RTx	69		67[b]		73	56*	
Eichhorn 2003 [19]: 1 institution (Germany) 1975–1995	484	8 median	50–60 Gy; TB, CL, UM	DTC	TT+I	355						
					TT+I-RTx	129						
				DTC pT4 M0	TT+I	40	94		20	89		
					TT+I-RTx	53	96			96		

Table 8.1 *Continued*

Study	Patients (*n*)	Follow-up years	RTx	Inclusion criteria	Groups	Patients in groups (*n*)	Outcomes					Comment
							5 years		*n* years			
							Survival (%)	Freedom from recurrence (%)	n	Survival (%)	Freedom from recurrence (%)	
Kim 2003 [40]: 1 institution (S Korea) 1981–1997	94		^{60}Co/ 4 MV LA 50–70 Gy; TB, CL, UM	PTC pT4 or N1	R+I	68	100[b]	68[b]	7	98	68*	
					R+RTx	11	97[b]	95[b]		90	95*	
					R+I+RTx	12						

The columns are defined as follows: Study: number of institutions, country, time of initial therapy; Patients: number of patients reported on (number may differ from sum in groups column); Follow-up years: in years
TC thyroid cancer, *PTC* papillary carcinoma, *FTC* follicular carcinoma, *DTC* differentiated carcinoma, *pT4* locally invasive cancer, *N1* lymph node positive), *RTx* RTx protocol, *iRTx* inadequate RTx, *RM* radium mould, *XR* X-rays, *uh* ultrahigh voltage, *MV* megavolt, *LA* linear accelerator, *el.* electrons, *ph.* photons, absorbed dose in Gy; target volumes: *TB* thyroid bed, *CL* cervical lymph nodes, *UM* upper mediastinum; + means that therapy was performed, – that it was not performed and ± that it was performed in some patients; *I* ^{131}I therapy, *I(a)* ablative I, *I(r)* for recurrence, *L-T₄* thyroid hormone therapy, *R* resection, *iR* incomplete R, *uR* unilateral R, *R1* microscopically iR, *R2* macroscopically iR, *TT* total thyroidectomy
[a] Cumulative survival/freedom from recurrence
[b] Estimated from graph
* Statistically significant: $p<0.05$

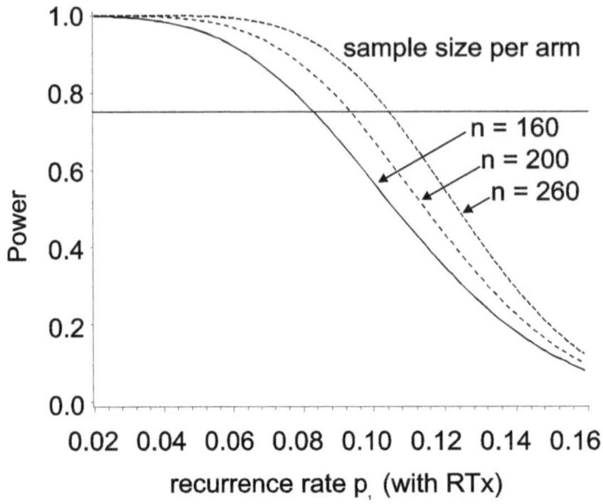

Fig. 8.1 Power calculation underlying the Multicenter Study Differentiated Thyroid Cancer (MSDS) trial. The assumption was that the recurrence rate without RTx was 19% over a recruitment period of 5 years and a further 3-year follow-up and that a reduction the recurrence rate to p_1 through RTx should be detected with 80% power (Fisher's exact test, $P<0.05$, two-tailed). For a recurrence rate of 8% in the RTx arm, this required 2 × 160 randomised patients, for a recurrence rate of 11%, 2 × 250 patients [6]

papillary thyroid cancer (PTC) in Germany in 1996 received RTx, but no data on outcomes); Hundahl 2000 [36] (128/5310 patients in US in 1996 received RTx, no data on outcomes); Chow 2002 [15] (only 10/215 patients with RTx); Foote 2003 [22] (18 patients with RTx for Hürthle cell carcinoma, without control group); Chebotareva 2002 [13] (article in Russian; 218 patients); Jarzab 2001 [38] (article in Polish; only preliminary results from 800 patients); Ford 2003 [23] (41 patients with RTx, without control group); Lin 2003 [48] (18/910 patients with DTC received RTx; no comparison with and without RTx); Kim 2004 [39] (no data on RTx). A number of papers focused on radiation technique rather than outcomes [29, 30]. One report described an afterloading technique [56], one intensity-modulated RTx [57]. There were three reports on RTx of canine thyroid carcinoma [10, 59, 91].

8.3.2
Methodological Quality of the Studies

Nearly all authors tried their best to get the maximum information from the available historical data. The need to accumulate a sufficient number of patients with sufficiently long follow-up for the slow-growing tumour means that a single-institution survey needs to go back at least 10 years. Most early studies did not include statistical methods in the Methods section [49, 84, 95, 99] and used cumulative survival [49, 61]. The first studies to use life-table analysis at least for some endpoints were Simpson's of 1978 [84] and Leisner's of 1982 [45]. Most of the studies were underpowered. With DTC it generally takes more than 200 patients in each arm for an evaluation even of strong treatment effects (cf. Fig. 8.1) [6, 96].

As with all historical data, inconsistencies are frequent. For example, Simpson's paper included 137 patients registered between 1958 and 1977 at the Princess Margaret Hospital in Toronto, ON, Canada, for the treatment of DTC, but reports one case of skin necrosis "developed from an overdose of radiation when the operator was removed by the Gestapo while the patient was under a radiotherapy machine" [84].

Common to all the studies were the following limitations inherent in historical data:

- Changes in diagnostics: CT, sonography and serum thyroglobulin (Tg) and even thyroid function testing evolved over the years and were not available before the 1980s. Likewise ^{131}I scintigraphy cameras became more sensitive. Thus the chance of diagnosing local and distant failures was limited in the early trials and the beginning of the observation periods of later trials.
- Differences in pathological staging: Over the years, the classification of tumour types changed [32], as well as staging systems such as TNM [98].
- Changes in treatment: Surgery, and in particular radiotherapy [orthovoltage (150–200 kV), supervoltage (~500 kV), and supravoltage X-ray; linear accelerators (>>1 MV) with photon and electron beams; two-dimensional (2-D) versus 3-D planning; and intensity-modulated radiotherapy; lower absorbed doses in early trials] underwent major changes. As Portmann admitted in 1941: "According to modern standards the [RTx] technique would be considered antequated [sic] and the dosage inadequate." [65]. This makes a meaningful comparison between studies very difficult.
- Information that was not recorded in hospital records, e.g. acute toxicity under RTx, is lost and cannot be regained.
- Allocation bias. While in some studies risk factors between RTx and non-RTx groups are evenly balanced, the more aggressive therapy is generally allocated to patients with the worse disease. In this comparison, RTx is therefore at a disadvantage.

8.3.3 Rationale of RTx

PTC in particular is often multifocal [89] and tends to metastasise into the regional lymph nodes of the neck and the upper mediastinum [24]. Most but not all cervical lymph node metastases show ^{131}I uptake on pre- or post-therapeutic ^{131}I scintigraphies [63]. It may, however, be difficult to demonstrate ^{131}I uptake on post-therapeutic scans in the present of intense thyroid bed uptake and to distinguish between scattered thyroid remnant tissue and uptake in lymph node metastases. In comparison with histology after neck dissection, lymph node metastases are probably underdiagnosed by conventional staging [19].

The rationale underlying adjuvant RTx in addition to ^{131}I therapy is that micrometastases in cervical lymph nodes are frequent especially in locally invasive carcinomas, that they cause clinically relevant recurrences if left untreated, and that they can be sterilised by RTx but not ^{131}I. Monte-Carlo simulations by Sautter-Bihl et al. showed that the energy of the beta particles emitted by ^{131}I deposited their energy outside micrometastases, and Sautter-Bihl argued that this "therapeutic gap" could be closed by RTx [72]. Another simulation was performed by Li et al. [47] to elucidate the microdosimetry in micronodular

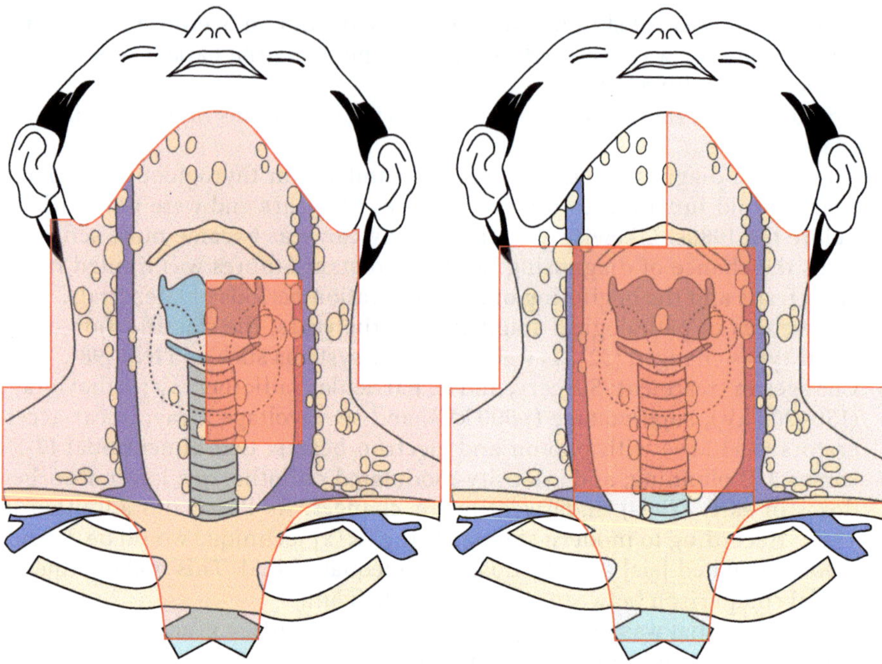

Fig. 8.2 RTx protocols. On the *left* is the German protocol. First-order target volume (*dark*) is the thyroid bed, 2nd-order volume (*grey*) the entire neck from the mastoid process and mandible down to the upper mediastinum and the tracheal bifurcation. The Toronto protocol on the *right* includes an involved field with the entire thyroid bed, including a 2-cm safety margin (*dark*). The extended field includes only those cervical lymph nodes that are assumed to be involved and always spares the contralateral submandibular region in order to protect the salivary glands. See text for further details

metastases of PTC, which have sizes ranging from less than 0.1 to 1 mm [87]. The new simulations indicate that energy deposition is adequate even around lesions of 0.1 mm. This result appears plausible because, despite the small size of the pulmonary lesions, ^{131}I therapy is known to be curative [12]. Therefore, the debate for the effectiveness of ^{131}I therapy for treating occult micrometastases in the neck is open at least for tissue that does take up ^{131}I. The effectiveness of ^{131}I treatment for macrometastatic disease in cervical lymph nodes has been demonstrated [50].

8.3.4 RTx Protocols

Past radiotherapy protocols were highly variable (cf. Table 8.1). Even the two major current RTx protocols (German vs North American) have important differences:

1. The irradiated target volumes. Simpson et al. limit RTx to the thyroid bed with a 2- to 3-cm safety margin around the pre-operative extent of the tumour [86], with typical upper and lower field margins at the hyoid bone and the lower portion of the suprasternal notch. Only in the case of lateral neck lymph node involvement is the volume extended to the mid-mastoid and inferior to the carina (J.D. Brierley, personal communication). Current German practice is to include lymph node regions from the mastoid process to the tracheal bifurcation (Fig. 8.2) [81].
2. Delivered tissue doses. Simpson et al. deliver 50 Gy in 2-Gy fractions over 5 weeks to the entire target volume(s) with a 10-Gy boost in 2-Gy fractions over one more week to the thyroid bed [86]. The German radiotherapy guidelines recommend slightly higher tissue doses to the regional lymph nodes of 50–60 Gy and to the thyroid bed of 60–70 Gy (ICRU 50), the higher doses being reserved for nodal positive disease (pN1/x) and incomplete resections (R1/2), respectively [81].
3. Timing of RTx in relation to ablative ^{131}I therapy. In many institutions RTx is begun soon after the first fraction of ablative radioiodine therapy. In contrast, current German guidelines recommend adjuvant RTx only after completion of ablative ^{131}I, with elimination of all therapeutically relevant ^{131}I uptake [17, 81]. This is based on the rationale that ^{131}I therapy can achieve much higher doses in tumour tissue (>300 Gy; [2]) than external beam RTx alone and that the lower tissue doses delivered through external RTx may inhibit subsequent ^{131}I uptake. There is no evidence that delaying adjuvant RTx by the time necessary to complete ^{131}I therapy is associated with an adverse prognosis [45].

There is consensus that 3-D or quasi 3-D planning of RTx is mandatory so that doses to risk organs such as the spinal cord (40–45 Gy) are not exceeded.

8.3.5 Retrospective Studies

Of the 19 post-1970-studies listed in Table 8.1, 6 demonstrated a statistically significant benefit of RTx in terms of local control: Esik 1994 in PTC [20]; Simpson 1988 and Tsang 1998 in PTC after R1 resection [85, 93]; Farahati 1996 in PTC pT4 N1 over age 40 [21]; Kim 2003 in PTC pT4 or N1 [40]; and Chow 2002 in PTC R2 [14]. In all but the last 3 studies, patients did not receive ^{131}I therapy or only inconsistently. Two studies found improved local control after RTx with doses above 50 Gy versus doses below 50 Gy with older RTx techniques: Tubiana 1985 [94] (10% vs 15% local recurrences; n.s.) and Esik 1994 [20] (both better local control and survival). In the first of these, ^{131}I was inconsistently used; in the latter, there was no ^{131}I therapy.

Five studies were able to demonstrate a survival benefit: Esik 1999 in PTC [20]; Leisner 1992 in locally invasive DTC (pT4) despite no difference in local control [45]; Kim 2003 in PTC pT4 or N1 [40]; Tsang 1988 after R1 and Chow 2002 after R2 resection of PTC [14, 93]; and Wu 1987 after incomplete resection of TC [99]. In two of these, patients had received no ^{131}I therapy at all [20, 99], and in two only inconsistently [40, 93].

Two studies found statistically significant poorer local control after RTx: Mazzaferri 1994 [51] and Samaan 1992 [70]; three found worse survival: the latter two [51, 70] and Rossi 1998 [69], all presumably due to allocation bias. The remaining studies produced inconclusive results due to allocation bias, limited effects of therapy or too-small patient numbers.

8.3.6 Prospective Studies

The National Thyroid Cancer Treatment Cooperative Study included 385 patients with high-risk PTC and FTC from 1987 to 1997. Mean patient follow-up was 3.1 years. Only 46 patients received RTx, generally those with poorer risk factors such as gross residual disease after surgery. The relative risk (RR) of dying was higher for irradiated patients than for patients without RTx (RR 4.55; CI 1.79–11.6) as well the RR of recurrence (RR 4.46; CI 1.5–13.0) [90].

The Multicenter Trial Differentiated Thyroid Carcinoma (MSDS) [6, 7] is an ongoing study in Germany and Austria. From 2000, it recruited patients between 18 and 70 years, with locally invasive DTC (pT4 pN0/1/x R0/1 M0/x) and without secondary malignancies or serious medical conditions. Four weeks after surgery, ^{131}I ablation was to be performed with 3–5 GBq, and TSH-suppression therapy with L-thyroxine begun. After diagnostic ^{131}I whole-body scintigraphy 3–4 months later, patients were to be randomised to receive or not to receive RTx. Until 31 March 2003, only 36 of 279 patients had been randomised. Based on the power calculation in Fig. 8.1, the trial's steering committee therefore decided to continue MSDS as a purely observational trial in April 2003 [6]. Data on the acute toxicity of RTx for DTC have been published [78]. So far the event rate in the non-RTx arm is far below the expected cumulative 19% recurrence over a 5- to 7-year follow-up in the power calculation of the trial.

A similar trial under the auspices of the American College of Surgeons Oncology Group was not funded out of concern that recruitment of the 2 × 200 patients required was not feasible (J.D. Brierley, personal communication).

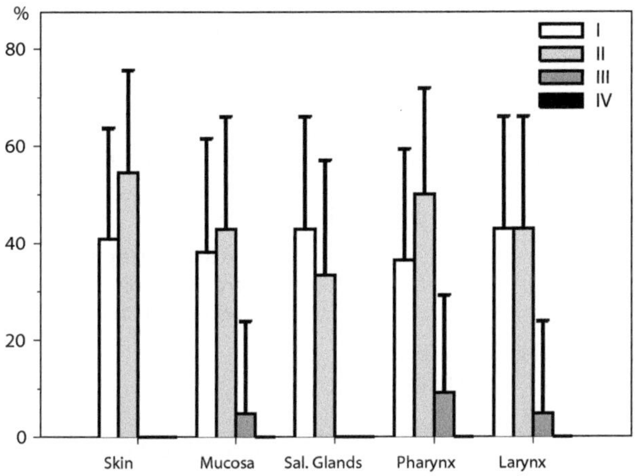

Fig. 8.3 Maximum acute RTx toxicity in the MSDS trial (n = 22 patients). All symptoms were fully reversible. Grade III toxicity occurred in 2 patients. Error bars indicate the upper limit of the 95% confidence interval (exact binomial distribution; SAS V. 8, SAS). Data from [78]. RTOG III toxicity in the oral mucosa represents confluent mucositis, which may require narcotics; in the pharynx, dysphagia leading to dehydration or >15% weight loss; in the larynx, whispered speech or pain, requiring narcotics [80]. (Sal. Salivary)

8.3.7 Toxicity

Acute and chronic toxicity [80] reported in the literature are listed in Table 8.2. Data from the MSDS trial are depicted in Fig. 8.3. Radiation myelopathy of the cervical spinal cord no longer occurs with modern planning techniques [86].

Two more aspects are of note. First, surgeons report that soft-tissue fibrosis makes repeat operations more difficult [74]; however, there are no controlled data. Second, in our experience in the follow-up of more than 1,500 DTC patients at our own institution, tissue fibrosis after RTx may make the sonographic diagnosis of recurrent disease very demanding, because even [^{18}F]fluorodeoxyglucose (FDG)-positive viable tumour may have the same echogenicity as the surrounding tissue. This potential cause of bias in the diagnosis of recurrences after RTx should not affect the above analysis, as most studies were from the presonographic era or from countries in which sonography is not routinely utilised in the follow-up of DTC patients.

8.3.8 Guidelines

Current German interdisciplinary guidelines recommend RTx for undifferentiated TC limited to the thyroid gland, and after incomplete resection of DTC with

Table 8.2 RTx toxicity

Study	Patients irradiated (*n*)	Acute toxicity	Chronic toxicity
Simpson 1978 [84] 1958–1977	91	10% severe oesophagitis/tracheitis; 2% Lhermitte's syndrome; 1% tracheal chondritis	3% fibrosis of neck tissues; 1% skin necrosis; 1% brain necrosis
Tubiana 1985 [94]	186		1% brachial plexopathy; 0.5% tracheal constriction; 0.5% carotid obstruction
Simpson 1988 [85] 13 institutions (Canada)	110	2% spinal cord necrosis (both ✝); 1% infected tracheostomy (✝)	
Glanzmann 1993 [27] 1960–1988	68		3% laryngitis (both ✝); 1% tracheostoma (all before 1969)
Phlips 1993 [62] 1974–1989	38	3% grade 3 dysphagia	3% severe skin fibrosis
Esik 1994 [20] 1961–1991	>91		3% severe neck fibrosis; 1% Lhermitte's syndrome; 1% dry mouth
Farahati 1996 [21] 1997–1992	99	33% local erythema, lymphoedema, pharyngitis	None
Adamietz 1998 [1]	138	74% grade I/II; 3% grade III/IV	2% subcutaneous fibrosis
Tsang 1998 [93] 1986–1996	185	7% acute oesophagitis and tracheitis; 0.6% spinal chord necrosis in patient with metastasis in vertebral column	5% significant neck fibrosis; 0.6% acute myel. leukaemia (✝); 0.6% aspiration pneumonia (✝); 0.6% postop. infection (✝); 0.6% perforated peptic ulcer due to analgesics (✝)
Kim 2003 [40]	23	100% mild oesophagitis and tracheitis	None
MSDS 2003 [6, 78] 2000–2003	22	See Fig. 8.3	

Patients irradiated: total number of patients receiving RTx. Lhermitte's sign: sudden paresthesias when the patient flexes their head

microscopic (R1) or macroscopic (R2) tumour residues if a repeat-operation and/or elimination by ^{131}I-therapy are not possible. For locally invasive DTC pT4 R0, RTx is no longer recommended except in controlled trials such as MSDS and assuming negative results from ^{131}I scintigraphy before start of RTx [17]. Guidelines published by German radio-oncologists recommend RTx routinely in the case of locally invasive DTC independent of nodal status (pT4 N0/1/x) and, based on a judgement of the patient's risk profile, in nodal-positive disease (T1–3 N1) [81] in line with the 1995 Freiburg consensus [68]. In contrast, American guidelines merely state that RTx "may be beneficial" in patients with poorly differentiated tumours that do not concentrate ^{131}I and "may be considered" in patients who have gross evidence of local invasion and who are presumed to have microscopic residual disease after primary surgical treatment [31]. None of the guidelines are evidence-based, i.e. based on a systematic literature review [3].

8.4 Discussion

Only 2 of 19 studies found a statistically significant improvement in local control *in the presence of ^{131}I therapy*: Farahati et al., from Germany, in 1996 in PTC pT4 N1 over 40 years [21], and Kim et al., in South Korea, in PTC pT4 or N1 [40]. It this context it is of note that Tsang et al. found that ^{131}I therapy was more effective than RTx in preventing recurrences in the thyroid bed [93].

Only 3 of 19 studies demonstrated a statistically significant benefit in terms of survival *in the presence of ^{131}I therapy*: Leisner et al., from Germany, in 1982 in pT4 DTC [45], Chow et al., from Hong Kong, in 2002 in R2-resected PTC [14], and Kim et al., in South Korea, in 2003 in pT4 or N1 PTC [40]. In Farahati's study in 1996, the number of patients in each arm was too small (21 vs 20) for the effect of RTx on mortality to (no versus five deaths) to reach statistical significance [21]. It is unclear why none of the North American trials could reproduce the German and South Korean results in patients with pT4 DTC. Both the inconsistent use of ^{131}I therapy, the more limited RTx target volumes and the lower tissue doses may have contributed to this. Two studies indicate that doses should be more than 50 Gy [20, 95], as stipulated by current guidelines.

It is subject to debate how far the studies which show a benefit of RTx represent the same diagnostic and therapeutic standard as in today's specialised centres in central Europe or North America. Recent data from the MSDS trial indicate that endocrine surgery as a whole has noticeably improved in Germany since 1996 [5]. In our own cohort of more than 1,000 patients treated and followed up at the Department of Nuclear Medicine since 1988, we have achieved excellent long-term results without the addition of RTx to our treatment protocol [46] except for patients with lowly differentiated or inoperable R2-resected DTC. Increased sensitivity in diagnosing recurrences may also mean that a recurrence in today's terms of a 10-mm lesion in the thyroid bed discovered by high-resolution ultrasound no longer represents the same risk to the patient's wellbeing as a symptomatic or palpable recurrence diagnosed in the 1980s, then responsible for 38 % of all tumour-related deaths [70].

However, the outlined wait-and-see approach requires meticulous follow-up in a specialised centre [9, 43] by means of serum hTg under TSH stimulation, possibly hTg under TSH suppression [4], high-resolution ultrasound, ^{131}I whole-body scanning and – in selected cases – FDG-PET [8], so that recurrences, particularly those in the thyroid bed, are recognised before the patient becomes symptomatic. If recurrences are operated at a leading centre for endocrine surgery, local control can be achieved with minimal morbidity. Where this level of care is unavailable, however, we still see a role for RTx in DTC pT4 and/or R1 in addition to ^{131}I therapy. We do not see a role in nodal-positive disease pT1–3 N1. First, only one study with very small patient numbers has indicated potential benefit [40]. Second, clinically relevant lymph node metastases in the lateral cervical compartments are as a rule palpable and can be operated before they cause serious complications. In contrast, symptoms from disease in the thyroid bed or central compartment usually indicate that significant complications such as recurrent laryngeal nerve invasion have already occurred.

The benefits of RTx have to be balanced against the toxicity. With modern 3-D-planning techniques, serious chronic toxicity such as in the spinal cord is the exception. However, significant acute toxicity occurs (cf. Fig. 8.3), if somewhat less frequently than for RTx of oral cancer [44]. Regardless of further improvements in planning techniques, acute toxicity in the pharynx and oesophagus is unavoidable because these are directly adjacent to the target volume. If one takes the assumptions underlying the MSDS trial's power calculation (Fig. 8.1) for granted – better data will be available after long-term follow-up of the MSDS cohort – only 1 in 10 patients receiving RTx will benefit in terms of one avoided recurrence. Views on what constitutes acceptable toxicity in DTC differ in the medical community. Admittedly, the acute side-effects are fully reversible [78]. Ultimately, the patient decides.

Regrettably, none of the two planned randomised trials on RTx was able to recruit a sufficient number of patients. Discussion on inaugurating a randomised trial in Germany began in 1982 [45]. The MSDS experience suggests that the window of opportunity for such a trial is now closed and that the definitive answer on the clinical benefit of RTx for the treatment of DTC will never be reached.

Acknowledgements. We thank the Deutsche Krebshilfe, sponsor of the MSDS trial (project No. 70–2294), and all members of the MSDS study group for their cooperation. A full list of all trial participants has been published [6].

References

1. Adamietz IA, Schiemann MS, Petkauskas JG, Schemmann F, Bottcher HD (1998) Prognostic factors and the effect of radiotherapy in the treatment of differentiated thyroid carcinomas. Strahlenther Onkol 174:618–623
2. Bal C, Padhy AK, Jana S, Pant GS, Basu AK (1996) Prospective randomised clinical trial to evaluate the optimal dose of ^{131} I for remnant ablation in patients with differentiated thyroid carcinoma. Cancer 77:2574–2580
3. Belin RM, Ladenson PW, Robinson KA, Powe NR (2002) Development and use of evidence-based clinical practice guidelines for thyroid disease. Endocrinol Metab Clin North Am 31:795–817
4. Biermann M, Nofer JR, Riemann B, Lu J, Wilde J, Schober O (2004) Clinical evaluation of a new highly sensitive thyroglobulin assay (Nichols Advantage) in 99 patients with differentiated thyroid cancer (DTC) after total thyroidectomy (abstract). Clin Chem 50: A73

5. Biermann M, Pixberg MK, Schober O (2003) Changing patterns of care for locally advanced differentiated thyroid carcinoma (DTC) in German-speaking Europe since 1996 (abstract). Eur J Nucl Med 30:S155
6. Biermann M, Pixberg MK, Schuck A, Heinecke A, Köpcke W, Schmid KW, Dralle H, Willich N, Schober O, for the MSDS study group (2003) Multicenter Study Differentiated Thyroid Carcinoma (MSDS): diminished acceptance of adjuvant external beam radiotherapy for differentiated thyroid carcinoma. Nuklearmedizin 42:244–250
7. Biermann M, Schober O (2002) GCP-compliant management of the Multicentric Study Differentiated Thyroid Carcinoma (MSDS) with a relational database under Oracle 8i. Inform Biom Epidemiol Med Biol 33:441–459
8. Biermann M, Schober O (2003) Should High hTG levels in absence of iodine uptake be treated? Eur J Nucl Med 30:160–163
9. Biermann M, Schober O (2002) How many high-risk patients with differentiated thyroid carcinoma does a "tumor center" need per year? (Editorial) Nuklearmedizin 41:61–62
10. Brearley MJ, Hayes AM, Murphy S (1999) Hypofractionated radiation therapy for invasive thyroid carcinoma in dogs: a retrospective analysis of survival. J Small Anim Pract 40:206–210
11. Brierley JD, Tsang RW (1999) External-beam radiation therapy in the treatment of differentiated thyroid cancer. Semin Surg Oncol 16:42–49
12. Casara D, Rubello D, Saladini G, Masarotto G, Favero A, Girelli ME, Busnardo B (1993) Different features of pulmonary metastases in differentiated thyroid cancer: natural history and multivariate statistical analysis of prognostic variables. J Nucl Med 34:1626–1631
13. Chebotareva ED, Shishkina VV, Siniuta BF, Dzhuzha DA, Cheren'ko SM, Sheptukha AI, Gorobeiko MB, Ivanov NA (2002) Analysis of efficacy of complex treatment of patients with differentiated forms of the thyroid gland cancer using distant radiation therapy. Klin Khir pp 25–28
14. Chow SM, Law SC, Mendenhall WM, Au SK, Chan PT, Leung TW, Tong CC, Wong IS, Lau WH (2002) Papillary thyroid carcinoma: prognostic factors and the role of radioiodine and external radiotherapy. Int J Radiat Oncol Biol Phys 52:784–795
15. Chow SM, Law SC, Mendenhall WM, Au SK, Yau S, Yuen KT, Law CC, Lau WH (2002) Follicular thyroid carcinoma: prognostic factors and the role of radioiodine. Cancer 95:488–498
16. Chung CT, Sagerman RH, Ryoo MC, King GA, Yu WS, Dalai PS, Emmanuel IG (1980) External irradiation for malignant thyroid tumors. Radiology 136:753–756
17. Deutsche Krebsgesellschaft (2002) Malignant thyroid tumors. In: Concise interdisciplinary guidelines 2002. Zuckschwerdt, Germering
18. Egger M, Davey Smith G, Schneider M, Minder C (1997) Bias in meta-analysis detected by a simple, graphical test. BMJ 315:629–634
19. Eichhorn W, Tabler H, Lippold R, Lochmann M, Schreckenberger M, Bartenstein P (2003) Prognostic factors determining long-term survival in well-differentiated thyroid cancer: an analysis of four hundred eighty-four patients undergoing therapy and aftercare at the same institution. Thyroid 13:949–958
20. Esik O, Nemeth G, Eller J (1994) Prophylactic external irradiation in differentiated thyroid cancer: a retrospective study over a 30-year observational period. Oncology 51:372–379
21. Farahati J, Reiners C, Stuschke M, Muller SP, Stuben G, Sauerwein W, Sack H (1996) Differentiated thyroid cancer. Impact of adjuvant external radiotherapy in patients with perithyroidal tumor infiltration (stage pT4). Cancer 77:172–180
22. Foote RL, Brown PD, Garces YI, McIver B, Kasperbauer JL (2003) Is there a role for radiation therapy in the management of Hurthle cell carcinoma? Int J Radiat Oncol Biol Phys 56:1067–1072

23. Ford D, Giridharan S, McConkey C, Hartley A, Brammer C, Watkinson JC, Glaholm J (2003) External beam radiotherapy in the management of differentiated thyroid cancer. Clin Oncol (R Coll Radiol) 15:337–341
24. Gimm O, Rath FW, Dralle H (1998) Pattern of lymph node metastases in papillary thyroid carcinoma. Br J Surg 85:252–254
25. Glanzmann C, Horst W (1979) Treatment and prognosis of follicular and papillary thyroid carcinoma. Strahlentherapie 155:223–229
26. Glanzmann C, Lütolf UM (1992) Long-term follow-up of 92 patients with locally advanced follicular or papillary thyroid cancer after combined treatment. Strahlenther Onkol 168:260–269
27. Glanzmann C, Lütolf UM (1992) Papillary and follicular thyroid carcinoma: Long-term follow-up of 339 patients at Zurich University Hospital between 1960 and 1988, and review. Schweiz Rundsch Med 81:457–467
28. Hare HF (1941) Radiation treatment of carcinoma of the thyroid. Am J Roentgenol 46:451–453
29. Harmer C, Bidmead M, Shepherd S, Sharpe A, Vini L (1998) Radiotherapy planning techniques for thyroid cancer. Br J Radiol 71:1069–1075
30. Harmer CL (1977) External beam radiotherapy for thyroid cancer. Ann Radiol Paris 20:791–800
31. Hay ID, Thompson GB, Grant CS, Bergstralh EJ, Dvorak CE, Gorman CA, Maurer MS, McIver B, Mullan BP, Oberg AL et al (2002) Papillary thyroid carcinoma managed at the Mayo Clinic during six decades (1940–1999): temporal trends in initial therapy and long-term outcome in 2444 consecutively treated patients. World J Surg 26:879–885
32. Hedinger C, Williams ED, Sobin LH (1989) The WHO histological classification of thyroid tumors: a commentary on the second edition. Cancer 63:908–911
33. Heinze HG, Schmeis E (1976) Malignome der Schilddrüse. Behandlungsergebnisse bei 305 Patienten. Strahlentherapie 152:114
34. Hölzer S, Reiners C, Mann K, Bamberg M, Rothmund M, Dudeck J, Stewart AK, Hundahl SA (2000) Patterns of care for patients with primary differentiated carcinoma of the thyroid gland treated in Germany during 1996. Cancer 89:192–201
35. Hölzer S, Steiner D, Bauer R, Reiners C, Farahati J, Hundahl SA, Dudeck J (2000) Current practice of radioiodine treatment in the management of differentiated thyroid cancer in Germany. Eur J Nucl Med 27:1465–1472
36. Hundahl SA, Cady B, Cunningham MP, Mazzaferri EL, McKee R, Rosai J, Shah JP, Fremgen AM, Stewart AK, Hölzer S (2000) Initial results from a prospective cohort study of 5583 cases of thyroid carcinoma treated in the United States during 1996. Cancer 89:202–217
37. Jacobson F (1954) Treatment of carcinoma of the thyroid. Acta Radiol 41:169–192
38. Jarzab B (2001) Indications for adjuvant therapy of thyroid cancer with radioiodine therapy. Wiad Lek 54 [Suppl 1]:254–265
39. Kim S, Wei JP, Braveman JM, Brams DM (2004) Predicting outcome and directing therapy for papillary thyroid carcinoma. Arch Surg 139:390–394
40. Kim TH, Yang DS, Jung KY, Kim CY, Choi MS (2003) Value of external irradiation for locally advanced papillary thyroid cancer. Int J Radiat Oncol Biol Phys 55:1006–1012
41. Kleinert G (1989) Results of external beam radiotherapy for thyroid cancer. Radiobiol Radiother 30:473–480
42. Kuijpens JL, Hansen B, Hamming JF, Ribot JG, Haak HR, Coebergh JW (1998) Trends in treatment and long-term survival of thyroid cancer in southeastern Netherlands, 1960–1992. Eur J Cancer 34:1235–1241
43. Kumar H, Daykin J, Holder R, Watkinson JC, Sheppard MC, Franklyn JA (2001) An audit of management of differentiated thyroid cancer in specialist and non-specialist clinic settings. Clin Endocrinol (Oxf) 54:719–723

44. Lee D, Cosmatos D, Marcial V (1995) Results of an RTOG phase III trial (RTOG 85–27) comparing radiotherapy plus etonidazole with radiotherapy alone for locally advanced head and neck cancer. Int J Radiat Oncol Biol Phys 32:567–576
45. Leisner B, Degelmann G, Dirr W, Kanitz W, Bull U, Langhammer H, Lissner J, Pabst HW (1982) Therapeutic results of malignant goiter 1960–1980. Significance of percutaneous radiotherapy in well differentiated carcinomas. Dtsch Med Wochenschr 107:1702–1707
46. Lerch H, Schober O, Kuwert T, Saur HB (1997) Survival of differentiated thyroid carcinoma studied in 500 patients. J Clin Oncol 15:2067–2075
47. Li WB, Friedland W, Pomplun E, Jacob P, Paretzke HG, Lassmann M, Reiners C (2001) Track structures and dose distributions from decays of (131)I and (125)I in and around water spheres simulating micrometastases of differentiated thyroid cancer. Radiat Res 156:419–429
48. Lin JD, Liou MJ, Chao TC, Weng HF, Ho YS (1999) Prognostic variables of papillary and follicular thyroid carcinoma patients with lymph node metastases and without distant metastases. Endocr Relat Cancer 6:109–115
49. Mabille JP (1961) Résultats thérapeutiques des cancers throidiens. Ann Radiol 4:477–491
50. Maxon HR, Englaro EE, Thomas SR, Hertzberg VS, Hinnefeld JD, Chen LS, Smith H, Cummings D, Aden MD (1992) Radioiodine-^{131} therapy for well-differentiated thyroid cancer – a quantitative radiation dosimetric approach: outcome and validation in 85 patients. J Nucl Med 33:1132–1136
51. Mazzaferri EL, Jhiang SM (1994) Long-term impact of initial surgical and medical therapy on papillary and follicular thyroid cancer. Am J Med 97:418–428
52. Mazzaferri EL, Kloos RT (2001) Current approaches to primary therapy for papillary and follicular thyroid cancer. J Endocrinol Metab 86:1447–1463
53. Mazzaferri EL, Young RL (1981) Papillary thyroid carcinoma: a 10-year follow-up report of the impact of therapy in 576 patients. Am J Med 70:511–518
54. Mazzaferri EL, Young RL, Oertel JE, Kemmerer WT, Page CP (1977) Papillary thyroid carcinoma: the impact of therapy in 576 patients. Medicine (Baltimore) 56:171–96
55. Müller-Gärtner H-W, Brzac HT, Rehpenning W (1991) Prognostic indices for tumor relapse and tumor mortality in follicular thyroid carcinoma. Cancer 67:1903–1911
56. Nakashima T, Yano G, Nomura Y, Tomita K, Wada S, Hata K (1994) Use of a remote controlled radiotherapy afterloading system to manage unresectable, metastatic thyroid cancer in the trachea. Eur Arch Otorhinolaryngol 251 [Suppl 1]:S73–S75
57. Nutting CM, Convery DJ, Cosgrove VP, Rowbottom C, Vini L, Harmer C, Dearnaley DP, Webb S (2001) Improvements in target coverage and reduced spinal cord irradiation using intensity-modulated radiotherapy (IMRT) in patients with carcinoma of the thyroid gland. Radiother Oncol 60:173–180
58. O'Connell ME, RP AH, Harmer CL (1994) Results of external beam radiotherapy in differentiated thyroid carcinoma: a retrospective study from the Royal Marsden Hospital. Eur J Cancer 30A:733–739
59. Pack L, Roberts RE, Dawson SD, Dookwah HD (2001) Definitive radiation therapy for infiltrative thyroid carcinoma in dogs. Vet Radiol Ultrasound 42:471–474
60. Pape E (2002) External beam radiotherapy for medullary carcinoma with metastases. In: Feldkamp J, Scherbaum WA (eds) Medullary thyroid cancer. De Gruyter, Berlin, pp 83–63
61. Pemberton JdJ, Black BM (1939) Malignant lesions of the thyroid gland: review of 774 cases. Surg Gynaecol Obstet 69:417–430
62. Phlips P, Hanzen C, Andry G, van Houtte P, Fruuling J (1993) Postoperative irradiation for thyroid cancer. Eur J Surg Oncol 19:399–404
63. Pineda JD, Lee T, Ain K, Reynolds JC, Robbins J (1995) Iodine-131 therapy for thyroid cancer patients with elevated thyroglobulin and negative diagnostic scan. J Endocrinol Metab 80:1488–1492

64. Pollinger B, Duhmke E (2001) External radiotherapy of thyroid cancer. Onkologie 24:134–138
65. Portmann UV (1941) Experience in the treatment of malignant tumors of the thyroid gland. Am J Roentgenol 46:454–466
66. Puskás C, Biermann M, Willich N, Schober O (2001) Percutaneous radiation therapy. In: Biersack H-J, Grünwald F (eds) Thyroid cancer. Springer, Berlin Heidelberg New York, pp 121–129
67. Reiners C (2003) Radioiodtherapie des differenzierten Schilddrüsenkarzinoms. Arzneimitteltherapie 2:39–47
68. Reinhardt M, Guttenberger R, Slanina J, Frommhold H, Moser E (1995) Indications for external beam radiotherapy in thyroid carcinoma. The Freiburg consensus. Radiologe 35:535–539
69. Rossi RL, Cady B, Silverman M, Wool S, ReMine SG, Hodge MB, Salzman FA (1988) Surgically incurable well-differentiated thyroid carcinoma. Prognostic factors and results of therapy. Arch Surg 123:569–574
70. Samaan NA, Schultz PN, Hickey RC, Goepfert H, Haynie TP, Johnston DA, Ordonez NG (1992) The results of various modalities of treatment of well differentiated thyroid carcinomas: a retrospective review of 1,599 patients. J Clin Endocrinol Metab 75:714–720
71. Sautter-Bihl ML, Heinze HG (1992) External radiotherapy of differentiated thyroid carcinoma. Dtsch Med Wochenschr 117:665–668
72. Sautter-Bihl ML, Herbold G, Heinze HG, Bihl H (1991) Postoperative external beam radiation in differentiated thyroid cancer: situations in which radioiodine is insufficient? Some dosimetric considerations with Monte Carlo techniques. Strahlenther Onkol 167:267–272
73. Sautter-Bihl M-L, Raub J, Hetzel-Sesterheim M, Heinze HG (2001) Differentiated thyroid cancer: prognostic factors and influence of treatment on the outcome in 441 patients. Strahlenther Onkol 177:125–131
74. Scheumann GFW, Dralle H (1992) External radiotherapy of differentiated thyroid carcinoma (letter). Dtsch Med Wochenschr 117:1576–1577
75. Schlumberger M, Challeton C, de Vathaire F, Travagli JP, Gardet P, Lumbroso JD, Francese C, Fontaine F (1996) Radioactive iodine treatment and external radiotherapy for lung and bone metastases of differentiated thyroid carcinoma. J Nucl Med 37:398–605
76. Schlumberger M, Pacini F (2003) Thyroid tumors. Éditions Nucléon, Paris
77. Schuck A, Biermann M, Müller S, Schober O, Willich N (2001) Adjuvant percutaneous radiotherapy in the treatment of differentiated thyroid cancer. Nuklearmediziner 24:225–229
78. Schuck A, Biermann M, Pixberg MK, Müller S, Schober O, Willich N (2003) Acute toxicity of adjuvant radiotherapy in locally advanced differentiated thyroid cancer: First results of the Multicenter Study Differentiated Thyroid Cancer (MSDS). Strahlenther Onkol 179:821–827
79. Schümichen C, Schmitt E, Scheuffele C, Blattmann H, Pauli-Harnasch C (1983) Einfluss des Therapiekonzepts auf die Prognose des Schilddrüsenkarzinoms. Nuklearmedizin 23:87–105
80. Seegenschmidt MH, Sauer R (1993) The systematics of acute and chronic radiation sequelae. Strahlenther Onkol 169:83–95
81. Seegenschmiedt MH, Sautter-Bihl ML, Schmitt G, Willich N, Müller R-P (1998) Guidelines in radiooncology. External beam radiotherapy of malignant struma. AWMF-Guideline registry no. 052/001. http://www.awmf-online.de
82. Sheline GE, Galante M, Lindsay S (1966) Radiation therapy in the control of persistent thyroid cancer. Am J Roentgenol 97:923–930
83. Simpson WJ (1990) Radioiodine and radiotherapy in the management of thyroid cancers. Otolaryngol Clin North Am 23:509–521
84. Simpson WJ, Carruthers JS (1978) The role of external radiation in the management of papillary and follicular thyroid cancer. Am J Surg 136:457–460

85. Simpson WJ, Panzarella T, Carruthers JS, Gospodarowicz MK, Sutcliffe SB (1988) Papillary and follicular thyroid cancer: impact of treatment in 1,578 patients. Int J Radiat Oncol Biol Phys 14:1063–1075
86. Simpson WJ, Sutcliffe SB, Gospodarowicz MK (1994) The thyroid. In: Cox JD (ed) Moss' radiation oncology: rationale, technique, results, 7th edn. Mosby International, St. Louis, pp 280–304
87. Sisson JC, Jamadar DA, Kazerooni EA, Giordano TJ, Carey JE, Spaulding SA (1998) Treatment of micronodular lung metastases of papillary thyroid cancer: are the tumors too small for effective irradiation from radioiodine? Thyroid 8:215–21
88. Smedal MI, Salzman FA, Meissner WA (1967) The value of 2 mV roentgen-ray therapy in differentiated thyroid carcinoma. Am J Roentgenol Radium Ther Nucl Med 99:352–364
89. Sugg SL, Ezzat S, Rosen IB, Freeman JL, Asa SL (1998) Distinct multiple RET/PTC gene rearrangements in multifocal papillary thyroid neoplasia. J Endocrinol Metab 83:4116–4122
90. Taylor T, Specker B, Robbins J, Sperling M, Ho M, Ain K, Bigos ST, Brierley J, Cooper D, Haugen B et al (1998) Outcome after treatment of high-risk papillary and non-Hurthle-cell follicular thyroid carcinoma. Ann Intern Med 129:622–627
91. Theon AP, Marks SL, Feldman ES, Griffey S (2000) Prognostic factors and patterns of treatment failure in dogs with unresectable differentiated thyroid carcinomas treated with megavoltage irradiation. J Am Vet Med Assoc 216:1775–1779
92. Thomusch O, Dralle H (2000) Endocrine surgery and evidence-based medicine. Chirurg 71:635–645
93. Tsang RW, Brierley JD, Simpson WJ, Panzarella T, Gospodarowicz MK, Sutcliffe SB (1998) The effects of surgery, radioiodine, and external radiation therapy on the clinical outcome of patients with differentiated thyroid carcinoma. Cancer 82:375–388
94. Tubiana M, Haddad E, Schlumberger M, Hill C, Rougier P, Sarrazin D (1985) External radiotherapy in thyroid cancers. Cancer 55:2062–2071
95. Tubiana M, Tacour J, Monnier J, Bergiron C, Gerard-Marchand R, Roujeau J, Bok B, Parmentier C (1975) External radiotherapy and radioiodine in the treatment of 359 thyroid cancers. Br J Radiol 48:894–907
96. Udelsman R, Lakatos E, Landenson P (1996) Optimal surgery for papillary thyroid carcinoma. World J Surg 20:88–93
97. Windeyer BW (1954) Cancer of the thyroid and radiotherapy. Br J Radiol 27:537–552
98. Wittekind C, Wagner G (1997) TNM classification of malignant tumors. Springer, Berlin Heidelberg New York
99. Wu XL, Hu YH, Li QH, Guo JR, Sun D, Yan JH, Xu GZ, Qin DX, Ha XW, Gu XZ (1987) Value of postoperative radiotherapy for thyroid cancer. Head Neck Surg 10:107–112
100. Young RL, Mazzaferri EL, Rahe AJ, Dorfman SG (1980) Pure follicular thyroid carcinoma: impact of therapy in 214 patients. J Nucl Med 21:733–737

Chapter 9

Thyroid Cancer: Treatment with Thyroid Hormone 9

P.-M. Schumm-Draeger

9.1 Introduction

All patients with thyroid cancer must be treated with thyroid hormone after thyroidectomy for correction of surgically induced hypothyroidism and to suppress stimulated growth of persistent or recurrent thyroid cancer by reducing thyroid-stimulating hormone (TSH) levels.

TSH mainly controls growth and differentiation of normal thyroid follicular cells. Secreted by the pituitary gland it is a glycoprotein composed of an alpha and a beta subunit (normal serum TSH concentrations: 0.4–4 μU/ml). After binding with its membrane receptor, TSH stimulates follicular cell proliferation and differentiation functions, including iodine uptake, thyroglobulin synthesis and thyroid hormone production. Thyrotropin releasing hormone (TRH) stimulates TSH secretion, increases thyroid hormones (thyroxin, T4) and decreases TSH secretion by means of a feedback mechanism mainly at the pituitary level after local conversion into T3 by the enzyme 5'-deiodinase type 2.

The main principles of thyroid hormone treatment and its clinical implications (monitoring and adjustment of hormone dosage to clinical situations, side effects) will be summarized here.

9.2 Rationale of Thyroid Hormone Therapy

Experimental and clinical data have shown that thyroid cell proliferation and differentiation is mainly TSH dependent. Therefore, TSH secretion has to be inhibited via thyroid hormone therapy in all patients treated for differentiated thyroid cancer.

Thyroid hormone therapy decreases TSH secretion and expression of characteristic signs of follicular cell differentiation. Before administration of radioiodine, thyroid hormone therapy must be interrupted (4 weeks on average) for diagnosis or treatment of thyroid cancer. Radioiodine uptake, thyroglobulin synthesis and its secretion by thyroid cancer cells will be stimulated by increased TSH levels.

9.3 Effects on Thyroid Growth

The rationale for thyroid hormone therapy in patients with differentiated thyroid cancer has been evaluated by numerous studies.

Experimental studies have shown that conditions of increased TSH (e.g., goitrogens, iodine deficiency or partial thyroidectomy) enhance the development of thyroid cancer especially in irradiated animals. Thyroid cancer also occurs in rats chronically fed with the goitrogen thiouracil [10, 19]. Reduction of TSH secretion (thyroid hormone therapy, hypophysectomy in animals) can prevent thyroid tumor development [24].

In vitro, TSH stimulates thyroid cell proliferation. Functional TSH receptor has been found in the majority of differentiated thyroid carcinomas [8].

Clinical studies have demonstrated that TSH is correlated with the progression of thyroid cancer. Dunhill et al. [11] were the first to observe a regression of papillary thyroid cancer in two patients treated with thyroid hormone. Dramatic regression of metastatic thyroid cancer in a patient with thyroid hormone therapy was later reported by Balme. [1]. Since then thyroid hormone has been a basic principle that is included in the guidelines of thyroid cancer therapy. In many cases lymph node or distant metastases increase in size during prolonged periods of thyroid hormone withdrawal, while shrinkage is found after thyroid hormone therapy. In addition, thyroid hormone treatment has been found to reduce the recurrence rate and cancer-related mortality in clinical studies [9, 22, 25].

9.4 Effects on Differentiation of Thyroid Cells

Thyroid cell differentiation is TSH dependent. Metastases from differentiated thyroid cancer retain several biological functions characteristic of the normal thyroid cell (iodine uptake, thyroglobulin, synthesis and secretion). As with normal thyroid cells, also thyroid cancer cells' differentiation is TSH dependent; radioiodine uptake of metastases correlates with high serum TSH levels. Serum thyroglobulin concentration also correlates with hypothyroidism and high serum TSH levels in patients with persistent/recurrent disease, even without radioiodine uptake. In conclusion, TSH stimulates functional properties and probably growth of differentiated thyroid carcinomas after long-term withdrawal of thyroid hormone therapy [29, 30, 32].

9.5 Optimal Level of TSH Suppression in Patients with Differentiated Thyroid Cancer

Suppression of endogenous secretion should always be maintained in patients with differentiated thyroid cancer. In persistent/recurrent disease an undetectable TSH level is seen to be beneficial [25]. Up to now it has not been proven, however, whether an undetectable TSH level is superior to a detectable TSH level [3]. Reduction of serum thyroglobulin (Tg) concentration is achieved with doses of thyroid hormone that reduce serum TSH to very low but not undetectable levels [6].

In contrast, undifferentiated thyroid carcinomas and medullary thyroid carcinomas derived from parafollicular C cells, which are not TSH dependent, do not benefit from TSH suppression and only require replacement therapy after thyroidectomy.

9.6 Treatment with Thyroid Hormones

The drug of choice for the long-term treatment of thyroid carcinoma is levothyroxine (L-T4). L-T4 is the main hormone produced by the thyroid gland and converted to the active form of thyroid hormone, triiodothyronine (T3), mainly in the liver. This mechanism also operates after oral administration of L-T4, thereby reproducing the physiological situation. As serum T3 levels are stable following L-T4 administration in contrast to direct oral administration of T3, hormone therapy with T3 is not indicated [2, 7, 21].

9.7 Pharmacology of Thyroid Hormones (Levothyroxine, L-T4)

The optimal dose of L-T4 has to be well defined for each patient, can remain constant over time in most patients and can be achieved without repeated blood tests. The actual purity of T4 preparations is close to 100% with a variation of 3%. Bioavailability may vary between different preparations. If possible each patient should always receive the same preparation.

Several old preparations of thyroid hormone extracts have no place in the treatment of thyroid carcinoma and no particular advantages over L-T4. The recommendation of replacement doses of L-T4 combined with TRIAC (tri-iodo-acetic acid), a thyromimetic drug, has not been found to be an improvement on the therapy as TRIAC has similar effects both at the pituitary level and on peripheral tissues [23].

L-T3 is not indicated in long-term treatment of thyroid carcinoma. Before administration of diagnostic or therapeutic doses of ^{131}I or for a few days when L-T4 therapy is resumed after withdrawal, L-T3 therapy has been found to be useful [7].

As L-T4 has a blood half-life of 6–8 days, a single daily dose is sufficient. After oral administration, up to 80% of L-T4 is absorbed from the gut with interindividual variability [14]. Food intake is an important factor that reduces L-T4 absorption, and patients should be informed that they should ingest their L-T4 dose on an empty stomach, preferably early in the morning, 20–30 min before breakfast. Several substances are known to interfere with L-T4 absorption in the gut [14, 34], which has to be considered in patients who instead of a suppressive dose of L-T4, present with inappropriate serum TSH concentrations. Several chronic diseases (regional enteritis, pancreatic disease, cirrhosis) can induce decreased L-T4 absorption. Elevated serum TSH, due to anti-mouse antibody interference in the assay system, has also been described [16].

9.8 Optimal Dosage and Adjustment of L-T4 in Thyroid Cancer Patients According to Disease Status

After total thyroidectomy and ^{131}I ablation in patients with thyroid cancer the daily L-T4 dose to suppress TSH secretion is higher than the L-T4 dose needed in patients with spontaneous hypothyroidism [2, 6]. The L-T4-dose is correlated with body weight and ranges between 1.8 and 2.8 µg/kg/day. Age also has an effect on the dose. Younger patients, and especially children, require higher doses per kilogram of body weight. The mean dose of L-T4 necessary to suppress serum TSH in athyreotic patients, progressively decreases from 3.4 µg/kg in patients aged 6–20 years to 2.8 µg/kg in those aged 21–40 years, 2.6 µg/kg in those aged 41–60 years, and 2.4 µg/kg in subjects aged 61 and older. Further reduction of L-T4 dose often is needed in patients with severe heart disease [27, 28].

The effectiveness of L-T4 therapy is controlled by serum TSH measurement with ultra-sensitive assays, 3 months after surgical and radioiodine therapy. The suppressive L-T4 dose is achieved with serum TSH values less than 0.1 µU/ml and serum free T3 (FT3) concentrations within the normal range [2, 21]. Iatrogenic thyrotoxicosis has to be avoided.

Serum tetraiodothyronine (T4; FT4) is often increased by a factor of about 25% at 3–4 h after ingestion of the daily L-T4 dose. Therefore, patients should be advised not to take their medication in the morning before blood testing.

The daily dose of L-T4 has to be increased or decreased by 25 µg respectively in the case of either unsuppressed TSH levels or over-suppressed levels. Animal controls are sufficient after the suppressive L-T4 dose has been determined.

Adjustment of L-T4 dose is necessary during pregnancy [20] and in several chronic diseases. During pregnancy, blood determinations are performed every 2–3 months; frequently the L-T4 dosage has to be increased. L-T4 treatment does not affect the outcome of pregnancy, and pregnancy does not affect the outcome of thyroid cancer [31].

As ultrasensitive assays for TSH determination clearly define hypo-, eu- and hyperthyroidism, measurement of TRH-stimulated TSH gives no further information and is not required.

L-T4 suppressive therapy is safe and normally free of long-term adverse effects, provided the described guidelines for treatment are followed.

An important and controversial issue is whether L-T4 therapy initially given in suppressive doses to thyroid cancer patients should be continued throughout the patient's life or whether the degree of TSH suppression and L-T4 dose should be adapted to the clinical status. There is no doubt that patients with no evidence of persistent or recurrent disease or high risk of recurrence should be kept on suppressive therapy, in order to decrease the risk of tumor progression or recurrence [9]. In patients with evidence of complete cure (i.e., negative ^{131}I total body scan, undetectable serum thyroglobulin) the L-T4 dose may be decreased with the aim of achieving serum TSH levels between 0.1 and 0.5 μU/ml. Whether low but detectable TSH concentrations induce a higher risk of tumor recurrence in patients with thyroid cancer when compared to suppressed serum TSH concentrations needs further investigation. Baudin et al. [3] described 106 patients considered to be in complete remission, who were given L-T4 replacement therapy. During the 10 years of follow-up the mean serum TSH concentration was below 0.1 μU/ml in 2% of measurements, with levels ranging between 0.1 and 0.3 μU/ml in 23% of cases and above this value in 76%: no relapse was observed in the cohort, and the serum TG level was undetectable in all patients at the end of the study. More than 80% of patients with thyroid cancer belong to this group. In summary long-term suppressive therapy is warranted only in a minority of patients who are not cured and those with high risk of tumor recurrence.

9.9 Important Side Effects of L-T4 Suppressive Therapy

Side-effects of L-T4 therapy on target organs, mainly heart and bone, in patients requiring long-term suppressive L-T4 therapy is still controversial. Whether suppression of TSH secretion by L-T4 therapy induces an increase in circulating T4 levels and consequently leads to clinical or overt hyperthyroidism has to be further evaluated [15, 26].

9.9.1 Side Effects of L-T4 Therapy: Bone

Whereas early studies have shown that L-T4 suppressive therapy may be associated with variable degrees of bone loss (particularly at the cortical level and in postmenopausal women) subsequent studies have failed to demonstrate any decrease in bone mass in patients submitted to long-term L-T4 treatment [12, 21], nor any documented increase in a risk of fractures [18]. Calcium metabolism and markers of bone turnover in women on L-T4 were no different either with or without TSH suppression [13].

As presented by a meta-analysis of 15 available studies in women with subnormal L-T4 induced TSH levels a significant degree of bone loss was found in postmenopausal, but not in premenopausal women. No convincing evidence exists that patients with a history of thyroid hormone suppressive therapy have a higher incidence of fractures [18, 33]. Obviously the skeleton is not particularly affected by L-T4 suppressive therapy, although in postmenopausal women TSH suppression may contribute to bone loss. Estrogen replacement therapy should be considered particularly in postmenopausal women with simultaneous long-term suppressive L-T4 treatment.

9.9.2 Side Effects of L-T4 Therapy: Heart

Long-term TSH suppression has been associated with an increased nocturnal and daytime heart rate [4, 5, 17], frequent premature atrial beats, increased left ventricular regular mass index and systolic function, higher values of fractional shortening and rate-adjusted velocity of shortening [4]. Beta-blocker therapy has led to a substantial improvement of these abnormalities [5]. The clinical significance of these findings is not clear for young individuals who are on L-T4 therapy but otherwise healthy. In young individuals with long-term treatment no side effects to the heart have been demonstrated (no change in: morbidity, mortality, quality of life, incidence of cardiovascular diseases). However, in patients with severe heart disease L-T4 treatment has to be started at a low dose (25 μg/day) and increased very slowly (25 μg L-T4 every 2–3 weeks) in order to avoid deterioration of heart disease. In patients over 50 years old the daily L-T4 dose often has to be reduced and must be monitored carefully to avoid cardiac side effects [27, 28].

Is has to be emphasized that L-T4 suppressive therapy is safe and has no adverse effect on bone maturation, final height and pubertal development in children.

9.10 Conclusion

L-T4 treatment is a life-long therapy in patients with thyroid cancer. It is to be adapted for each patient according to their clinical status. In cured patients, the aim of therapy is to maintain serum TSH levels within a low but detectable range. In patients with persistent or recurrent disease, the aim is to maintain suppression of TSH but to avoid overt hyperthyroidism. The minimal possible L-T4 suppressive dose should be used. Adverse effects of L-T4 therapy are minimal both on the heart and bone; however, L-T4 may aggravate other underlying disorders.

References

1. Balme HW (1954) Metastatic carcinoma of the thyroid successfully treated with thyroxine. Lancet 1:812–813
2. Bartalena L, Martino E, Pacciarotti A, Grasso L, Aghini-Lombardi F, Buratti L, Bambini G, Breccia M, Pinchera A (1987) Factors affecting suppression of endogenous thyrotropin secretion by thyroxine treatment: retrospective analysis in athyreotic and goitrous patients. J Clin Endocrinol Metab 64:849–855
3. Baudin E, Schlumberger M (1994) Levothyroxine treatment in patients with differentiated thyroid carcinoma. In: Orgiazzi J, Leclere J (eds) The thyroid and tissues. Schattauer, Stuttgart, pp 213–215
4. Biondi B, Fazio S, Carella C, Amato G, Cittadini A, Lupoli G, Sacca L, Bessastella A, Lombardi G (1993) Cardiac effects of long-term thyrotropin-suppressive therapy with levothyroxine. J Clin Endocrinol Metab 77:334–338

5. Biondi B, Fazio S, Carella C, Sabatini D, Amato G, Cittadini A, Bellastella A, Lombardi G, Sacca L (1994) Control of adrenergic overactivity by b-blockade improves the quality of life in patients receiving long-term suppressive therapy with levothyroxine. J Clin Endocrinol Metab 78:1028–1033
6. Burmeister LA, Goumaz MO, Mariash CN, Oppenheimer JH (1992) Levothyroxine dose requirements for thyrotropin suppression in the treatment of differentiated thyroid cancer. J Clin Endocrinol Metab 75:344–350
7. Busnardo B, Bui F, Girelli ME (1983) Different rates of serum thyrotropin suppression after total body scan in patients with thyroid cancer: effect of regular doses of thyroxine and triiodothyronine. J Endocrinol Invest 6:35–40
8. Carayon P, Thomas-Morvan C, Castanas E, Tubiana M (1980) Human thyroid cancer: membrane thyrotropin binding and adenylate cyclase activity. J Clin Endocrinol Metab 51:915–920
9. Cooper DS, Specker B, Ho M, Sperling M, Ladenson PW, Ross DS, Ain KB, Bigos T, Brierley JD, Haugen BR, Klein I, Robbins J, Sherman SL, Taylor T, Maxon HR (1998) Thyrotropin suppression and disease progression in patients with differentiated thyroid cancer: results from National Thyroid Cancer Treatment Cooperative Registry. Thyroid 8:737–744
10. Doniach I (1963) Effects including carcinogenesis of I-131 and x-rays on the thyroid of experimental animals: a review. Health Phys 9:1357–1362
11. Dunhill TP (1937) Surgery of the thyroid gland (The Lettsomian Lectures). Br Med J 1:460–461
12. Franklyn JA, Betteridge J, Daxkin J, Holder R, Oates GD, Parle JV, Lilley J Heath DA, Sheppard MC (1992) Long term thyroxine treatment and bone mineral density. Lancet 340:9–13
13. Gam AN, Jensen GF, Hasselstrom K, Olsen M, Sierbaek Nielsen K (1991) Effect of thyroxine therapy on bone metabolism in substituted hypothyroid patients with normal or suppressed levels of TSH. J Endocrinol Invest 14:451–455
14. Hays MT (1989) Intestinal absorption and secretion of the thyroid hormones. Thyroid Today 12:1–9
15. Jennings PE, O'Malley BP, Griffin KE, Northover B, Rosenthal FD (1984) Relevance of increased serum thyroxine concentrations associated with normal serum triiodothyronine values in hypothyroid patients receiving thyroxine: a case for "tissue" thyrotoxicosis. Br Med J 289:1645–1647
16. Kahn BB, Weintraub BD, Csako G, Zweig MH (1988) Factitious elevation of thyrotropin in a new ultrasensitive assay: implications for the use of monoclonal antibodies in "sandwich" immunoassay. J Clin Endocrinol Metab 66:526–533
17. Ladenson PW (1993) Editorial: thyrotoxicosis and the heart: something old and something new. J. Clin Endocrinol Metab 77:332–333
18. Leese GP, Jung RT, Guthrie C, Waugh N, Browning MCK (1992) Morbidity in patients on L-thyroxine: a comparison of those with a normal TSH to those with a suppressed TSH. Clin Endocrinol 37:500–503
19. Lindsay S, Chaikoff IL (1964) The effects of irradiation on the thyroid gland with particular reference to the induction of thyroid neoplasms: a review. Cancer Res 24:1099–1107
20. Mandel SJ, Larsen PR, Seely EW, Brent GA (1990) Increased need for thyroxine during pregnancy in women with primary hypothyroidism. N Engl J Med 323:91–96
21. Marcocci C, Golia F, Bruno-Bossio G, Vignali E, Pinchera A (1994) A carefully monitored levothyroxine suppressive therapy is not associated with bone loss in premenopausal women. J Clin Endocrinol Metab 78:818–823
22. Mazzaferri EL, Jhiang SM (1994) Long-term impact of initial surgical and medical therapy on papillary and follicular thyroid cancer. Am J Med 97:418–428
23. Mechelany C, Schlumberger M, Challeton C, Comoy E, Parmentier C (1991) TRIAC (3,5,34-triiodothyroacetic acid) has parallel effects at the pituitary and peripheral tissue levels in thyroid cancer patients treated with L-thyroxine. Clin Endocrinol 35:123–128

24. Nadler NJ, Mandavia M, Goldberg M (1970) The effect of hypophysectomy on the experimental production of rat thyroid neoplasms. Cancer Res 30:1909–1911
25. Petersen K, Bengtsson C, Lapidus L, Lindstedt G, Nystrom E (1990) Morbidity, mortality and quality of life for patients treated with levothyroxine. Arch Intern Med 150:2077–2081
25. Pujol P, Daures JP, Nsakala N, Baldes L, Bringer J, Jaffiol C (1998) Degree of thyrotropin suppression as a prognostic determinant in differentiated thyroid cancer. J Clin Endocrinol Metab 81:4318–4323
26. Ross DS (1991) Monitoring L-thyroxine therapy: lessons from the effects of L-thyroxine on bone density. Am J Med 91:1–4
27. Sawin CT, Herman, T, Molitch ME, London MH, Kramer SM (1983) Aging and the thyroid. Decreased requirement of thyroid hormone in older hypothyroid patients. Am J Med 75:206–209
28. Sawin CT, Geller A, Wolf PA, Belanger AJ, Baker E, Bacharach P, Wilson PWF, Benjamin EJ, D'Agostino RB (1994) Low serum thyrotropin concentrations as a risk factor for a trial fibrillation in older persons. N Engl J Med 331:1249–1252
29. Schlumberger M, Charbord P, Fragu P, Lumbroso J, Parmentier C, Tubiana M (1980) Circulating thyroglobulin and thyroid hormones in patients with metastases of differentiated thyroid carcinoma: relationship to serum thyrotropin levels. J Clin Endocrinol Metab 51:513–519
30. Schlumberger M, Charbord P, Fragu P, Gardet P, Lumbroso J, Parmentier C, Tubiana M (1983) Relationship between TSH stimulation and radioiodine uptake in lung metastases of differentiated thyroid carcinoma. J Clin Endocrinol Metab 57:148–151
31. Schlumberger M, De Vathaire F, Ceccarelli C, Delisle MJ, Francese C, Couette JE, Pinchera A, Parmentier C (1996) Exposure to radioiodine (I-131) for scintigraphy or therapy does not preclude pregnancy in thyroid cancer patients. J Nucl Med 37:606–612
32. Schneider AB, Line BR, Goldman JM, Robbins J (1981) Sequential serum thyroglobulin determinations, 131-I scans and 131-I uptakes after tri-iodothyronine withdrawal in patients with thyroid cancer. J Clin Endocrinol Metab 53:1199–1206
33. Solomon BL, Wartofsky L, Burman KD (1993) Prevalence of fractures in postmenopausal women with thyroid disease. Thyroid 3:17–23
34. Uzzan B, Campos J, Cucherat M, Nony B, Boissel JP, Perret JY (1996) Effects on bone mass of long-term treatment with thyroid hormone: a meta-analysis. J Clin Endocrinol Metab 81:4278–4279
35. Wartofsky L (2000) Thyroid cancer. A comprehensive guide to clinical management. Humana Press, Totowa, New Jersey

Chapter 10

Treatment with Cytotoxic Drugs 10

B. Saller

10.1 Introduction

Experience with chemotherapy in patients with differentiated and undifferentiated thyroid cancer is limited, because most recurrent tumors respond well to surgery, radioiodine therapy, or external beam radiation. Cytotoxic drugs are almost exclusively used in patients with tumors that are not surgically resectable, not responsive to ^{131}I, and have already been treated by or are not amenable to external beam radiotherapy. The majority of patients with distant metastases that have lost their ability to concentrate ^{131}I die within 5 years. However, even those patients may stabilize over a period of months or even several years without specific therapy. Chemotherapy in differentiated thyroid cancer should therefore only be given in cases of progressive metastatic disease refractory to radioiodine treatment. Only in poorly differentiated and anaplastic carcinoma can chemotherapy following conventional treatment be approved from the beginning.

10.2 Results of Chemotherapy in Differentiated Thyroid Carcinoma

Clinical studies investigating the effect of chemotherapy in thyroid carcinoma are limited and mostly include only small numbers of patients. Moreover, data from patients with different histological types of thyroid cancer have been included in single series. As a result, some studies not only include patients with differentiated thyroid carcinoma in whom the usual therapeutic alternatives have been exhausted, but also patients with poorly differentiated and anaplastic carcinoma.

10.2.1 Monotherapy

Doxorubicin is an anthracycline and is the cytotoxic drug that has been most extensively studied in chemotherapy of thyroid cancer. It is rapidly eliminated from plasma and is metabolized by the liver. Doxorubicin, like all anthracyclines, is myelosuppressive and causes gastrointestinal toxicity. Long-term administration is limited by cumulative, dose-dependent cardiotoxicity. Irreversible cardiomyopathy is a significant risk in patients who have received total doses in excess of 500–550 mg/m^2. However, cardiac toxicity may also be induced by lower cumulative doses. Doxorubicin is contraindicated in patients with major cardiac diseases and in patients with impaired liver function.

In 1970, Bonadonna et al. first reported on the effectiveness of chemotherapy with doxorubicin in two patients with thyroid carcinoma [13]. Five years later, a series of 43 patients was published by Gottlieb et al. [29]. The patients had been treated by doxorubicin 75 mg/m^2 every 3 weeks, and complete or partial tumor responses were seen in 35% of patients. In 1978, this group reported the results in 53 patients, with 32% showing a partial or even complete tumor response [17]. During the following years, the effectiveness of doxorubicin was evaluated in several other studies. In a review of all published data [1], the overall response rate to doxorubicin was 38%, defined as a reduction in tumor mass. The usual effective dose was between 60 and 90 mg/m^2 every 3 weeks. Alternatively, 10 mg/m^2 once a week was given. The highest response can be observed in the case of pulmonary metastases, followed by bone metastases and local tumor growth. If thyroid carcinomas respond to chemotherapy, even by no change of tumor mass only, a prolongation of median survival rates from 3–5 months in nonresponders to 15–20 months in responders is suggested [1]. Doxorubicin at a dose below that used as monotherapy in cancer chemotherapy has been used as adjunctive therapy with external beam radiotherapy, but in differentiated thyroid cancer this approach may be no better than radiotherapy alone [37].

There is one report on the use of aclarubicin, a newer agent less cardiotoxic than doxorubicin, in the treatment of thyroid cancer [47]. Aclarubicin (25–30 mg/m^2) was given daily for 4 days and treatment was repeated every 3 weeks. A 22% response rate was seen in a group of 24 patients.

Bleomycin has been used as monotherapy in a limited number of patients with differentiated thyroid cancer [10, 33] and seems to be less effective than doxorubicin. A phase II evaluation of mitoxantrone in patients with advanced non-anaplastic thyroid cancer shows no beneficial effect. This is also the case with cisplatin monotherapy [21] and monotherapy with etoposide (VP-16) [41]. Somatostatin analogs have also failed to yield any tumor response in a small series of patients with advanced thyroid cancer [67].

10.2.2 Combination Chemotherapy

Doxorubicin as the cytotoxic drug with the best established effect in monotherapy has also been investigated in several combination therapy protocols.

10.2.2.1
Doxorubicin and Cisplatin

There have been two randomized studies on the effectiveness of a combination of doxorubicin and cisplatin compared with doxorubicin alone in patients with advanced thyroid carcinoma including some cases with anaplastic carcinoma. In the first study, 41 patients received doxorubicin (60 mg/m^2 every 3 weeks) as a single agent and partial response was seen in 7 patients (17%) [54]. With 3-weekly applications of doxorubicin (60 mg/m^2) and cisplatin (40 mg/m^2), 11 of 43 patients had either a partial or complete response (26%). The overall response rate was not significantly different between the two groups. However, complete tumor responses were seen only in the combined therapy group and lasted more than 2 years in 4 of 5 patients, leading the authors of this study to conclude that a combination of doxorubicin and cisplatin was superior to doxorubicin monotherapy. The second prospective study with doxorubicin and cisplatin was carried out in 22 patients with all cell types of advanced thyroid cancer [63]. In contrast to the first study, in this series there were only brief partial tumor responses in two cases (10%). Similarly, the combination of doxorubicin and cisplatin was found to be ineffective in a study reporting on chemotherapy results in 94 patients with metastatic differentiated thyroid carcinoma from the Institute Gustave-Roussy [21]. In all studies, life-threatening toxicities from chemotherapy occurred more often in patients treated with the combination of drugs and there was one case of a drug-related death while under treatment with doxorubicin and cisplatin [63].

Morris et al. [42] reported on a patient treated with cisplatin and doxorubicin in whom a repeat ^{131}I imaging after three cycles of chemotherapy showed significant ^{131}I uptake in previously non-iodine-concentrating lesions. The patient was subsequently treated with 200 mCi ^{131}I. This effect may either be due to a differentiating effect of chemotherapy on the tumor cells or to a selective cytotoxicity against nonfunctional, less-differentiated thyroid cancer cells.

10.2.2.2
Doxorubicin and Bleomycin

The combination of doxorubicin (75 mg/m^2 every 3 weeks) with bleomycin (intramuscular application of 30 mg once a week) did not appear to be superior to doxorubicin monotherapy [10]. In this study, an overall tumor response to doxorubicin alone or in combination with bleomycin was seen in 16 of 47 patients (34%) – the series included not only differentiated carcinoma but also 10 patients with medullary thyroid cancer and 15 patients with anaplastic carcinoma. Interestingly, therapy was least effective in patients with locally invasive tumor growth and a reduced state of general health, as well as in anaplastic carcinoma. Best results were obtained in follicular and medullary thyroid cancer.

10.2.2.3 Doxorubicin and Other Cytotoxic Drugs

There are several reports of small series treated with other combination protocols including doxorubicin. Almost all of them failed to show a therapeutic effect that was superior to doxorubicin monotherapy.

Partial tumor response was seen in 4 of 11 patients treated with doxorubicin, vincristine, and 5-fluorouracil and in 7 out of 21 patients treated with doxorubicin, etoposide, fluorouracil, and cyclophosphamide [5]. In the study from the Institute Gustave-Roussy, the combination of doxorubicin, etoposide, 5-fluorouracil and cyclophosphamide, as well as all other treatment regimens tested were found to be ineffective [21]. Another study investigated the effect of combination chemotherapy with doxorubicin, bleomycin, vincristine, and melphalan in 11 patients with metastatic thyroid cancer. Six of eleven patients responded, 5 with a partial, and 1 with a complete and long-lasting response [16]. A combination chemotherapy of doxorubicin (50 mg/m^2), cisplatin (60 mg/m^2), and vindesine (3 mg/m^2) resulted in three minor responses in 8 patients with differentiated thyroid carcinoma [51]. A good and long-lasting response has been reported in a single case of a patient resistant to therapy with doxorubicin and cyclophosphamide to a combination therapy with doxorubicin, lomustine, and methotrexate [11].

10.3 Results of Chemotherapy in Poorly Differentiated and Anaplastic Thyroid Carcinoma

In poorly differentiated and anaplastic carcinoma, chemotherapy seems to be even less effective than in advanced differentiated thyroid cancer. Most of these tumors are very resistant to anticancer agents [6]. Due to this poor effect of chemotherapy and since survival seems also to be rarely altered by treatment with surgery or radiotherapy alone, various protocols have recently investigated the effect of a combination of surgery, external beam radiotherapy, and chemotherapy. This multimodal approach seems currently to be the most promising strategy in patients with anaplastic thyroid cancer.

10.3.1 Chemotherapy

The cytotoxic drug that has been most commonly used in anaplastic thyroid carcinoma is doxorubicin, but monotherapy with this drug has given quite disappointing results [10, 27, 54]. Partial responses may be seen in some patients, but there is little evidence of complete responses [2]. In the series from Gottlieb et al., there were two partial remissions in nine patients with anaplastic carcinoma (doxorubicin 75 mg/m^2, every 3 weeks) [27, 28]. In a review of all published studies, a 22% total response rate was reported for 77 patients [1]. Other chemotherapeutic agents have been even less effective as monotherapy, although minimal effects have been claimed for bleomycin [44], etoposide [34], cisplatin [34], and methotrexate [35].

Studies on combination chemotherapy for poorly differentiated and anaplastic thyroid carcinoma typically included doxorubicin. In a prospective study, three complete and three partial responses were found with doxorubicin (60 mg/m^2) in combination with cisplatin (40 mg/m^2) in 19 patients with anaplastic thyroid carcinoma [54]. However, these promising results were not seen in another prospective trial published by Williams et al. [63], which included patients with advanced differentiated and anaplastic carcinoma and which was terminated due to a lack of efficacy and serious side-effects. A combined regimen of bleomycin (30 mg/day, day 1–3), doxorubicin (60 mg/m^2, day 5), and cisplatin (60 mg/m^2, day 5) resulted in two complete responses and one partial response as well as in a long median survival time of 16 months in five patients with anaplastic thyroid carcinoma [19]. Doxorubicin, bleomycin, and vincristine induced a partial response in four out of five anaplastic carcinoma patients from a larger series of patients with advanced thyroid cancer [56]. Partial tumor responses have also been reported from combination therapy with doxorubicin, vincristine, bleomycin, and melphalan [16]. Recently, the results of a pilot study investigating the effect of an aggressive combination therapy with cisplatin (40 mg/m^2, day 1), doxorubicin (60 mg/m^2, day 1), etoposide (100 mg/m^2/day, days 1–3), peplomycin (5 mg/body/day subcutaneously, days 1–5) and granulocyte colony-stimulating factor (G-CSF; 2 µg/kg/day subcutaneously, days 6–14) were reported [18]. The regimen was repeated every 3 weeks and local radiotherapy was added if indicated. A partial tumor response lasting between 2 and 11 months was seen in 5 of 17 patients. The toxicities of the chemotherapy were acceptable and were mainly bone marrow suppression, despite G-CSF support.

Two studies investigated the effects of chemotherapy combinations that did not include doxorubicin. Therapy with cisplatin (100 mg/m^2), vincristine (1.5 mg/m^2), and mitoxantrone (20 mg/m^2) resulted in four complete and six partial remissions in 15 patients with anaplastic thyroid carcinoma and a prolonged median survival time of 20.8 months in responders, compared with 4.5 months in non-responders [39]. A good response rate of 7 responders out of 9 anaplastic carcinoma patients was also reported with a combination of bleomycin, cyclophosphamide, and 5-fluorouracil [23].

Santini et al. [48] investigated whether increasing the metabolic rate of thyroid cancer cells by TSH stimulation might result in a higher response rate to chemotherapy. A combination of carboplatinum and epirubicin at 4- to 6-week intervals for six courses resulted in a 37% response rate, which rose to 81% when including patients with stable disease. However, response rate did not differ between patients with TSH stimulation – either by reduction of levothyroxine replacement or by recombinant TSH – and those without.

Recently, very promising results of a phase-2 clinical trial on the activity of paclitaxel against anaplastic thyroid carcinoma in patients with persistent or metastatic disease despite surgery or local radiation therapy have been reported [4]. Twenty patients were treated with 96-h continuous infusion of paclitaxel every 3 weeks for 1–6 cycles (120–140 mg/m^2 per 96 h). Nineteen evaluable patients demonstrated a 53% total response rate with one complete response and nine partial responses. Peripheral neuropathy was the only higher-grade toxicity.

10.3.2
Combined Modality Treatment

10.3.2.1
Treatment Protocols Including Chemotherapy with Single Cytotoxic Drugs

A combined treatment regimen consisting of once-weekly administration of doxorubicin (10 mg/m^2) before hyperfractionated radiotherapy (1.6 Gy per treatment, twice a day for 3 days per week up to a total dose of 57.6 Gy in 40 days) was used in 19 patients with anaplastic thyroid carcinoma [37]. There was an 84% complete local tumor response after completion of therapy and 68% retained local disease control until their death. The median survival was 1 year, and 4 patients survived longer than 20 months. The deaths were due to lung or brain metastases. Patients whose tumor volume exceeded 200 ml at presentation did not respond to this therapy. The patients surviving longer than 1 year were those who had undergone radical surgery and minimal residual disease at the time of irradiation. In another study, a combination of hyperfractionated radiotherapy (1 Gy or 1.3 Gy twice a day for 5 days per week to a total dose of 30 Gy) and doxorubicin (20 mg once a week) was followed by debulking surgery after 2 – 3 weeks, when feasible. Then an additional 16 Gy was given with concomitant doxorubicin and was followed by additional doxorubicin. Among 33 patients, surgery was possible in 23 cases (70%). There were no signs of local recurrence in 16 patients (48%). In only 8 patients (24%) was death attributed to local failure. In 4 patients, survival with no evidence of disease exceeded 2 years [61]. Sauerwein et al. [50] reported on the results with a similar approach combining hyperfractionated radiotherapy (1.5 Gy twice a day to a total dose of 54 Gy) with chemotherapy with mitoxantrone (7 mg/m^2 once a week during radiotherapy for 4 weeks, followed by four applications of 16 mg/m^2 at 1-week intervals) in 19 patients with surgically treated anaplastic carcinoma and without evidence of metastatic disease. Sixteen patients died between 2 and 48 months after diagnosis (median 10 months), none of them from local recurrence, 3 patients were alive after 2, 20, and 74 months.

10.3.2.2
Treatment Protocols Including Combination Chemotherapy

Several studies have addressed the question of whether a multimodal approach with a combination chemotherapy regimen might be more effective than combined regimens including only a single cytotoxic drug. The combination of hyperfractionated radiotherapy (1 Gy twice a day for 5 days per week to a total dose of 30 Gy in 3 weeks) and combination chemotherapy (bleomycin 5 mg daily, cyclophosphamide 200 mg daily, and 5-fluorouracil 500 mg every 2nd day) was followed by surgery after 2–3 weeks, when feasible. Then radiotherapy was continued following the same protocol to an additional total dose of 16 Gy with concomitant chemotherapy and was followed by additional chemotherapy [60]. Out of 20 patients, 15 had an objective tumor remission and 3 survived for more than 1 year. Seven patients died from local tumor growth. One third of the patients in this series suffered severe toxicity. In another study, doxorubicin (60 mg/m^2) and cisplatin (90 mg/m^2) was given every 4 weeks and radiotherapy (17.5 Gy in seven fractions to the neck and the upper mediastinum) was performed between days 10 and 20 of the first four courses of chemotherapy [52]. The study included 12 patients aged less than 65 years. Complete tumor control was obtained in 5 patients and 2 patients survived longer than 20 months. All the patients suffered from severe pharyngoesophagitis and tracheitis. The same chemotherapeutic drugs combined with postoperative radiotherapy in 5 patients with anaplastic carcinoma resulted in an average survival of 11 months, with 1 long-term survivor at 31 months [53].

In a study from Japan [33], 37 patients with anaplastic thyroid carcinoma were treated with different chemotherapeutic regimens in combination with radiotherapy and surgery. Treatment resulted in an increased median survival of 8 months compared with a group receiving palliative therapy alone (2 months). The most favorable results were seen in patients with primary lesions less than 5 cm in diameter who had undergone complete resection. Similar results have been reported with chemotherapy with bleomycin, cyclophosphamide, and 5-fluorouracil in combination with hyperfractionated radiotherapy and surgery in 19 patients [52]. The 10 patients with local, non-invasive disease had a significantly longer survival (median 12 months), and 3 of them were alive after 31, 61, and 80 months.

Recently, a 61-year-old woman who presented with a massive and unresectable tumor was treated with a combination of hydroxyurea (1 g twice daily for 11 doses), 5-fluorouracil (800 mg/m^2 per day continuously over 5 days), paclitaxel (20 mg/m^2 continuously over 5 days), and radiotherapy (2 Gy daily for 5 days) [59]. Although the patient suffered from severe side effects, the tumor regressed sufficiently to allow a near-total thyroidectomy to be performed 6 months after the beginning of treatment. Subsequently, the patient was tumor free for at least 38 months [2].

10.4 Drugs with In Vitro Anti-Tumor Effects

Cell lines of differentiated and undifferentiated thyroid cancer offer attractive models for investigating molecular biology and growth regulation of this malignancy. In addition, when grown in culture dishes or as xenograft tumors in athymic mice, the cells provide an opportunity to study the potential of new antineoplastic agents. Some drugs that have not yet been investigated for their in vivo efficacy in patients with thyroid carcinoma have shown in vitro antitumor actions, indicating a potential beneficial clinical effect. Nevertheless, since cell lines do not fully reflect the properties of the tumors from which they are derived, and their properties may change during culture time, data from in vitro experiments on chemosensitivity cannot fully predict the in vivo response to chemotherapy.

Antineoplastic activity against anaplastic thyroid carcinoma in vitro and in vivo in xenograft tumors in nude mice was found with paclitaxel [3]. As recently shown, this effect is enhanced by the application of manumycin, a farnesyl-protein transferase inhibitor [66]. In addition, the angiogenesis inhibitor O-(chloroacetyl-carbamoyl)-fumagillol was shown to be therapeutically effective in human anaplastic thyroid carcinoma xenografts [32].

Other substances with in vitro activity include combretastatin A4 phosphate [22], gemcitabine [45], gemcitabine monophosphate [40], the specific tyrosine kinase inhibitor STI571 [43], and endostatin, a potent antiangiogenic factor [65].

10.5 Mechanisms of Resistance Against Cytotoxic Drugs

Thyroid tumors exhibit a wide spectrum of neoplastic pathology, varying from well-differentiated tumors to highly malignant anaplastic carcinomas. Malignant transformation has been demonstrated to be caused by several factors, including the activation of proto-oncogenes and the inactivation of tumor suppressor genes [24].

The clinical refractoriness to chemotherapy in thyroid carcinomas is mostly characterized by resistance to multiple cytostatic drugs. Multidrug resistance (MDR) is a phenomenon that was first described in the 1970s and is well known in many human malignancies. It is defined as the protection of a tumor cell population against numerous drugs differing in chemical structure and mechanisms of influence on the cells. It is one of the major causes of failures of chemotherapy in human cancer.

Recent studies have shown that the molecular mechanisms of MDR are numerous. Cellular drug resistance is mediated by different mechanisms operating at different steps of the cytotoxic action of the drug from a decrease in drug accumulation in the cell to the abrogation of apoptosis induced by the chemical substance. Sometimes several different mechanisms are switched on in the cells. The most investigated mechanisms with known clinical significance in various malignancies are the activation of transmembrane proteins effluxing different chemical substances from the cells (P-glycoprotein is the most well-known efflux pump), the activation of the enzymes of the glutathione detoxification system, and alterations of genes and proteins involved into the control of apoptosis.

Several in vitro models have been used to clarify why most thyroid carcinomas are chemoresistant [7, 57, 58]. The data that are currently available on the origin of cytotoxic drug resistance of thyroid cancer cells indicate that different mechanisms, including drug efflux functions and alterations in the regulation of apoptosis may be involved.

10.5.1
Overexpression of P-glycoprotein and Multidrug Resistance-Associated Protein.

Many chemoresistant cells overexpress a membrane glycoprotein of 170 kDa termed 'P-glycoprotein,' which is encoded by the multiple drug resistance 1 gene (*ABCB 1*), or a 190-kDa membrane protein termed the 'multidrug resistance-associated protein' (MRP), the product of the *ABCB 1* gene. Although these proteins both belong to the ATP-binding cassette superfamily of transporters, they are only distantly related. Despite their low homology, these proteins mediate resistance by the expulsion of a similar range of cytotoxic drugs out of resistant cancer cells [36].

There are some data on P-glycoprotein and MRP expression in human thyroid cancer cells. Satake et al. [49] investigated ten anaplastic carcinoma cell lines by immunohistochemistry for protein expression and reverse-transcriptase polymerase chain reaction (RT-PCR) for mRNA expression of multidrug resistance proteins. All the cell lines expressed MRP, and 6 expressed P-glycoprotein (*ABCB 1*). In another study, P-glycoprotein seems to be expressed only by a minority of anaplastic tumors [7, 64]. Similarly, Sugawara et al. [58] recently reported on a low frequency of P-glycoprotein expression in anaplastic thyroid carcinoma. However, MRP expression was found in 52% of anaplastic carcinoma investigated and was significantly higher than in other thyroid cancer types. Overall, these data indicate that an increased expression of MRP and P-glycoprotein may at least partly explain the failure of chemotherapy in patients with thyroid cancer.

10.5.2
Alterations of DNA Topoisomerases.

DNA topoisomerase II is an essential enzyme that plays a role in virtually every cellular DNA process. Beyond this critical physiological function, topoisomerase II is the target for some of the most successful anticancer drugs, including adriamycin, etoposide, and mitoxantrone [26]. Data from various human malignancies suggest that a reduction in DNA topoisomerase II-alpha activity and/or expression may contribute to the resistance of cancer cells to topoisomerase II-targeted drugs. In one study, multiple anticancer drug-resistant anaplastic thyroid carcinomas were examined for mutations of DNA topoisomerase II by RT-PCR and subsequent DNA sequencing [49]. No mutation was found in a variety of cell lines and tumor tissues. In addition, there was no significant difference in DNA topoisomerase II-alpha content among the cell lines and tissues. These experimental data indicate that alterations of DNA topoisomerases play no major role in resistance to anticancer agents in anaplastic thyroid carcinoma. No data are currently available on differentiated thyroid carcinoma.

10.5.3 Alterations of Glutathione and Glutathione S-transferases.

It is well established that elevated levels of glutathione and glutathione S-transferases in tumor cells are associated with the development of resistance to alkylating agents as well as anthracyclines by an increase in drug detoxification [31]. Moreover, glutathione (GSH) has been considered to play an important role in the MRP1-mediated multidrug resistance. No data are currently available on a possible contribution of this mechanism to the resistance of thyroid cancer to cytotoxic drugs. There is only one study that indicates a possible role of glutathione by showing that glutathione levels are higher in thyroid carcinomas than in benign thyroid tissues [46].

10.5.4 Control of Apoptosis.

In the normal thyroid gland, total cell mass is maintained constant by a balance between cell proliferation and apoptosis. In thyroid cancer cells, this equilibrium is disrupted, resulting in an increased growth rate and tumor formation. Broecker et al. [15] recently demonstrated that cytotoxic drugs increase the expression of the pro-apoptotic protein bax and decrease the expression of the antiapoptotic protein bcl-2 in benign primary thyroid cells, but not in undifferentiated thyroid carcinoma cells. Therefore, the poor response of thyroid cancer cells to cytotoxic drugs may at least partly be explained by an altered regulation of apoptosis in thyroid cancer.

10.6 Future Directions in Chemotherapy of Thyroid Cancer

There have been major advances in cellular biology, genetics, pharmacology, and immunology in the past decade, which might be translated into progress in the treatment of advanced thyroid cancer in the near future.

One important step is manifested by new cytotoxic drugs that are currently in clinical practice. Paclitaxel is a drug with in vitro and in vivo evidence for a therapeutic efficacy in undifferentiated thyroid cancer [3, 4, 59, 66]. Possible immunotherapeutic approaches include monoclonal antibody therapies [8]. Several new drugs under development are targeted at reversal or prevention of the multidrug resistance mechanism, which has been suggested as playing an important role in chemotherapy resistance in thyroid cancer [49, 57, 58, 64]. Tumor angiogenesis as a target is being studied in several early clinical trials in patients with nonthyroid cancer and these substances may also be effective in thyroid cancer patients [20, 32].

The emerging field of gene therapy will also provide opportunities for the discovery of new therapeutic strategies [9, 14]. For example, in anaplastic thyroid carcinoma cell lines expressing the nonfunctional tumor suppressor gene p53, infection with a p53-expressing adenovirus was shown to exert a cytotoxic effect. Moreover, the p53 wild-type-expressing cell lines became much more sensitive to chemotherapy with adriamycin [12]. Another way would be to use gene therapeutic methods to reinduce iodine uptake in cancer cells that are no longer responsive to ^{131}I therapy [25]. The restoration of iodine accumulation into thyroid cancer cells can also be achieved by redifferentiation therapy with retinoic acid. This approach is already being investigated in clinical trials and is reviewed in Chap 11 [30, 55].

10.7 Current Suggestions for Management

In summary, there has not yet been any chemotherapeutic agent or combination of agents developed with sufficient antineoplastic activity against differentiated and undifferentiated thyroid cancer.

10.7.1 Differentiated Thyroid Cancer.

In differentiated thyroid cancer, partial responses can be seen in one-third of patients, and there have only been rare cases of complete tumor responses. Doxorubicin is the cytotoxic drug that has been most extensively studied and still provides the best clinical results with overall response rates of 30–40%. According to the existing data, combination therapy is not definitely superior to doxorubicin monotherapy in these patients.

Based on these overall poor results, chemotherapy should only be given to patients:

- With tumors or metastases that are not surgically resectable
- Who are not responsive to ^{131}I
- Who are not amenable to external radiotherapy
- Who have rapidly progressive disease as documented by repeated imaging studies and thyroglobulin measurements

The first choice of treatment for these patients is monotherapy with doxorubicin at either 3-weekly or weekly intervals (Table 10.1). If a patient is not responsive to this regimen, combination chemotherapy may be initiated (Table 10.1). Certainly, any opportunity to enroll such patients into clinical therapy trials should be taken. An overview of ongoing clinical trials in different countries is given on-line by the National Cancer Institute.

Table 10.1. Monotherapy and combination chemotherapy protocols in advanced thyroid cancer

	Dose		
Doxorubicin	(21-day cycle)	[1, 13, 17, 29]	
Doxorubicin	60 mg/m^2	IV	Day 1
Doxorubicin	(7-day cycle)		
Doxorubicin	10 mg/m^2	IV	Day 1
Doxorubicin and cisplatin	(21-day cycle)	[54]	
Doxorubicin	60 mg/m^2	IV	Day 1
Cisplatin	40 mg/m^2	IV	Day 1
Doxorubicin, cisplatin and bleomycin	(21-day cycle)	[19]	
Bleomycin	30 mg	IV	Day 1–3
Doxorubicin	60 mg/m^2	IV	Day 5
Cisplatin	60 mg/m^2	IV	Day 5
Cisplatin, vincristine, and mitoxantrone	(21-day cycle)	[39]	
Cisplatin	60 mg/m^2	IV	Day 1
Vincristine	1.5 mg/m^2	IV	Day 1
Mitoxantrone	20 mg/m^2	IV	Day 1

Table 10.2. Chemotherapy protocols in combined modality treatment of anaplastic thyroid carcinoma

Doxorubicin [37]

Debulking surgery, followed by:

Doxorubicin 10 mg/m^2 IV once a week in combination with hyperfractionated radiotherapy

Doxorubicin [61]

Doxorubicin 20 mg/m^2 IV once a week in combination with hyperfractionated radiotherapy and debulking surgery

Mitoxantrone [50]

Debulking surgery, followed by:

Mitoxantrone 7 mg/m^2 IV once a week for 4 weeks in combination with hyperfractionated radiotherapy, followed by:

Mitoxantrone 16 mg/m^2 IV once a week for 4 weeks

Doxorubicin and cisplatin [52, 53]

Debulking surgery, followed by:

Doxorubicin 60 mg/m^2 IV every 4 weeks

Cisplatin 90 mg/m^2 IV every 4 weeks in combination with hyperfractionated radiotherapy

10.7.2
Poorly Differentiated and Anaplastic Thyroid Carcinoma.

In poorly differentiated and anaplastic thyroid carcinoma, multimodality treatment protocols are obviously more effective than chemotherapy alone. Initially, debulking surgery should be performed whenever possible and should be followed by a combined protocol of hyperfractionated radiotherapy and chemotherapy without delay (Table 10.2). Combination chemotherapeutic protocols might be advantageous to therapy with doxorubicin or mitoxantrone as a single agent; however, acute toxicity seems to be higher. Although the local response with all combined modality treatment protocols published so far appears good, the systemic response is still poor and the few long-term survivors were among the few patients who presented with local, noninvasive disease and underwent complete local surgical resections. Recent data from a clinical trial justifies the use of paclitaxel in cases of progressive disease [4].

References

1. Ahuja S, Ernst H (1987) Chemotherapy of thyroid carcinoma. J Endocrinol Invest 10:303–310
2. Ain KB (1998) Anaplastic thyroid carcinoma: behavior, biology, and therapeutic approaches. Thyroid 8:715–726
3. Ain KB, Tofiq S, Taylor KD (1996) Antineoplastic activity of taxol against human anaplastic thyroid carcinoma cell lines in vitro and in vivo. J Clin Endocrinol Metab 81:3650–3653
4. Ain KB, Egorin MJ, DeSimone PA (2000) Treatment of anaplastic thyroid carcinoma with paclitaxel: phase 2 trial using ninety-six-hour infusion. Collaborative Anaplastic Thyroid Cancer Health Intervention Trials (CATCHIT) group. Thyroid 10:587–594
5. Alexieva-Figusch J, Van Gilse HA, Treurniet RE (1977) Chemotherapy in carcinoma of the thyroid: retrospective and prospective. Ann Radiol (Paris) 20:810–813
6. Asakawa H, Kobayashi T, Komoike Y, et al. (1997) Chemosensitivity of anaplastic thyroid carcinoma and poorly differentiated thyroid carcinoma. Anticancer Res 17:2757–2762
7. Asakawa H, Kobayashi T, Komoike Y, et al. (1996) Establishment of anaplastic thyroid carcinoma cell lines useful for analysis of chemosensitivity and carcinogenesis. J Clin Endocrinol Metab 81:3547–3552
8. Baba M, Kobayashi T, Oka Y, et al. (1993) Preparation of a human monoclonal antibody derived from cervical lymph nodes of a patient with anaplastic carcinoma of the thyroid. Hum Antibodies Hybridomas 4:181–185
9. Barzon L, Pacenti M, Boscaro M, Palu G (2004) Gene therapy for thyroid cancer. Expert Opin Biol Ther 4:1225–1239
10. Benker G, Reinwein D (1983) Ergebnisse der Chemotherapie des Schilddrüsenkarzinoms. Dtsch Med Wochenschr 108:403–406
11. Bernhardt B (1981) Follicular thyroid carcinoma: response to chemotherapy. Am J Med Sci 282:45–46
12. Blagosklonny MV, Giannakakou P, Wojtowicz M, et al. (1998) Effects of p53-expressing adenovirus on the chemosensitivity and differentiation of anaplastic thyroid cancer cells. J Clin Endocrinol Metab 83:2516–2522
13. Bonadonna G, Monfardini S, DeLena M, Fossate F, Bellani-Fossati F, Beretta G (1970) Phase I and preliminary phase II evaluation of adriamycin (NSC 123 127). Cancer Res 30:2572

14. Braga-Basaria M, Ringel MD (2003) Clinical review 158: Beyond radioiodine: a review of potential new therapeutic approaches for thyroid cancer. J Clin Endocrinol Metab 88:1947–1960
15. Broecker M, de Buhr I, Mann K, Derwahl M (1999) The resistance of undifferentiated thyroid carcinoma cells to chemotherapeutic treatment with doxorubicin, cisplatin and camptothecin is due to a diminished rate of apoptosis. J Endocrinol Invest 22 [Supp]:73
16. Bukowski RM, Brown L, Weick JK, Groppe CW, Purvis J (1983) Combination chemotherapy of metastatic thyroid cancer. Phase II study. Am J Clin Oncol 6:579–581
17. Burgess MH, Stratton Hill C (1978) Chemotherapy in the management of thyroid cancer. In: Greenfield LD (ed) Thyroid cancer. CRC Press, Palm Beach, p 233
18. Chemotherapy Committee TJSoTS (1995) Intensive chemotherapy for anaplastic thyroid carcinoma: combination of cisplatin, doxorubicin, etoposide and peplomycin with granulocyte granulocyte colony-stimulating factor support. Jpn J Clin Oncol 25:203–207
19. De Besi P, Busnardo B, Toso S, et al. (1991) Combined chemotherapy with bleomycin, adriamycin, and platinum in advanced thyroid cancer. J Endocrinol Invest 14:475–480
20. Dowlati A, Robertson K, Cooney M, Petros WP, Stratford M, Jesberger J, Rafie N, Overmoyer B, Makkar V, Stambler B, Taylor A, Waas J, Lewin JS, McCrae KR, Remick SC (2002) A phase I pharmacokinetic and translational study of the novel vascular targeting agent combretastatin A-4 phosphate on a single-dose intravenous schedule in patients with advanced cancer. Cancer Res 62:3408–3416
21. Droz JP, Schlumberger M, Rougier P, Ghosn M, Gardet P, Parmentier C (1990) Chemotherapy in metastatic nonanaplastic thyroid cancer: experience at the Institut Gustave-Roussy. Tumori 76:480–483
22. Dziba JM, Marcinek R, Venkataraman G, Robinson JA, Ain KB (2002) Combretastatin A4 phosphate has primary antineoplastic activity against human anaplastic thyroid carcinoma cell lines and xenograft tumors. Thyroid 12:1063–1070
23. Ekman ET, Lundell G, Tennvall J, Wallin G (1990) Chemotherapy and multimodality treatment in thyroid carcinoma. Otolaryngol Clin North Am 23:523–527
24. Farid NR, Shi Y, Zou M (1994) Molecular basis of thyroid cancer. Endocr Rev 15:202–232
25. Filetti S, Bidart JM, Arturi F, Caillou B, Russo D, Schlumberger M (1999) Sodium/iodide symporter: a key transport system in thyroid cancer cell metabolism. Eur J Endocrinol 141:443–457
26. Fortune JM, Osheroff N (2000) Topoisomerase II as a target for anticancer drugs: when enzymes stop being nice. Prog Nucleic Acid Res Mol Biol 64:221–253
27. Gottlieb JA, Hill CS Jr, (1974) Chemotherapy of thyroid cancer with adriamycin. Experience with 30 patients. N Engl J Med 290:193–197
28. Gottlieb JA, Hill CS Jr, Ibanez ML, Clark RL (1972) Chemotherapy of thyroid cancer. An evaluation of experience with 37 patients. Cancer 30:848–853
29. Gottlieb JA, Stratton Hill C (1975) Adriamycin (NSC 123 127) therapy in thyroid carcinoma. Cancer Chemother Rep 6:283–296
30. Grunwald F, Pakos E, Bender H, et al. (1998) Redifferentiation therapy with retinoic acid in follicular thyroid cancer. J Nucl Med 39:1555–1558
31. Hall AG (1999) Glutathione and the regulation of cell death. Adv Exp Med Biol 457:199–203
32. Hama Y, Shimizu T, Hosaka S, Sugenoya A, Usuda N (1997) Therapeutic efficacy of the angiogenesis inhibitor O-(chloroacetyl-carbamoyl) fumagillol (TNP-470; AGM-1470) for human anaplastic thyroid carcinoma in nude mice. Exp Toxicol Pathol 49:239–247
33. Harada T, Nishikawa Y, Suzuki T, Ito K, Baba S (1971) Bleomycin treatment for cancer of the thyroid. Am J Surg 122:53–57
34. Hoskin PJ, Harmer C (1987) Chemotherapy for thyroid cancer. Radiother Oncol 10:187–194
35. Jereb B, Stjernsward J, Lowhagen T (1975) Anaplastic giant-cell carcinoma of the thyroid. A study of treatment and prognosis. Cancer 35:1293–1295

36. Kavallaris M (1997) The role of multidrug resistance-associated protein (MRP) expression in multidrug resistance. Anticancer Drugs 8:17–25
37. Kim JH, Leeper RD (1987) Treatment of locally advanced thyroid carcinoma with combination doxorubicin and radiation therapy. Cancer 60:2372–2375
38. Kobayashi T, Asakawa H, Umeshita K, et al. (1996) Treatment of 37 patients with anaplastic carcinoma of the thyroid. Head Neck 18:36–41
39. Kober F, Heiss A, Keminger K, Depisch D (1990) Chemotherapie hochmaligner Schilddrüsentumore. Wien Klin Wochenschr 102:274–276
40. Kotchetkov R, Groschel B, Gmeiner WH, Krivtchik AA, Trump E, Bitoova M, Cinatl J, Kornhuber B, Cinatl J (2000) Antineoplastic activity of a novel multimeric gemcitabine-monophosphate prodrug against thyroid cancer cells in vitro. Anticancer Res 20:2915–2922
41. Leaf AN, Wolf BC, Kirkwood JM, Haselow RE (2000) Phase II study of etoposide (VP-16) in patients with thyroid cancer with no prior chemotherapy: an Eastern Cooperative Oncology Group Study (E1385). Med Oncol 17:47-51
42. Morris JC, Kim CK, Padilla ML, Mechanick JI (1997) Conversion of non-iodine-concentrating differentiated thyroid carcinoma metastases into iodine-concentrating foci after anticancer chemotherapy. Thyroid 7:63–66
43. Podtcheko A, Ohtsuru A, Tsuda S, Namba H, Saenko V, Nakashima M, Mitsutake N, Kanda S, Kurebayashi J, Yamashita S (2003) The selective tyrosine kinase inhibitor, STI571, inhibits growth of anaplastic thyroid cancer cells. J Clin Endocrinol Metab 88:1889–1896
44. Poster DS, Bruno S, Penta J, Pina K, Catane R (1981) Current status of chemotherapy in the treatment of advanced carcinoma of the thyroid gland. Cancer Clin Trials 4:301–307
45. Ringel MD, Greenberg M, Chen X, Hayre N, Suzuki K, Priebat D, Saji M, Burman KD (2000) Cytotoxic activity of 2',2'-difluorodeoxycytidine (gemcitabine) in poorly differentiated thyroid carcinoma cells. Thyroid 10:865–869
46. Sadani GR, Nadkarni GD (1996) Role of tissue antioxidant defence in thyroid cancers. Cancer Lett 109:231–235
47. Samonigg H, Hossfeld DK, Spehn J, Fill H, Leb G (1988) Aclarubicin in advanced thyroid cancer: a phase II study. Eur J Cancer Clin Oncol 24:1271–1275
48. Santini F, Bottici V, Elisei R, Montanelli L, Mazzeo S, Basolo F, Pinchera A, Pacini F (2002) Cytotoxic effects of carboplatinum and epirubicin in the setting of an elevated serum thyrotropin for advanced poorly differentiated thyroid cancer. J Clin Endocrinol Metab 87:4160–4165
49. Satake S, Sugawara I, Watanabe M, Takami H (1997) Lack of a point mutation of human DNA topoisomerase II in multidrug-resistant anaplastic thyroid carcinoma cell lines. Cancer Lett 116:33–39
50. Sauerwein W, Reiners C, Lederbogen S (1996) Kombinierte Strahlen-Chemotherapie beim anaplastischen Schilddrüsenkarzinom. In: Usadel K-H, Weinheimer B (eds) Schilddrüse 1995. de Gruyter, Berlin, pp 401–408
51. Scherubl H, Raue F, Ziegler R (1990) Combination chemotherapy of advanced medullary and differentiated thyroid cancer. Phase II study. J Cancer Res Clin Oncol 116:21–23
52. Schlumberger M, Parmentier C, Delisle MJ, Couette JE, Droz JP, Sarrazin D (1991) Combination therapy for anaplastic giant cell thyroid carcinoma. Cancer 67:564–566
53. Serrano M, Monroy C, Rodriguez-Garcia JL, Pais JR, Fernandez-Garrido M (1994) Tratamiento combinado del carcinoma anaplásico de tiroides. Ann Med Interna 11:288–290
54. Shimaoka K, Schoenfeld DA, DeWys WD, Creech RH, DeConti R (1985) A randomized trial of doxorubicin versus doxorubicin plus cisplatin in patients with advanced thyroid carcinoma. Cancer 56:2155–2160
55. Simon D, Korber C, Krausch M, Segering J, Groth P, Gorges R, Grunwald F, Muller-Gartner HW, Schmutzler C, Kohrle J, Roher HD, Reiners C (2002) Clinical impact of retinoids in redifferentiation therapy of advanced thyroid cancer: final results of a pilot study. Eur J Nucl Med Mol Imaging 29:775–782

56. Sokal M, Harmer CL (1978) Chemotherapy for anaplastic carcinoma of the thyroid. Clin Oncol 4:3–10
57. Sugawara I, Arai T, Yamashita T, Yoshida A, Masunaga A, Itoyama S (1994) Expression of multidrug resistance-associated protein (MRP) in anaplastic carcinoma of the thyroid. Cancer Lett 82:185–188
58. Sugawara I, Masunaga A, Itoyama S, Sumizawa T, Akiyama S, Yamashita T (1995) Expression of multidrug resistance-associated protein (MRP) in thyroid cancers. Cancer Lett 95:135–138
59. Sweeney PJ, Haraf DJ, Recant W, Kaplan EL, Vokes EE (1996) Anaplastic carcinoma of the thyroid. Ann Oncol 7:739–744
60. Tallroth E, Wallin G, Lundell G, Lowhagen T, Einhorn J (1987) Multimodality treatment in anaplastic giant cell thyroid carcinoma. Cancer 60:1428–1431
61. Tennvall J, Lundell G, Hallquist A, Wahlberg P, Wallin G, Tibblin S (1994) Combined doxorubicin, hyperfractionated radiotherapy, and surgery in anaplastic thyroid carcinoma. Report on two protocols. The Swedish Anaplastic Thyroid Cancer Group. Cancer 74:1348–1354
62. Werner B, Abele J, Alveryd A, et al. (1984) Multimodal therapy in anaplastic giant cell thyroid carcinoma. World J Surg 8:64–70
63. Williams SD, Birch R, Einhorn LH (1986) Phase II evaluation of doxorubicin plus cisplatin in advanced thyroid cancer: a Southeastern Cancer Study Group Trial. Cancer Treat Rep 70:405–407
64. Yamashita T, Watanabe M, Onodera M, et al. (1994) Multidrug resistance gene and P-glycoprotein expression in anaplastic carcinoma of the thyroid. Cancer Detect Prev 18:407–413
65. Ye C, Feng C, Wang S, Liu X, Lin Y, Li M (2002) Antiangiogenic and antitumor effects of endostatin on follicular thyroid carcinoma. Endocrinology 143:3522–3528
66. Yeung SC, Xu G, Pan J, Christgen M, Bamiagis A (2000) Manumycin enhances the cytotoxic effect of paclitaxel on anaplastic thyroid carcinoma cells. Cancer Res 60:650–656
67. Zlock DW, Greenspan FS, Clark OH, Higgins CB (1994) Octreotide therapy in advanced thyroid cancer. Thyroid 4:427–431

Chapter 11

Redifferentiation Therapy of Thyroid Carcinomas with Retinoic Acid

11

D. Simon

11.1 Introduction

Therapy of differentiated thyroid cancer is mainly constituted under three therapeutic arms: (1) surgical removal of the tumor-bearing thyroid gland and extraglandular tumor spread in lymph nodes or distant sites; (2) radioiodide therapy mainly for distant metastases; and (3) thyrotropin suppressive thyroxine therapy. In the course of tumor progression differentiated morphological and functional characteristics of differentiated thyroid carcinomas (DTC) disappear. This applies to about one third of thyroid carcinomas documented by change of histological grading and altered iodide uptake [16]. Clinically it corresponds to more aggressive growth and metastatic spread.

Experimental data give evidence that differentiated functions of thyrocytes and of iodide metabolism can be reinduced by retinoic acids [40, 43, 51]. Retinoic acids (RA) are biologically active metabolites of vitamin A that play an important role in morphogenesis, differentiation and proliferation of many cell types [24, 34]. Retinoic acid signals are transduced by specific receptors, the RA receptors RARs and RXRs, which belong to the superfamily of nuclear receptors [15, 33, 42]. Similar to nuclear receptors they act as ligand-binding transcription factors switching on RA responsive genes. Retinoids have been administered for anti-cancer and preventive cancer treatment in various clinical trials and promising results have been achieved in therapy of acute promyelocytic leukemia, head and neck cancers and skin tumors [9, 14, 20, 25, 52]. Various partly tumor-specific mechanisms lead to redifferentiation or prevent further dedifferentiation of tumor cells.

Experimental studies indicate that retinoids have similar effects on thyroid tumor cells [12]. In follicular thyroid tumor cells retinoids have been found to be able to inhibit tumor growth and induce iodide uptake. A redifferentiating effect on follicular thyroid cancer cells has been shown by induction of type I iodothyronine-5'-deiodinase (5'-DI) and alkaline phosphatase as well as by stimulation of intercellular adhesion molecule-1 (ICAM-1) in thyroid carcinoma cell lines [3, 28, 40, 43, 56]. Furthermore, treatment of follicular thyroid tumor cells with retinoic acid (RA) leads to loss of tumorigenicity in athymic nude mice. The redifferentiating effects of RAs are confined to at least partly differentiated thyroid cancers and are not seen in anaplastic thyroid cancer.

Loss of differentiation is a common event in tumor progression and means loss of thyroid specific functions such as reduced or missing expression of thyrotropin receptor or the possibility of iodide accumulation. Thus, these tumors may no longer be amenable to standard treatment protocols including thyroid-stimulating hormone (TSH) suppression and radioiodide therapy. Therefore, the promising experimental results prompted clinical studies to be carried out with administration of 13-cis-RA in patients with advanced thyroid cancer. The effects and results of clinical application will be discussed in the context of our own experience with 49 patients.

11.2 Biological Effects of RAs

Retinoic acids or retinoids are natural or synthetic derivatives of vitamin A. Their biologically active metabolites are responsible for growth, differentiation and morphogenesis in vertebrates [54]. RAs are known to be teratogenic leading among other problems to limb malformation and are therefore contraindicated during pregnancy [20, 24, 34]. In adults retinoids maintain functional integrity of lung epithelium, testes, skin, and eyes [10, 14, 52]. Differentiating effects have been shown in various cell culture models of promyelocytic leukemia, pheochromocytoma (PC12), neuroblastoma, and others [6, 19, 38].

RA signals are transduced by specific receptors, the RA receptors RARs and RXRs, which belong to the superfamily of nuclear receptors such as T3, vitamin D3, glucocorticoids, steroid hormones, and others [15, 33]. The retinoid receptors have specificity for various ligands, e.g., all-trans-RA binds to RAR, and RXR, 9-cis-RA to RXR only. Similarly to nuclear receptors they act as ligand-binding transcription factors switching on RA responsive elements (RAREs) and thus regulate and modulate gene expression.

11.3 Retinoids in Cancer Treatment

As early as in the 1960s anticancer activity of retinoids was demonstrated in lung tumors. Since then, many studies have been performed to treat patients with solid tumors as well as with hematological diseases [25]. Acute promyelocytic leukemia (APL) was the most prominent example of successful cancer treatment [9]. The retinoic effect is very specific in this disease. Chromosomal translocation leads to a fusion protein that blocks normal RAR-alpha function, which is overcome by treatment with RA.

Thus, the APL model is not transferable to RA treatment of other solid tumors. However, experimental studies have shown a prevention or repression of tumor progression in chemically induced tumors of the skin, vulva, lung, esophagus, oral cavity, liver, among others [31, 35]. Based on the fact that reduced dietary intake of vitamin A might lead to an increased risk of cancer development, various studies on chemopreventive effects of RAs have been performed. At least, premalignant skin lesions regressed under RA therapy and the incidence of second primary tumors could be reduced in tumors of the head and neck, vulva, cervix, etc. Numerous studies using RAs alone or in combination for therapy of various cancers have been performed and are ongoing.

11.4 Thyroid-Specific Effects of Retinoids

Redifferentiation therapy of thyroid cancer with RAs requires intact receptor pathways in the tumor tissues. The presence of retinoid receptors RARs and RXRs and their subgroups has been studied in tumor cell lines. Functionality of the RA receptors was proven by ligand binding assays and electrophoretic mobility shift analyses showing high affinity binding sites for RA and DNA binding of RAR-alpha, RAR-chi, RXR-alpha, and RXR-beta [26, 42]. Reverse transcriptase-polymerase chain reaction (RT-PCR) revealed expression of all receptor subtypes RAR-alpha, RAR-beta, RAR-chi, RXR-alpha, and RXR-beta at various expression levels. RAR-beta was strongly reduced in a follicular thyroid carcinoma cell line and not stimulated by RA. In tumor tissues most receptor subtypes could be demonstrated except RXR-beta, which was undetectable in most of the examined tissues. These findings indicate a possible role of RAR-beta in thyroid carcinogenesis and would be in accordance with results found in other carcinomas [32].

11.4.1 Thyroid-Specific Functions

Iodide uptake and iodide metabolism are specific thyroid functions. Redifferentiation of thyroid cancer aims, among other things, at reinducing these functions, which are lost during tumor progression. A key role is played by deiodinases and the sodium/iodide symporter (NIS).

Type I 5'-deiodinase (5'-DI) is an enzyme that catalyzes deiodination of T4 to its biologically active form of T3 and inactivates T3 by deiodination to T2. The enzyme is mainly expressed in the liver, kidney, and pituitary gland. 5'-DI has been shown to be a differentiation marker in thyroid tumors displaying high activity and expression in normal thyroid tissue, low activity in differentiated thyroid cancer and absent activity in anaplastic thyroid cancer [28]. In thyroid carcinoma cell lines its activity can be stimulated by RA treatment. The well-differentiated follicular carcinoma cell line FTC-133 is stimulated 100-fold, the poorly differentiated cell line FTC-238 only 10-fold [40, 43]. Further experiments have revealed that 2 RAREs in the 5'-DI promoter mediate the RA effect in a cell-specific manner [26, 55].

The NIS was cloned in 1996 [11, 47] and since then has undergone intensive investigation because of its central role not only in iodide metabolism but also in diagnosis and treatment of thyroid cancer. As one would expect, NIS expression is lost in many of thyroid cancers thus preventing radioiodide therapy [2, 7, 8, 27, 30, 41, 47, 48]. However, our own investigations and others demonstrate the presence of NIS mRNA and protein despite a lack of iodide transport [37]. Induction of NIS expression by RA treatment in cell culture could be shown [41]. Surprisingly anaplastic carcinomas also had detectable NIS mRNA, which was not stimulated by RA. NIS protein was not stimulated either in differentiated or anaplastic carcinoma cell lines. The same applied to iodide uptake, which was not increased by RA, TSH, or forskolin. This is in contrast to studies from van Herle who found increased iodide accumulation in thyroid carcinoma cells [51].

11.4.2 Differentiation

Retinoic acid treatment induces significant phenotypic alterations in thyrocyte cell culture. This might indicate a potential role for cell adhesion molecules in the response to RA treatment. E-Cadherin is a well-established differentiation marker in various carcinomas. Loss of E-cadherin expression correlates with dedifferentiation, increased invasiveness, and poor prognosis, which has also been shown in thyroid carcinoma [5]. In thyroid cell culture RA was able to induce E-cadherin expression [21]. In one patient induction of E-cadherin expression in a lymph node metastasis was demonstrated following RA treatment (unpublished data).

Intercellular adhesion molecule-1 (ICAM-1), a glycoprotein of the immunoglobulin supergene family, is another possible candidate for the effects of RA. ICAM-1 is a mediator of cellular cytotoxic action against cancer cells. Normal thyrocytes do not exhibit ICAM-1, but it can be stimulated by various proinflammatory cytokines and RA [3]. Up-regulation might thus offer better interaction with immune competent cells.

11.4.3 Proliferation

Besides redifferentiating effects, RAs have been shown to have antiproliferative effects. Follicular thyroid carcinoma cells (FTC-133) decreased in number by 33% after 3 days' treatment with RA [23, 39]. Induced expression of fas-protein in thyroid carcinoma cell line FTC-236 might indicate that RA takes effect via apoptotic pathways [22].

Tumorigenicity of follicular thyroid carcinoma cells (FTC-133) was reduced after pretreatment with all-trans-RA prior to xenotransplantation into nude rats. RA-treated cells showed significantly decreased tumor growth after 9 weeks and no measurable serum thyroglobulin (Tg) levels, in contrast to untreated control cells. Interestingly, RA pretreatment of the cells had a long-lasting effect at least for several weeks after xenotransplantation.

11.5 Basis for Therapeutic Approach

Differentiated thyroid cancer is a malignant tumor with a fairly good prognosis and long-term survival over many years. Multimodal therapy with surgery, radioiodide therapy, and TSH suppressive therapy are the main therapeutic options with proven efficacy. However, tumor recurrence and dedifferentiation occur in up to one third of the tumors [16]. Various genetic alterations are known in the development of thyroid cancer. In contrast to the Vogelstein model of colon carcinoma genetic alterations neither clearly delineate benign from malignant thyroid lesions nor the stepwise tumor progression and dedifferentiation. P53 is the only genetic change that clearly correlates with poor prognosis, loss of differentiation and frequent association with anaplastic carcinoma of the thyroid. Nevertheless, there are some well-known markers of differentiation in thyroid carcinoma. Loss of TSH receptor explains the insensitivity to TSH and the lack of effectiveness of TSH suppressive therapy with thyroxine [4]. Reduction or loss of NIS expression corresponds to the clinical phenomenon of loss of radioiodide uptake [13]. In addition tumor dedifferentiation accompanies more aggressive tumor growth leading to extensive and infiltrative local tumor growth or much more frequently to distant metastatic spread so that surgical removal is neither sensible nor feasible. Thus, one is deprived of all standard and basic therapeutic modalities.

This is the scenario where redifferentiation therapy with retinoids has been studied and might have a place in the treatment of advanced thyroid cancer. The approach is a palliative one based on the discussed theoretical and experimental results. The therapeutic implications would at least be threefold:

- Thyroid tumor cells would regain former thyroid-specific properties such as iodide uptake, which allows reapplication of radioiodide therapy.
- Antiproliferative activity via proapoptotic pathways or improved immune response via cytotoxic activity.
- Reestablishment of TSH responsivity via reinduction of TSH receptor.

11.6 Results of a Clinical Pilot Study

Loss of differentiation is a common event in tumor progression and is observed in up to one third of patients with differentiated thyroid cancer [16]. Histomorphological dedifferentiation, assessed by tumor grading, means loss of thyroid-specific functions such as reduced or missing expression of thyrotropin receptor or the ability of iodide accumulation. Thus, these tumors may no longer be amenable to standard treatment protocols, including TSH suppression and radioiodide therapy. Therefore, the earlier discussed promising experimental results have prompted various clinical studies with administration of 13-cis retinoic acid in patients with advanced thyroid cancer [17, 18, 44–46]. In Germany a protocol has been developed for retinoid therapy of thyroid cancer. A multicenter pilot study was performed in university hospitals in Duesseldorf, Essen, Bonn, Wuerzburg, Rostock, and Innsbruck. This study presents the largest series of RA-treated patients with thyroid cancer.

Seventy-five patients were enrolled in this study by 1998. Only patients with advanced thyroid carcinoma of papillary or follicular origin were recruited. Most of the tumors had undergone partial dedifferentiation but had retained some differentiated thyroid-specific properties. Indication for redifferentiation therapy was inoperable tumor mass defined by locally invasive cervical and/or mediastinal tumor and/or, as in most cases, distant metastatic tumor spread. Radioiodine uptake was insignificant or absent so that radioiodide therapy was not possible. Exclusion criteria were anaplastic carcinomas and pregnancy.

For further evaluation of response to RA therapy 49 patients with comparable and completely documented data sets were included. Data included in the analysis were Tg levels under stimulating conditions (TSH >30 ng/ml) before and after RA treatment, a radioiodide scan before and after RA treatment, and assessment of tumor size by CT or MRI before and after RA treatment. Diagnostic imaging for assessment of tumor size and quantitative scintigraphy were not performed in all patients due to lack of quantifiable tumor mass (e.g., diffuse pulmonary metastases or bone metastases). 18-FDG-PET was not available in all cases but was considered to be useful especially in verification of iodide-negative metastases.

Histology demonstrated papillary origin in 24 patients, follicular origin in 14 patients, oxyphilic tumors in 6 patients, and mixed follicular/papillary in 5 patients. Tumor stages showed variable primary tumor stage (pT2–4) and lymph node involvement. All but 2 patients had distant metastases either in lung or bone or both. All the patients had undergone previous radioiodine therapy at variable dosages (3.7–59.4 GBq). All of the patients had undergone one or multiple operations (range 1 to 8), some had undergone additional external radiation therapy.

Treatment was performed with 13-cis-RA (Roaccutane) at an oral dosage of 1 –1.5 mg per kilogram body weight per day. Therapy was given for 5 weeks. During RA medication thyroid hormone therapy was continued with T3 for 3 weeks and discontinued for the final 2 weeks. After the RA treatment was complete radioiodide scan and assessment of serum Tg levels were performed under TSH-stimulating conditions.

Side effects occurred in 50% of patients and were well tolerated, with one exception where therapy had to be disrupted because of a significant increase in liver enzymes. In none of the other patients significant changes in blood count, liver enzymes, cholesterol or triglycerides were registered. The most frequent side effects were dryness of skin, lips, mucosa, and conjunctiva (60%), nausea (7%), and pruritus (5%); other rare side effects included hair loss, arthritis, and nose bleed [46].

Serum Tg levels increased in 37 patients (76%), were unchanged in 2 patients (4%) and decreased in 10 patients (20%) (Table 10.1). Radioiodide uptake increased in 24 patients (49%) with a marked increase in 10 patients (20%), was unchanged in 25 patients (51%) and decreased in none of the patients (Table 10.2). Tumor size was assessable in 22 patients as explained before showing an increase in tumor size in 16 patients (33%), no change in 6 (12%) and decrease in no patient (Table 10.3). With regard to clinical outcome patients were assigned to three categories defined as responders with increased radioiodide uptake and decrease of Tg level or tumor size, stable disease with no or insignificant changes in any of the parameters, and progressive disease with failure of radioiodide uptake and increase of tumor size or Tg levels. In terms of these parameters there were 5 responders and 8 patients with stable disease accounting for 13 (27%) of the patients (Tables 10.1–10.3). In this group radioiodide increased in 7 patients. Progressive disease was seen in 23 patients (47%). This group included 11 patients who progressed despite increased radioiodide uptake.

Table 11.1. Correlation of serum thyroglobulin (Tg) levels and outcome

Serum Tg levels	N	Responder	Stable	Progress	Not assessed
Increase	37	4 (11%)	5 (13%)	17 (46%)	11 (30%)
No change	2	–	1	1	–
Decrease	10	1 (10%)	2 (20%)	5 (50%)	2 (20%)

Table 11.2. Correlation of iodide uptake and outcome

Radioiodide uptake	Responder	Stable	Progress	Not assessed
Marked increase	3	1	4	2
Flaw increase	2	1	7	4

Table 11.3. Response of radioiodide uptake and tumor size after retinoic acid treatment

Parameter	Increase	No change	Decrease
Iodide uptake	24 (49%)	25 (51%)	0
Tumor size	16 (33%)	6 (12%)	0
Outcome	Responder	Stable	Progress
	5 (10%)	8 (16%)	23 (47%)

Summarizing these data 13 patients (27%) including those with stable disease showed response to RA treatment. Inclusion of patients with stable disease after a mean follow-up of 16 months (median 18 months, range 5–46 months) seems justified bearing in mind that all of these patients had documented tumor progression before RA therapy. In a significant number of the patients (27 of 49; 55%) the hard criteria of tumor size was not assessable due to diffuse metastases, which are not amenable to quantification by means of CT scan or MRI. Improved radioiodide uptake per se does not necessarily preclude tumor progression. As seen in this series increased radioiodide accumulation was obviously insufficient with regard to effective tumor reduction. There was no correlation between RA response and histological subtypes.

11.7 Conclusion and Perspectives

Based on the experimental results the clinical pilot study of a series of 49 patients clearly demonstrated a response to RA treatment in some of the patients. Enhanced radioiodide uptake, reduction or stabilization of tumor size and Tg levels were the aims of the study. At this early stage of investigation the final benefit for the patient in terms of the parameters described is not always clear.

As was demonstrated increased radioiodide uptake does not always correspond to response of the disease. Despite improved iodide uptake tumor progression was seen in some of the patients. This indicates that accumulation of radioiodide was insufficient for effective reduction of tumor mass. Intracellular iodide trapping by inhibition of iodide efflux might offer perspectives in the future [1, 29]. NIS seems to play a key role in iodide uptake; however, increased mRNA expression does not always correspond to increased iodide uptake indicating that maybe the promoter activity is responsible and could be influenced by alteration of methylation [53].

Interpretation of serum Tg levels is difficult in some patients. Serum Tg level is accepted as a marker of tumor relapse and increase of Tg suggests increase of tumor mass. However, in the setting of redifferentiation increase of serum Tg might be interpreted as increase of tumor mass as well as increase of tumor differentiation with subsequent enhanced production and release of the thyroid-specific protein. In another study with long-term application of retinoids Tg levels showed a significant increase in patients who demonstrated increased radioiodide uptake [17, 18].

The most relevant parameter for therapeutic success would be the tumor size. However, this is only quantifiable in some of the patients, as shown above. Quantification of diffuse metastases that frequently occur in the lung is difficult for diagnostic imaging as well as for scintigraphy. 18-FDG-PET might play a role here in the future. Metabolic changes have been observed in patients after RA treatment [45]. Evaluation of iodide-negative tumors would be useful in this setting.

Increased iodide uptake is the primary goal of RA therapy and the straightforward approach of the therapy. However, as could be seen in the study retinoids also exert effects other than induction of iodide transport. As we know from experimental studies retinoids also have antiproliferative effects mediated via proapoptotic pathways or direct action on the cell cycle [36, 50]. In this context synthetic RAs might play a future role with their specific effects on growth regulation and apoptosis [49, 56].

Up to now, only tumors in advanced stages have been treated with retinoids. Suppression of NIS in normal thyrocytes and differentiation-dependent effects of RAs in experimental studies might offer application of retinoids in less advanced and dedifferentiated tumors [41, 42]. The encouraging results of recent studies and the low rate of side effects with good tolerability of retinoids suggest and justify further studies with altered inclusion criteria, employment of other redifferentiating agents or combination of agents, and other imaging techniques.

References

1. Amphoux-Fazekas T, Sanüh N, Hovsepian S, Aouani A, Beauwens R, Fayet G (1999) DIDS (4,4'-diisothiocyanatostübene-2,2'-disulfonic acid) increases iodide trapping, inhibits thyroperoxidase and antagonizes the TSH-induced apical iodide efflux in porcine thyroid cells. Mol Cell Endocrinol 141:129–140
2. Arturi F, Russo D, Schlumberger M, du Villard JA, Caillou B, Vigneri P, Wicker R, Chiefari E, Suarez HG, Filetti S (1998) Iodide symporter gene expression in human thyroid tumors. J Clin Endocrinol Metab 83:2493–2496

3. Bassi V, Vitale Nt, Feliciello A, De Riu S, Rossi G, Fenzi G (1995) Retinoic acid induces intercellular adhesion molecule-1 hyperexpression in human thyroid carcinoma cell lines. J Clin Endocrinol Metab 80:1129–1135
4. Brabant G, Maenhaut C, Köhrle J, Scheumann G, Dralle H, Hoang-Vu C, Hesch RD, von zur Mühlen A, Vassart G, Dumont JE (1991) Human thyrotropin receptor gene: Expression in thyroid tumors and correlation to markers of thyroid differentiation and dedifferentiation. Mol Cell Endocrinol 82:R7–R12
5. Brabant G, Hoang-Vu C, Cetin Y, Dralle H, Scheumann G, Mölne J, Hansson G, Jansson S, Ericson LE, Nilsson M (1993) E-Cadherin: a differentiation marker in thyroid malignancies. Cancer Res 53:4987–4993
6. Breitman TR, Selonick S, Collins SJ (1980) Induction of differentiation of the human promyelocytic leukemia cell line (IHL-60) by retinoic acid. Proc Natl Acad Sci USA 77:2936–2940
7. Caillou B, Troalen F, Baudin E, Talbot M, Filetti S, Schlumberger M, Bidart JM (1998) Na+/l-symporter distribution in human thyroid tissues: an immunohistochemical study. J Clin Endocrinol Metab 83:4102–4106
8. Castro MR, Bergert ER, Beito TG, Roche PC, Ziesmer SC, Jhiang SM, Goellner JR, Morris JC (1999) Monoclonal antibodies against the human sodium iodide symporter: Utility for immunocytochemistry of thyroid cancer. J Endocrinol 163:495–504
9. Chomienne C, Fenaux P, Degos L (1996) Retinoid differentiation therapy in promyelocytic leukemia. FASEB J 10:1025–1030
10. Chytil F (1996) Retinoids in lung development. FASEB J 10:986–992
11. Dai G, Levy O, Carrasco N (1996) Cloning and characterization of the thyroid iodide transporter. Nature 379:458–460
12. Del Senno L, Rossi R, Franceschetti P, degli Uberti EC (1994) Expression of all-trans-retinoic acid receptor RNA in human thyroid cells. Biochem Mol Biol Int 33:1107–1115
13. Filetti S, Bidart JM, Arturi F, Caillou B, Russo D, Schlumberger M (1999) Sodium/iodide symporter: A key transport system in thyroid cancer cell metabolism. Eur J Endocrinol 141:443–457
14. Fisher GJ, Voorhees JJ (1996) Molecular mechanisms of retinoid actions in skin. FASEB J 10:1002–1013
15. Giguere V (1994) Retinoic acid receptors and cellular retinoid binding proteins complex interplay in retinoid signalling. Endocrine Rev 15:61–79
16. Goretzki PE, Simon D, Frilling A, Witte J, Reiners C, Grussendorf M, Horster FA, Röher HD (1994) Surgical reintervention for differentiated thyroid carcinoma. Br J Surg 80:1131–1134
17. Grünwald F, Pakos E, Bender H, Menzel C, Otte R, Palmedo H, Pfeifer U (1998b) Redifferentiation therapy with retinoic acid in follicular thyroid cancer. J Nucl Med 39:1555–1558
18. Grünwald F, Menzel C, Bender H, Palmedo H, Otte R, Finimers R, Risse J, Biersack HJ (1998) Redifferentiation therapy-induced radioiodine uptake in thyroid cancer. J Nucl Med 39:1903–1906
19. Haussler M, Sidell N, Kelly M, Donaldson C, Altman A, Mangelsdorf DJ (1983) Specific high-affinity binding and biologic action of retinoic acid in human neuroblastoma cell lines. Proc Natl Acad Sci USA 80:5525–5529
20. Hinds TS, West WL, Knight EM (1997) Carotenoids and retinoids: A review of research, clinical, and public health applications. J Clin Pharmacol 37:551–558
21. Hoang-Vu C, Schmutzler C, Schwarz 1, Bull K, Aust G, Köhrle J, Dralle H (1998) Effects of retinoic acid on protein expression of CD 97 and E-cadherin in the human thyroid carcinoma cell line FTC 133. J Endocrinol Invest 21 [Suppl]:14 (Abstract)
22. Hoang-Vu C, Schumann H, Krause G, Bull K, Schwarz I, Goretzki PE, Schmutzler C, Köhrle J, Holtz J, Dralle H (1998) Retinoic induced expression of Fas protein in the human thyroid carcinoma cell line FTC-236. Exp Clin Endocr Diab 106 [Suppl 1]:S83 (Abstract)
23. Hoang-Vu C, Bull K, Schwarz l, Krause G, Schmutzler C, Aust G, Köhrle J, Dralle H (1999) Regulation of CD97 protein in thyroid carcinoma. J Clin Endocrinol Metab 84:1104–1109

24. Hofman C, Eichele G (1994) Retinoids in development. In: Sporn MB, Roberts AB, Goodman DS (eds) The retinoids: biology, chemistry, and medicine. Raven Press, New York, pp 387–441
25. Hong WK, Itri LM (1994) Retinoids and human cancer. In: Sporn MB, Roberts AB, Goodman DS (eds) The retinoids: biology, chemistry, and medicine. Raven Press, New York, pp 597–630
26. Jakobs TC, Schmutzler C, Meissner J, Köhrle J (1997) The promoter of the human type 1 5'-deiodinase gene: mapping of the transcription start site and identification of a DR+4 thyroid hormone responsive element. Eur J Biochem 247:288–297
27. Jhiang SM, Cho JY, Ryu KY, DeYoung BR, Smanik PA, McGaughy VR, Fischer AR Mazzaferri EL (1998) An immunohistochemical study of Na+/I- symporter in human thyroid tissues and salivary gland tissues. Endocrinology 139:4416–4419
28. Köhrle J (1999) Local activation and inactivation of thyroid hormones: the deiodinase family. Mol Cell Endocrinol 151:103–119
29. Koong SS, Reynolds JC, Movius EG, Keenan AM, Ain KB, Lakshrnan MC, Robbins J (1999) Lithium as a potential adjuvant to 131-I therapy of metastatic, well differentiated thyroid carcinoma. J Clin Endocrinol Metab 84:912–916
30. Lazar V, Bidart JM, Caillou B, Mahe C, Lacroix L, Filetti S, Schlumberger M (1999) Expression of the Na'/l- symporter gene in human thyroid tumors: a comparison study with other thyroid-specific genes. J Clin Endocrinol Metab 84:3228–3234
31. Lotan R (1996) Retinoids in cancer chemoprevention. FASEB J 10:1031–1039
32. Love JM, Gudas LJ 1994 Vitamin A, differentiation, and cancer. Curr Opin Cell Biol 6:825–831
33. Mangelsdorff DJ, Evans RE (1995) The RXR heterodimers and orphan receptors. Cell 86:841–850
34. Means AL, Gudas LJ (1995) The roles of retinoids in vertebrate development. Annu Rev Biochem 64:201–233
35. Moon RC, Mehta RG, Rao KVN (1994) Retinoids and cancer in experimental animals. In: Sporn MB, Roberts AB, Goodman DS (eds) The retinoids: biology, chemistry, and medicine. Raven Press, New York, pp 573–595
36. Nagy L, Thomazy VA, Heyman RA, Davies PJ (1998) Retinoid-induced apoptosis in normal and neoplastic tissues. Cell Death Differ 5:11–19
37. Saito T, Endo T, Kawaguchi A, lkeda M, Katoh R, Kawaoi A, Muramatsu A, Onaya T (1998) Increased expression of the sodium/iodide symporter in papillary thyroid carcinomas. J Clin Invest 10 1:1296–1300
38. Scheibe RJ, Ginty D, Wagner JA (1991) Retinoic acid stimulates the differentiation of PCI2 cells that are deficient in cAMP-dependent protein kinase. J Cell Biol 113:1173–1181
39. Schmutzler C, Schreck R, Bienert K, Köhrle J (1994) Retinoid treatment of thyroid carcinoma cells: A prospect for a re-differentiation therapy? Proceedings, EORTC Thyroid Study Group Annual Meeting, Vienna
40. Schmutzler C, Brtko J, Bienert K, Köhrle J (1996) Effects of retinoids and role of retinoic acid receptors in human thyroid carcinomas and cell lines derived therefrom. Exp Clin Endocrinol Metab 104 [Suppl 4]:16–19
41. Schmutzler C, Winzer R, Meissner-Weigl J, Köhrle J (1997) Retinoic acid increases sodium/iodide symporter mRNA levels in human thyroid cancer cell lines and suppresses expression of functional symporter in nontransformed FRTL-5 rat thyroid cells. Biochem Biophys Res Commun 240:832–838
42. Schmutzler C, Brtko J, Winzer R, Jakobs TC, Meissner J, Simon D, Goretzki PE, Köhrle J (1998) Functional retinoid and thyroid hormone receptors in human thyroid cell lines and tissues. Int J Cancer 76:368–376
43. Schreck R, Schnieders F, Schmutzler C, Köhrle J (1994) Retinoids stimulate type 1 iodothyronine 5'-deiodinase activity in human follicular thyroid carcinoma cell lines. J Clin Endocrinol Metab 79:791–798

44. Simon D, Köhrle J, Schmutzler C, Mainz K, Reiners C, Röher HD (1996) Redifferentiation therapy of differentiated thyroid carcinoma with retinoic acid: basics and first clinical results. Exp Clin Endocrinol Metab 104 [Suppl 4]:13–15
45. Simon D, Köhrle J, Reiners C, Boerner AR, Schmutzler C, Mainz K, Goretzki PE, Röher HD (1998) Redifferentiation therapy with retinoids: Therapeutic option for advanced follicular and papillary thyroid carcinoma. World J Surg 22:569–574
46. Simon D, Köhrle J, Reiners C, Groth P, Börner AR, Grünwald F, Riccabona G, Mainz K (1998) Redifferentiation therapy in thyroid cancer – results of a multicenter pilot study. Thyroid 8:217 (Abstract)
47. Smanik PA, Liu Q, Furminger TL, Ryu K, Xing S, Mazzaferri EL, Jhiang SM (1996) Cloning of the human sodium iodide symporter. Biochem Biophys Res Commun 226:339–345
48. Smanik P-A, Ryu KY, Theil KS, Mazzaferri EL, Jhiang SM (1997) Expression, exon-intron organization, and chromosome mapping of the human sodium iodide symporter. Endocrinology 138:3555–3558
49. Sun SY, Yue P, Wu GS, EI-Deiry WS, Shroot B, Hong WX, Lotan R (1999) Mechanisms of apoptosis induced by the synthetic retinoid CD437 in human non-small cell lung carcinoma cells. Oncogene 18:2357–2365
50. Teixeira C, Pratt MA (1997) CDK2 is a target for retinoic acid-mediated growth inhibition in MCF-7 human breast cancer cells. Mol Endocrinol 11:1191–1202
51. van Herle AJ, Agatep UL, Padua HI DN, Totanes TL, Canlapan DV, van Herle HML, Juillard GJF (1990) Effects of 13 cis-retinoic acid on growth and differentiation of human follicular carcinoma cells (UCLA RO 82 W-1) in vitro. J Clin Endocrinol Metab 71:755–763
52. Van Pelt AMM, De Rooij DG (1990) Synchronization of the seminiferous epithelium after vitamin A replacement in vitamin-A-deficient mice. Biol Reprod 43:363–367
53. Venkataraman GM, Yatin M, Marcinek R, Ain KB (1999) Restoration of iodide uptake in dedifferentiated thyroid carcinoma: Relationship to human Na/I symporter gene methylation status. J Clin Endocrionol Metab 84:2449–2457
54. Wolf G (1996) A history of vitamin A and retinoids. FASEB J 10:1102–1107
55. Zhang CY, Kim S, Hamey JW, Larsen PR (1998) Further characterization of thyroid hormone response elements in the human type 1 iodothyronine deiodinase gene. Endocrinology 139:1156–1163
56. Zhou XF, Shen X-Q, Shemshedini L (1999) Ligand-activated retinoic acid receptor inhibits AP-1 transactivation by disrupting c-Jun/c-Fos dimerization. Mol Endocrinol 13:276–285

Follow-up of Patients with Well-Differentiated Thyroid Cancer 12

B. Shapiro, J. Freitas, and M. Gross

12.1 Introduction

Although uncommon, thyroid cancer generates significant attention in the medical literature that is out of proportion to its incidence. Whether this interest is the result of its demographics, where thyroid cancer tends to affect both old and young, with a slight female predominance, or, more importantly, that thyroid cancer is linked to prior radiation exposure remains a mystery [1, 2]. The large number of cases of differentiated thyroid cancer in children in Belarus and Ukraine as a result of the Chernobyl disaster has provided a unique opportunity to study its etiology and genetics [3]. Although there are no universally accepted algorithms for either initial therapy or follow-up care of thyroid cancer, mortality rates in the USA have declined significantly by more than 20% in the last three decades, most likely attributable to early diagnosis and effective therapy. Since no prospective study has been performed to assess the effects of surgical excision completeness, the use of radioiodine ablation and treatment, or the degree of serum thyroid-stimulating hormone (TSH) suppression, these and other controversies continue in the management of the thyroid cancer patient (Table 12.1). Here we outline our current approach to the thyroid cancer patient that has evolved at the University of Michigan over the last five decades.

12.2 Follow-up of Patients with Thyroid Cancer

12.2.1 Assessing the Risk of Morbidity and Mortality

The approach to the patient with thyroid cancer begins with an assessment of tumor histology and the extent of disease. The majority of patients will have papillary tumors (65%), with follicular thyroid neoplasms in about 25% [1, 4]. Medullary thyroid cancer comprises about 10%, while other types (i.e., anaplastic, lymphoma) are less common and are seen in fewer than 5% of cases [5]. Most patients with papillary and some patients with follicular cancer are diagnosed by fine-needle aspiration (FNA) before surgical referral.

Table 12.1 Dilemmas in the follow-up of patients with thyroid cancer

^{131}I imaging postthyroidectomy:		
Preparation of the patient?	→	6 weeks off T4? 2–3 weeks of T3? rhTSH?
Imaging dose of ^{131}I?	→	>2–5 mCi to prevent "stunning"? ^{123}I?
Thyroglobulin (Tg):		
Reliability of many assays?	→	Accuracy with anti-TG antibodies?
Detectable Tg post-Tx?	→	Residual tumor?
"Stimulated" Tg levels	→	<2 ng/ml, is ^{131}I scan necessary?
Ablation of thyroid remnants:		
In whom?	→	Low- versus high-risk patient (i.e., MACIS score >8)
Dose of ^{131}I?	→	<100 mCi versus >100 mCi?
Follow-up intervals?	→	^{131}I WBS year 1, 2, 3, 5, 10, 15, etc?
Dose of thyroid hormone: TSH level	→	<0.1 IU/ml? 0.1–0.2 IU/ml?
^{131}I imaging as follow-up:		
Follow-up intervals?	→	^{131}I WBS year 1, 2, 3?, etc.? Need for scanning when Tg level low?
Preparation of the patient?	→	6 weeks off T4?, 2–3 weeks of T3?, rhTSH?
Imaging dose of ^{131}I?	→	<5 mCi to prevent "stunning"? ^{123}I?
^{131}I therapy for recurrent/metastatic thyroid cancer:		
Reoperation	→	Remove gross disease? (Palpable nodes?)
In whom?	→	Dose? Dosimetry? ^{131}I body clearance?
Preparation	→	Low-iodine diet, drugs to ↑ ^{131}I uptake
^{131}I-negative thyroid cancer:		
Optimal imaging modality	→	^{99m}Tc-sestamibi/tetrofosmin, ^{201}Tl, ^{18}F-FDG, ^{111}In-pentetreotide (papillary and medullary)
		Anti-CEA monoclonal antibody (medullary)
		^{99m}Tc-(V)-DMSA (medullary)
↑ TG level	→	^{131}I therapy? Dose?
^{18}F-FDG:		
Thyroid uptake	→	Incidentally discovered thyroid cancer? versus benign lesion

As with many endocrine tumors, histology alone may not disclose the malignant potential of a neoplasm. This is especially true in tumors with "mixed" characteristics, as not only the categorization, but also the assessment of prognosis and subsequent treatment planning are dependent upon correct histological identification. Often more sophisticated histopathological techniques are necessary to define the actual tumor type and prognosis.

Table 12.2 Variables influencing thyroid cancer recurrence and death

	Factors predictive of high risk	Factors predictive of moderate-to-low risk
Patient variables	Age <15 years or >45 years	Age 15–45 years
	Male	Female
	Family history of thyroid cancer	No family history of thyroid cancer
Tumor variables	Tumor >4 cm in diameter	Tumor <4 cm in diameter
	Bilateral disease	Unilateral disease
	Extrathyroidal extension	No extrathyroidal disease
	Vascular invasion (both papillary and follicular)	No vascular invasion
	Cervical or mediastinal lymph node metastases	No lymph node metastases
	Certain tumor subtypes (Hürthle, tall, columnar, insular)	Encapsulated papillary thyroid carcinoma, papillary microadenoma, cystic papillary thyroid carcinoma
	Marked nuclear atypia, tumor necrosis and vascular invasion (i.e., histological grade)	Absence of cellular atypia, tumor necrosis, vascular invasion
	Tumors/metastases that do not (or poorly) concentrate ^{131}I	Tumors/metastases that concentrate ^{131}I
	Distant metastases	No distant metastases

(with permission from [6])

Prognostic indices for thyroid cancer provide information that is important to the planning of follow-up care. Age at diagnosis, size of the primary tumor, and the presence of and extent of extrathyroidal disease are important considerations in assessing risk of recurrence and mortality from thyroid cancer (Table 12.2) [6]. These factors have been incorporated into scoring systems that have clinical utility in determining risk of recurrence and prognosis of papillary (Table 12.3) and follicular (Table 12.4) thyroid cancer [7, 8]. The follicular thyroid cancer risk factors are as follows:

- Age >50 years
- Primary tumor >3.9 cm
- Vascular invasion
- Malignant histology
- Metastases at diagnosis

Table 12.3 Prognosis of papillary thyroid cancer – MACIS scoring

Parameter	Score
<39 years	3.1
>39 years	0.8 × age
Diameter of primary	0.3 × diameter
Incomplete resection	1.0
Extrathyroid	1.0
Distant metastases	3.0
Low risk	<6.0
High risk	>8.0

(From [7])

Table 12.4 Follicular thyroid cancer risk factors and survival

Risk factors (*n*)	Survival	
	5 years	20 years
≥2	47%	8%
<2	99%	86%

(From [7])

12.2.2 Postoperative Evaluation of Thyroid Cancer

Although outside the scope of this discussion, the initial treatment for thyroid cancer will obviously affect subsequent follow-up. Thyroidectomy has been the most widely accepted treatment for thyroid cancer; however, the extent of surgical resection, lobectomy versus lobectomy plus isthmusectomy versus total thyroidectomy with or without local lymph node sampling to radical neck dissection, continues to be topic of lively debate amongst endocrine surgeons [1, 7, 9]. However, the majority of thyroidologists now favor total or near-total thyroidectomy as the procedure of choice and preferentially refer their cases to endocrine surgeons that share this opinion. It is estimated that 80% of patients with differentiated thyroid cancer will do well regardless of the initial procedure, and it is clear that the more extensive the surgical resection, the higher the morbidity. Since the majority of well-differentiated thyroid cancers are not particularly aggressive tumors, a balanced surgical approach of thyroidectomy and selected lymph node sampling with particular attention to preserving parathyroid gland(s) and sparing recurrent laryngeal nerves is a prudent and conservative course of action [1, 10]. A competent thyroid surgeon should accomplish such a procedure with a complication rate of less than 3%. This provides a thyroid bed that has been cleared of most, if not all, normal tissue and the bulk of obviously malignant thyroid tissues.

12.2.3 Postoperative Laboratory Evaluation and Imaging

12.2.3.1 Radioiodine

The detection of residual benign or malignant thyroid tissue is dependent on multiple patient factors such as the mass of tissue, its avidity for radioiodine, the iodine turnover rate of the tissues, the circulating level of TSH, and the endogenous inorganic iodine pool size. The last two factors are amenable to intervention. The majority of cases of thyroid cancer are referred for evaluation after recovery from surgery at a time when TSH values are significantly elevated to levels of >50 mIU/l, usually 6 weeks or more postoperatively [11]. In patients studied later or in whom thyroid hormone has already been started, opinions vary as to the optimal method of preparation for imaging [12–14]. In patients unable to tolerate 6 weeks or more abstinence from thyroid hormone, substitution of triiodothyronine (50–75 µg/day in divided doses) for 2–3 weeks and then 2 weeks of abstinence has been offered as an alternative [14, 15]. In selected patients with known locally invasive or metastatic thyroid cancer, rising TSH stimulation for 1–2 weeks can induce rapid growth in metastatic tumor tissue in brain or impinging on the spinal cord, which can lead to marked clinical deterioration or even death. With thyroid hormone withdrawal, patients with mild to moderate renal insufficiency can experience progressive, symptomatic azotemia, because glomerular filtration rate falls with the development of hypothyroidism with an increase in serum creatinine and blood urea nitrogen of 45–50%. Some elderly patients and patients with pituitary or hypothalamic disease fail to generate a sufficient rise in serum TSH for optimal imaging. Administration of recombinant human (rh) TSH (Thyrogen) obviates the need for a prolonged period of abstinence from thyroid hormone, and it has become a preferred method for the preparation of patients for long-term postthyroidectomy biochemical (e.g., thyroglobulin, Tg) and imaging evaluations [15–17]. Studies indicate that TSH levels exceed 30 mIU/l after two sequential intramuscular injections of rhTSH of 0.9 mg [16]. The agent is approved for diagnostic purposes and has been offered as a means to raise TSH in preparation for radioiodine therapy, but is not as yet approved for this latter indication.

Radioiodine uptake by benign and malignant thyroid tissue is increased by reduction of the endogenous, stable iodine pool [15]. This can be accomplished by lowering daily iodine intake to <100 µg/day with a low iodine diet for 10 days prior to radioiodine tracer dose administration. Although there has been a well-documented >50% decline in iodine intake in the USA over the past two decades, a low-iodine diet further reduces iodine intake in our patient population by approximately 70% (unpublished data). Obviously, other sources of iodine such as radiographic contrast media or drugs (i.e., amiodarone) must be avoided for at least 6 weeks prior to radioiodine scanning.

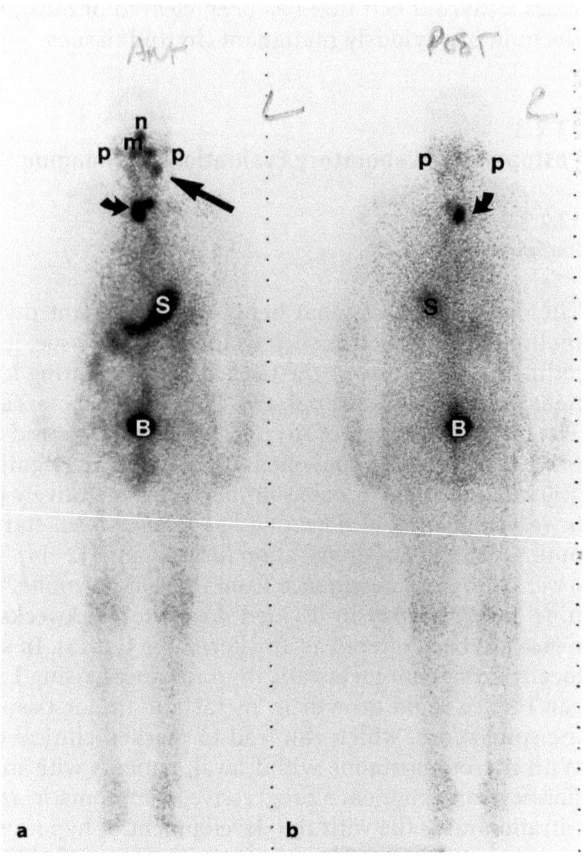

Fig. 11.1. Anterior (**a**) and posterior (**b**) whole body images 24 h after 2 mCi ^{131}I 8 weeks following near-total thyroidectomy for papillary thyroid cancer. Note: large thyroid bed remnant (*curved arrow*), normal uptake in nose (*n*), mouth (*m*), parotid glands (*p*), stomach (*S*), and bladder (*B*). There is increased ^{131}I in the left submandibular gland due to an obstructing calculus (*straight arrow*)

Radioiodine remains the primary diagnostic agent used to determine the presence of both normal and neoplastic thyroid tissues after surgery for thyroid cancer. It is clear that, with more extensive operations (i.e., thyroidectomy), the ability to detect disease outside of the thyroid bed is enhanced [18–21]. Despite total thyroidectomy, more than 95% of patients undergoing postoperative radioiodine scanning have residual normal tissue uptake in the neck, usually in the upper poles, ligament of Berry region, or embryonic thyroglossal duct remnant. Even small amounts of normal thyroid tissue left in the neck may result in sufficient accumulation radioiodine to make evaluation of the thyroid bed, neck and surrounding areas for thyroid cancer difficult (Fig. 12.1). Foci of uptake that lie outside the thyroid bed are suggestive of thyroid cancer [22]. It is important to image the chest, abdomen, and occasionally the extremities, especially in patients with follicular thyroid cancer (Fig. 12.2). At times delayed imaging, sometimes at 48–72 h after radio-iodine administration, is necessary to detect metastases of thyroid cancer [22]. Artifacts of ^{131}I imaging are an important consideration and must be excluded (Fig. 12.3) [23].

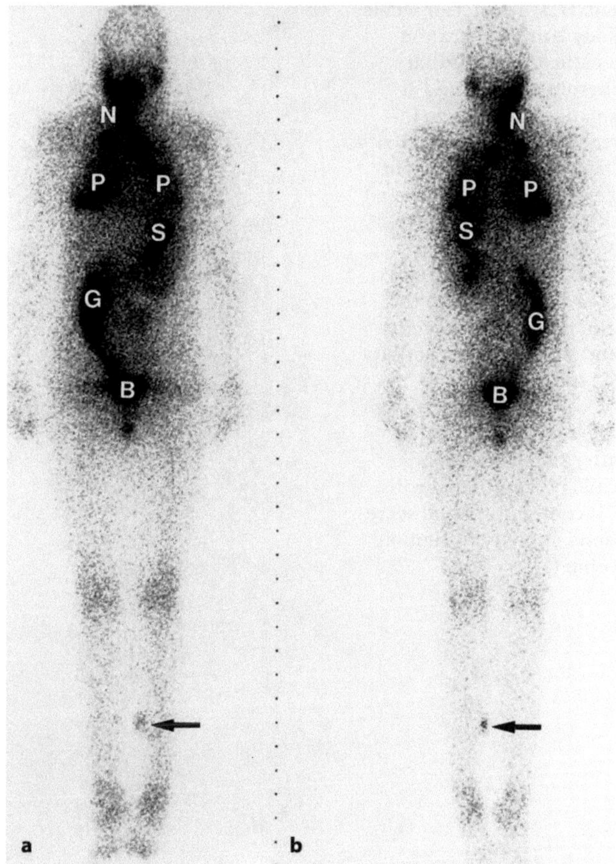

Fig. 11.2. Whole body diagnostic images (**a**, anterior; **b**, posterior) obtained 24 h following a 2 mCi dose of ^{131}I in a man with aggressive metastatic papillary thyroid carcinoma. There are extensive ^{131}I-avid lymph node metastases in the right lateral neck and superior mediastinum (*N*) and diffuse bilateral pulmonary metastases (*P*). There is also normal biodistribution of ^{131}I in the stomach (*S*), gut (*G*), and bladder (*B*). Gut uptake is intense due to hypothyroidism. *Arrow* identifies urine contamination on leg not to be confused with metastases

The diagnostic dose of ^{131}I used for scintigraphic studies has been shown to affect subsequent uptake of therapeutic doses of ^{131}I. This "stunning" effect of ^{131}I has been seen with imaging doses as low as 2–5 mCi in some studies, but the "effect" and its significance continues to be a topic of controversy [12, 15, 24, 25]. ^{123}I has been recommended as a substitute for ^{131}I, since it has not been demonstrated to induce stunning [24]. However, the availability and expense of ^{123}I as compared to ^{131}I have limited its use in the past. Recently, its price has significantly declined and it is supplanting ^{131}I as the radioiodine of choice for diagnostic studies in many centers. Alternatively, others advocate that doses of ^{131}I to be used for imaging of thyroid cancer should be limited to less than 5 mCi to avoid untoward effects of diagnostic doses upon the potential effectiveness of subsequent therapeutic radioiodine [25].

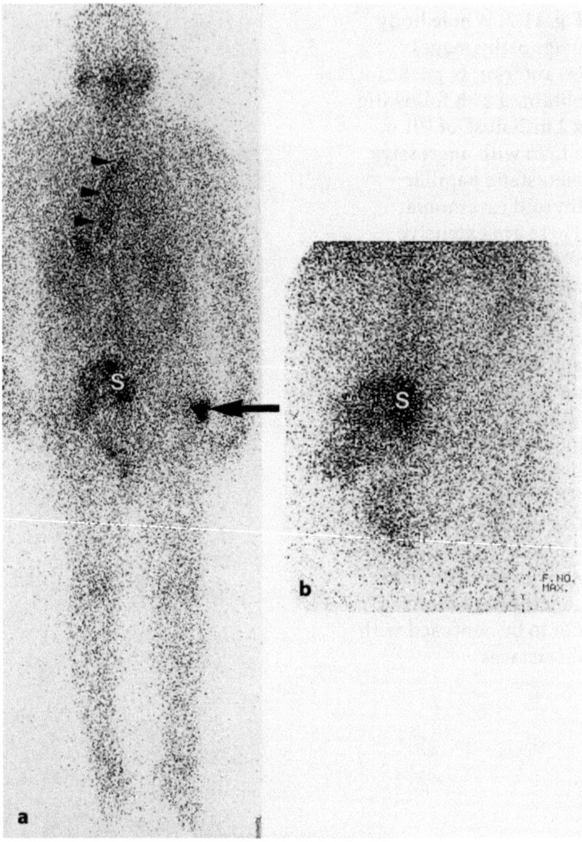

Fig. 11.3. a Posterior whole body 2 mCi ^{131}I scan in a patient with papillary thyroid cancer and ^{131}I ablation showing an intense focus of radioactivity in the region of the right greater trochanter (*arrow*) that might be interpreted as a skeletal metastasis. There is also some reflux of radioactivity into the esophagus (*arrowheads*) and sigmoid colon activity (*S*) in the pelvis. **b** Posterior spot view from the hip pocket of pelvis after removal of handkerchief contaminated with ^{131}I containing nasal secretions. Activity in sigmoid colon (*S*)

12.2.3.2 Alternative Thyroid Cancer Imaging Agents

Other imaging agents have been used to depict thyroid cancer. Technetium-99m (99mTc)-sestamibi, ^{99m}Tc-tetrofosmin, ^{201}Tl, ^{111}In-octreotide and ^{18}F-fluorodeoxyglucose have been used to image a large variety of neoplasms (Figs. 12.4 and 12.5) [26–29]. Although generally reserved for thyroid cancers that do not accumulate radioiodine, the cardiac agents ^{99m}Tc-sestamibi, ^{99m}Tc-tetrofosmin, ^{201}Tl, the somatostatin-receptor imaging agent ^{111}In-octreotide, and the glucose analog ^{18}F-fluorodeoxyglucose (18F-FDG) have been shown to localize many types of thyroid cancer [26–29]. They all have the benefit of not requiring abstinence from thyroid hormone before imaging, although recent studies indicate that ^{18}F-FDG accumulation by the thyroid is enhanced by an elevated TSH [30]. They allow tomography (either single photon emission tomography for ^{99m}Tc and ^{201}Tl or positron emission tomography with ^{18}F) to be performed. The more widespread use of FDG in patients with malignancies other than thyroid cancer has identified a significant number of patients with abnormal thyroid

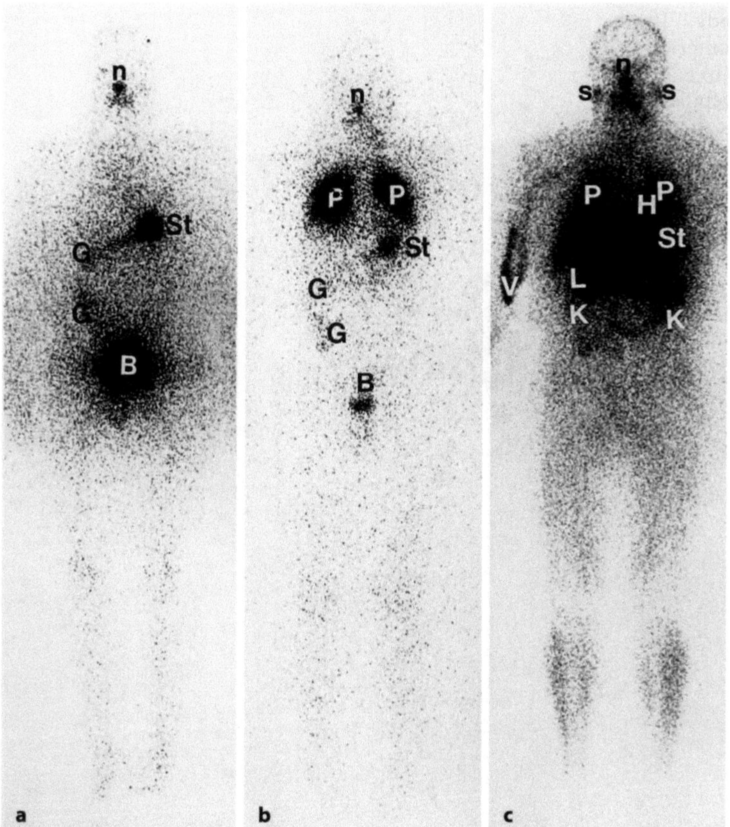

Fig. 12.4a-c Anterior whole body scans of a patient following total thyroidectomy. **a** Scan performed 24 h after administration of 2 mCi ^{131}I in error while the patient was still taking thyroid hormone (TSH<0.03 μU/ml). Note normal uptake in nasopharynx (*n*), stomach (*St*), gut (*G*), and bladder (*B*). **b** Scan repeated 6 weeks later after withdrawal of thyroid hormone (TSH 68 μU/ml). Note intense uptake in diffuse metastases not visualized while taking thyroid hormone and proving the TSH dependence of ^{131}I uptake by the lung metastases. **c** Scan performed 30 min after 2 mCi of ^{201}Tl while taking (TSH<0.03 μU/ml). Note that uptake of ^{201}Tl in the lung metastases is less TSH-dependent than the uptake of ^{131}I. Normal uptake is seen in the nasopharynx (*n*), salivary glands (*s*), heart (*H*), stomach (*St*), liver (*L*), and the injected vein (*V*)

accumulation of tracer and a subset of patients with unsuspected thyroid cancer [31] (Fig. 12.6). The diagnostic accuracy for these agents in the evaluation of thyroid cancer is variable. They are most useful in the evaluation of thyroid cancer patients previously ablated or treated with ^{131}I, which eliminates normal thyroid tissue. The somatostatin analog ^{111}In-octreotide has been shown to not only depict well-differentiated thyroid carcinomas that express somatostatin receptors, but also has enjoyed success as an agent to localize medullary thyroid carcinoma (Fig. 12.7) [32].

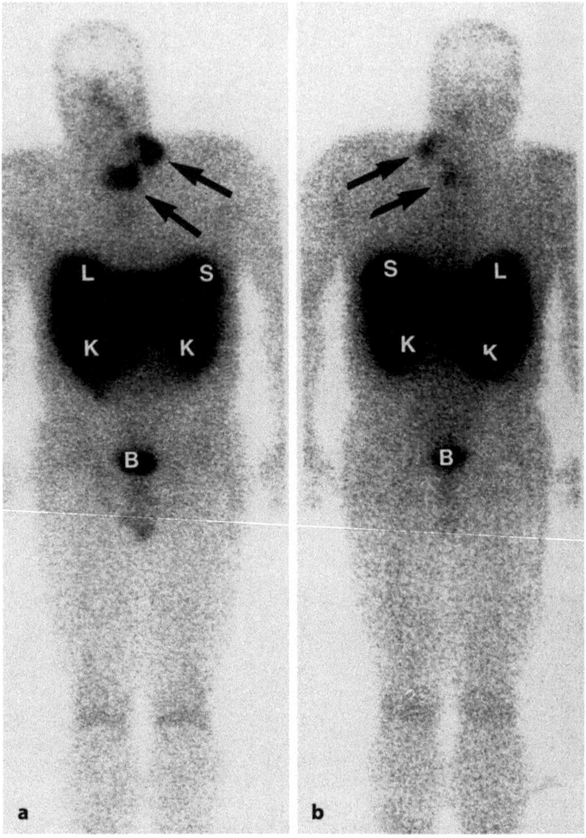

Fig. 12.5 Whole body ^{111}In-DTPA-octreotide anterior (**a**) and posterior (**b**) scans in a patient with papillary follicular thyroid cancer with left cervical lymph node metastases (*arrows*) showing the presence of extensive somatostatin-receptor binding. There is also normal ^{111}In-octreotide uptake in liver (*L*), spleen (*S*), kidneys (*K*), and bladder (*B*)

12.2.3.3 Thyroglobulin

The principal glycoprotein secreted by follicular epithelium, Tg, not only participates in the biosynthesis of thyroid hormone, but also has become a useful marker for the presence of thyroid tissue [33]. The postoperative evaluation of patients with thyroid cancer now includes measurement of serum Tg concentration [33, 34]. Serum Tg concentration (approximate 3-day circulating half-life) is affected by the degree of thyrotropin receptor stimulation (by hCG, TSH, or TSH receptor antibodies), any inflammation or injury to thyroid tissue (e.g., thyroiditis or FNA), the presence of residual normal thyroid tissue, and the thyroid cancer mass. Interpretation of individual and serial serum Tg concentrations requires knowledge of the conditions present at the time of sampling (i.e., on or off thyroid hormone suppression), the functional sensitivity of the particular Tg assay, and the athyrotic normal range of the assay. Serum Tg values from one assay cannot normally be compared with values from another assay, especially in determining cut-off values for the presence or absence of thyroid cancer,

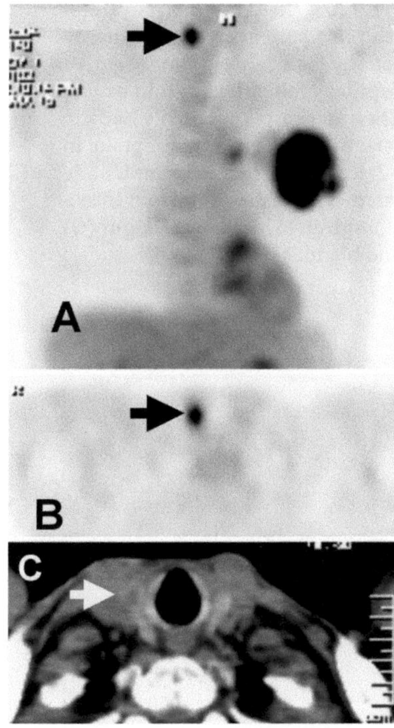

Fig. 12.6 a–c [^{18}F]fluorodeoxyglucose (FDG)/CT scan in a patient with recurrent, stage III non-Hodgkin's lymphoma, with an incidentally discovered Hürthle cell neoplasm in the neck (*arrow*)

which can vary between <1 and 30 ng/ml in commercial assays. The best Tg assay is one with a functional sensitivity <1 ng/ml with good interassay precision (<10% coefficient of variation). In the absence of interfering anti-thyroglobulin antibodies, a TSH-stimulated low or undetectable Tg is strong evidence against the need for a further search for the presence of metastases, while an elevated or rising Tg level indicates the presence of metastases or recurrence of thyroid cancer in the proper clinical setting [33–35]. An elevated Tg level may signal residual or recurrent disease in the face of negative ^{131}I imaging and is not an uncommon occurrence in many series [34].

12.2.4 Follow-up Therapy After Thyroidectomy

12.2.4.1 Ablation of Thyroid Remnants

The presence of remnant tissues in the bed of the thyroid after thyroidectomy is a commonly encountered finding ^{131}I scintigrams. In patients with low indices of recurrence (MACIS scores <6) and obvious small remnants, further therapy may not be warranted [7, 36]. However, there is little or no consensus and the

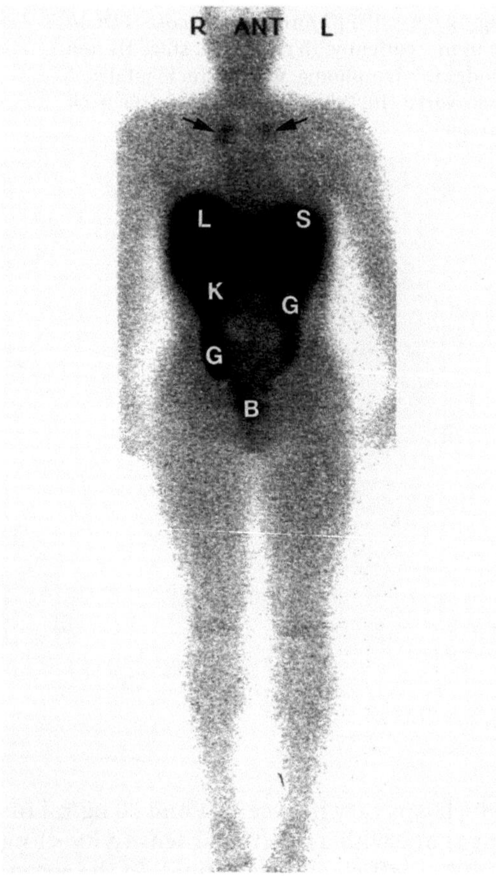

Fig. 12.7 ^{111}In-DTPA-octreotide scan in a patient after total thyroidectomy for a radioiodine-negative, papillary follicular thyroid cancer. The anterior planar whole body image depicts abnormal uptake in bilateral paratracheal lymph nodes (arrows). Normal uptake in liver (*L*), spleen (*S*), kidney (*K*), gut (*G*), and bladder (*B*)

treatment of thyroid remnants is yet another area of controversy [1]. Proponents of postoperative ^{131}I therapy point to data that suggests that recurrence rates are decreased, while others argue that small remnants pose little or no threat to patients [37]. Larger remnants, especially in patients with higher prognostic scores, may benefit from ablation not as a therapeutic maneuver, but as a means to remove normal tissues to allow subsequent diagnostic ^{131}I scans the best opportunity to detect recurrence or the presence of metastatic disease. The dose of radioiodine used for this purpose is controversial [38]. Higher doses of 100 mCi or more have a greater likelihood of ablation of remnants. Prior to 1997, the Nuclear Regulatory Commission (NRC) guidelines mandated in-patient hospitalization for any patient whose whole-body retention exceeded 30 mCi of ^{131}I (equivalent to >5 mrad/h at 1 m). New NRC guidelines are dose-based, rather than patient-activity based, and no longer require in-patient hospitalization for all patients retaining more than 30 mCi. Effective from 29 May 1997, patients can be released by the licensee when the total effective dose equivalent of a member of the general public exposed to the patient is not likely to exceed 5 mSv

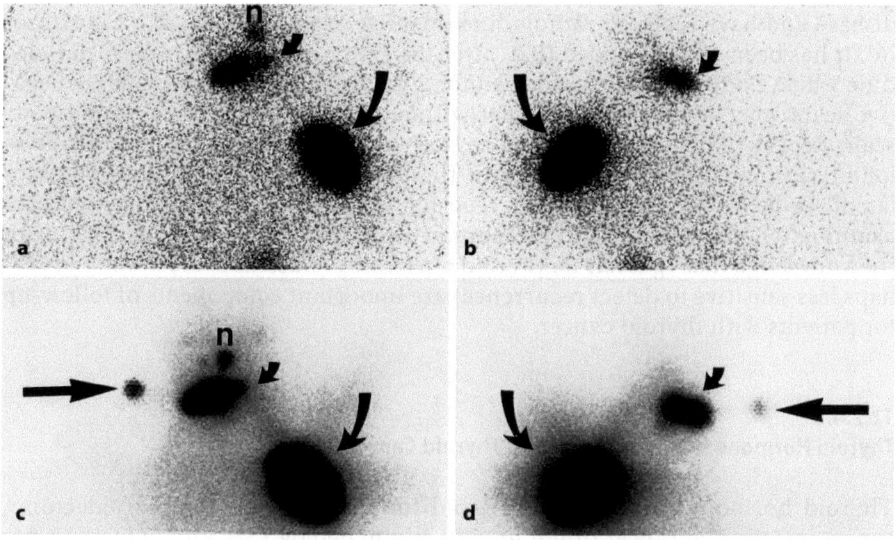

Fig. 12.8 Anterior (**a**, **c**) and posterior (**b**, **d**) views of the neck and chest of a 48-year-old female patient after complete thyroidectomy for papillary follicular thyroid cancer, with subsequent skeletal metastases to the second cervical vertebra and left scapula (*curved arrows*). Images were obtained 24 h after 1 mCi ^{131}I (**a**, **b**) and 72 h after a 302-mCi therapeutic dose of ^{131}I (**c**, **d**). *Straight arrow*, salivary contamination on a neurosurgical halo-shoulder support frame (*n* nasal uptake)

(0.5 rem). This so-called patient discharge rule has eliminated most but not all in-patient hospitalizations for ^{131}I ablation. Repeat imaging, usually not before 6 months after an ablative dose of ^{131}I, is used to assess the success of therapy. Imaging shortly after the administration of a therapeutic dose may disclose the presence of unexpected disease, but the value of early post-^{131}I therapy imaging has been recently questioned (Fig. 12.8). In patients with greater risk of metastases or recurrence, further therapy with ^{131}I directed specifically at thyroid cancer can be planned on the basis of repeat diagnostic imaging.

12.2.4.2 Follow-up Intervals After Successful Ablation

Successful ablation will result in the absence of radioiodine accumulation in the neck and a marked decrease in Tg levels. The delay in rescanning to assess the effects of radioiodine after therapy depends upon the overall risk of metastatic thyroid cancer. In patients at low risk, radioiodine whole-body scanning can be performed 1 year later. In patients at higher risk, repeat radioiodine scans can be performed as early as 4–6 months after therapy. With successful ablation, follow-up scanning intervals for patients with low-risk disease are controversial. Low Tg levels after TSH stimulation have been used to confirm the absence of disease and have replaced radioiodine imaging in some diagnostic algorithms [6]. It has been recommended that, after the first negative scan, repeat radioiodine whole-body scans be performed for 2 years [5, 33]. Two consecutive negative scans may be followed by a year without a repeat radioiodine whole-body scan. Repeat radioiodine scanning at later intervals may not be productive in long-term management, especially in the presence of low (<2 ng/ml) "stimulated" Tg levels [17, 39]. Whether seen for scanning or not, history, physical examination, chest X-ray, and measurements of thyroid hormone and Tg (with the knowledge that Tg levels on thyroid hormone replacement are lower and perhaps less sensitive to detect recurrence) are important components of follow-up for patients with thyroid cancer.

12.2.4.3
Thyroid Hormone Replacement in the Thyroid Cancer Patient

Thyroid hormone corrects hypothyroidism induced by total thyroidectomy, suppresses thyroid cancer tumor growth stimulated by TSH, and reduces tumor recurrence and death in long-term follow-up [6]. L-Thyroxine (L-T4) is most commonly used because of its long half-life and consistent T4 and T3 concentrations, mimicking normal thyroid gland production. The optimal degree of TSH suppression by exogenous L-T4 remains uncertain. Using a third-generation TSH assay that detects TSH concentrations to 0.01 mIU/l, most physicians suppress serum TSH to <0.1 mIU/l for the first few years after initial treatment. The L-T4 dose to achieve such suppression averages 2.5 µg/kg per day [40]. In patients with no evidence of recurrence or residual tumor after a few years of follow-up, the degree of thyroid hormone suppression is often reduced to allow serum TSH to rise to the 0.1–0.4 mIU/l range, lessening the impact of excessive thyroid hormone on the skeleton, especially in postmenopausal women [6, 41, 42]. In patients with recurrent or known residual tumor, continued TSH suppression of less than 0.1 mIU/l is recommended.

12.2.4.4
Radioiodine Therapy for Recurrent/Metastatic Thyroid Cancer

The demonstration of abnormal foci of radioiodine accumulation in the neck, chest, or elsewhere, once potential false positive areas are excluded, is evidence of metastases or recurrence. In patients with bulky disease in the form of palpable masses or lymph nodes, repeat operation may be recommended as a prelude to radioiodine therapy. In this instance debulking of gross tumor may facilitate the therapeutic effects of radioiodine. The dose of radioiodine used for therapy of this type is controversial [1, 5, 22, 37, 43–45]. The dose usually chosen for local disease in the neck is in the range of 150–175 mCi, and greater doses for disease in the lungs (200–250 mCi) or bone (>250 mCi) [1, 5, 22, 37, 43]. Others have advocated an approach that considers body retention with the goal of limiting bone marrow exposure to less than 200 mCi or lung retention of less than

75–80 mCi [44, 45]. This allows a significantly greater radioiodine dose to be given (300–400 mCi). Dosimetry can also be used to estimate the dose to tumor. This is a more cumbersome approach but can be used to safely administer even higher doses of radioiodine. These higher doses are accompanied with a greater risk of side-effects from radiation such as nausea, vomiting, cystitis, and sialadentitis early after treatment, and a greater degree of bone marrow depression and xerostomia seen later after radioiodine therapy. The recent liberalization of release rules by the US Nuclear Regulatory Commission after radioiodine allows many patients to be sent home immediately after therapy. It is important to carefully select which patients can be sent home early, as therapeutic doses of radioiodine of this magnitude may result in inadvertent exposure of members of the public in noncompliant patients. Repeat whole-body imaging early after therapeutic doses of radioiodine may be useful to assess for any unanticipated findings. Follow-up of patients after successful therapy is by repeat radioiodine whole-body scans for 2 consecutive years, and if negative then follow up with routine studies to include "stimulated" Tg levels in addition to measurements of TSH. A remote recurrence >10 years after successful therapy is not common, but must be kept in mind in the long-term follow up of these patients. The identification of recurrence would be followed by repeat radioiodine therapy up to a usually assumed maximum of 1,000 mCi cumulative dose.

12.2.4.5 Radioiodine-Negative Thyroid Cancer

Either as a result of dedifferentiation or with certain types of thyroid cancer, some thyroid tumors do not accumulate or lose the ability to accumulate radioiodine [46]. In the case of Hürthle cell or medullary thyroid carcinoma, other diagnostic and therapeutic approaches are necessary. Computed tomography, real-time ultrasound, magnetic resonance, ^{99m}Tc-sestamibi/tetrofosmin, ^{201}Tl, ^{111}In-octreotide, and ^{18}F-FDG can be used to depict metastases or recurrence (Fig. 12.9) [28–31, 47, 48]. External beam radiation therapy and chemotherapy with adriamycin and/or other agents has been used to induce partial remissions [49, 50]. Medullary thyroid cancers can be familial, and there are methods to identify susceptible members of affected families [51]. Medullary thyroid cancers produce calcitonin, carcinoembryonic antigen, and other markers that can be used to follow patients and the effects of surgery and chemotherapy [52]. Further, medullary thyroid cancers have been imaged with ^{99m}Tc (V)-dimercaptosuccinic acid, radiolabeled anti-CEA monoclonal antibodies, and ^{131}I- and ^{123}I-metaiodobenzylguanidine (MIBG), and, as this tumor also expresses somatostatin, receptors can be imaged with ^{111}In-octreotide [53–56]. Surgical extirpation of the primary neoplasm and metastases is the most successful therapeutic approach for Hürthle cell and medullary thyroid cancer, but is often incomplete as a result of early and distant spread of these tumors. In the case of medullary thyroid cancer, high-dose ^{131}I-MIBG has been used with some success [57]. Other radiopharmaceuticals based on somatostatin analogs have been

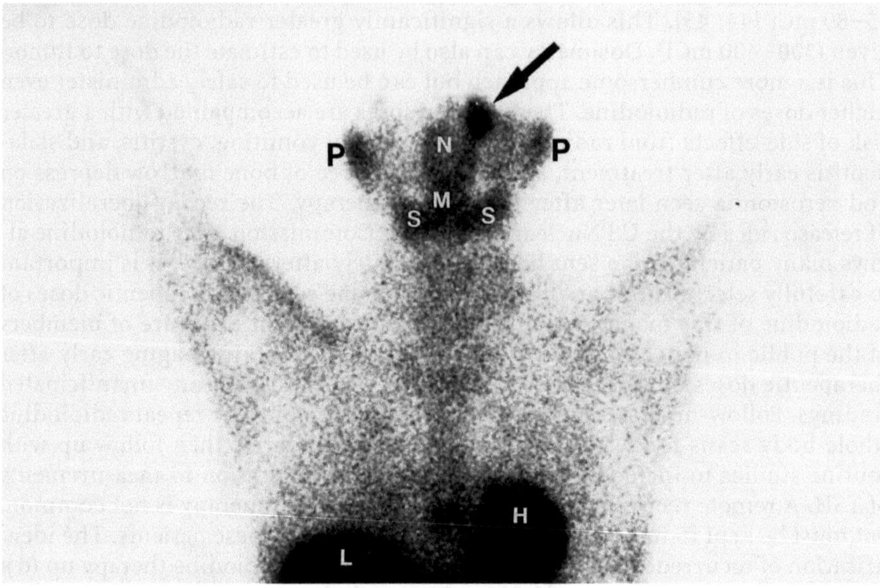

Fig. 12.9 ^{99m}Tc-MIBI anterior planar image of the head, neck, and chest after total thyroidectomy with surgical absence of thyroid bed activity and normal uptake in the parotid glands (*P*), nasopharynx (*N*), mouth (*M*), submandibular glands (*S*), heart (*H*), and liver (*L*). The patient has a solitary orbital metastasis of Hürthle cell thyroid cancer, which was negative on ^{131}I scintigraphy

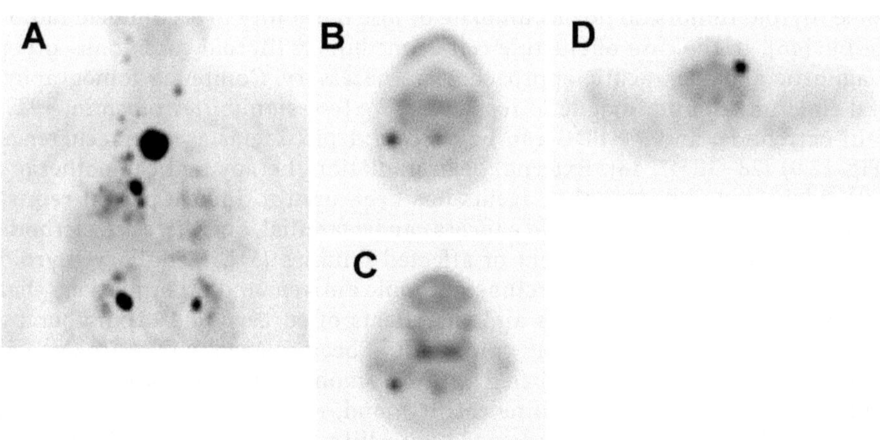

Fig. 12.10 a–d A 69-year-old man with recurrent, radioiodine-negative, papillary thyroid cancer with a rising Tg levels. ^{18}F-FDG scan depicts known, low cervical lymph node metastasis (**A, D**) and also multiple metastatic deposits in the neck (**B, C**) and chest (**A**)

suggested as potential radiotherapeutic agents for medullary thyroid cancer and other neuroendocrine neoplasms that express somatostatin receptors [58].

In some papillary and follicular thyroid cancers, loss of radioiodine uptake can be seen after ^{131}I therapy. Diagnostic radioiodine scans are negative, but Tg levels may be elevated or increasing. Many of these patients will have normal conventional imaging studies (CT, neck ultrasound, and MR). Confirmation of the presence of metastases/recurrence with other imaging agents (^{99m}Tc-sestamibi/tetrofosmin, ^{201}Tl, ^{111}In-octreotide, and ^{18}F-FDG) can be used to identify tumors (Fig. 12.10). FDG has shown high efficacy in the identification of metastases of thyroid cancer [59–61]. The avidity of FDG accumulation by thyroid cancer has been predictive of radioiodine resistance [62]. In patients with a TSH-stimulated serum Tg concentration >10 ng/ml but no localization of disease, some have advocated therapeutic administration of I-131 to simultaneously localize and treat occult metastases most commonly in lungs, thyroid bed or cervical or mediastinal nodes [63–65]. Many patients treated empirically in this fashion show ^{131}I localization in metastases on posttherapy scans and a subsequent fall in serum Tg over time, but not often to the normal athyrotic range [6]. It is desirable to treat and possibly cure microscopic metastases presumably early in their course (10-year, 100% survival) and prevent CT micronodules (10-year 63% survival) or chest X-ray-detectable lung disease (10-year, 11% survival), which is much more difficult to eradicate [66–68]. However, it is still not clear what is the natural course of such small metastatic deposits detected by elevated serum Tg measurements [69].

12.3 Summary

Despite the lack of consensus that surrounds almost all aspects of the treatment and follow up surveillance of patients with thyroid cancer, most if not all physicians would agree that initial adequate therapy begins with: (1) an appropriate surgical approach to remove as much abnormal and normal thyroid tissue as possible; (2) ablation of thyroid remnants and/or abnormal foci of ^{131}I accumulation in the neck and elsewhere if possible, and (3) surveillance at intervals sufficient to identify tumor recurrence. Many different algorithms have been offered as alternative methods for follow-up of patients with thyroid cancer and the "devil (as always) is found in the details" (Fig. 12.11). Whatever approach to management is chosen, however, each patient presents with a unique set of circumstances that often require a flexible approach to successful, individual care.

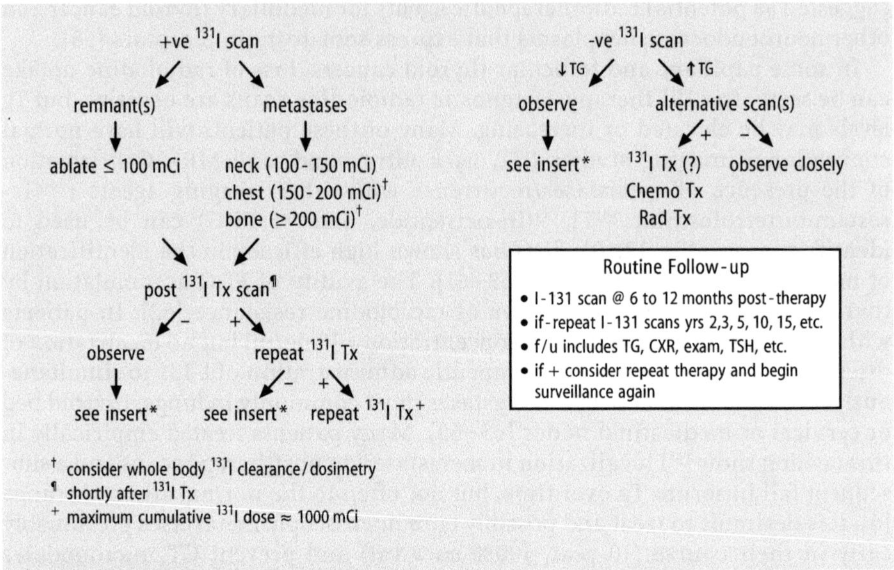

Fig. 12.11 Follow-up of patients with well-differentiated thyroid cancer

References

1. Mazzaferri E (1995) Impact of initial tumor features and treatment selected on the long term course of differentiated thyroid cancer. Thyroid Today 28:1–13
2. Ron E, Lubin JH, Shore RE et al (1995) Thyroid cancer after exposure to external radiation: a pooled analysis of seven studies. Radiat Res 141:259–277
3. Tuttle RM, Becker DV (2000) The chernobyl accident and its consequences: update at the Millenium. Semin Nucl Med 30:133–140
4. Samaan NA, Maheshwari YK, Nader S et al (1983) Impact of therapy for differentiated carcinoma of the thyroid: an analysis of 706 cases. J Endocrinol Metab 56:1131–1138
5. Clarke SEM (1998) Radioiodine therapy of the thyroid. In: Murray IPC, Ell PJ (eds) Nuclear medicine in clinical diagnosis and therapy. Churchill and Livingstone, Edinburgh, pp 1049–1062
6. Mazzaferri EL, Kloos RT (2001) Current approaches to primary therapy for papillary and follicular thyroid cancer. J Clin Endocrinol Metab 86:1447–1463
7. Hay ID (1989) Prognostic factors in thyroid carcinoma. Thyroid Today 12:1–9
8. Nygaards BJ, Hegedus L, Gervil M, Hjalgrim H, Soe-Jensen P, Hansen JM (1993) Radioiodine treatment of multinodular goiter. Br Med J 307:828–832
9. Mazzaferri E (1991) Treating differentiated thyroid carcinoma: where do we draw the line? Mayo Clin Proc 66:105–111
10. DeGroot LJ, Kaplan EL, McCormick M, Straus FH (1990) Natural history, treatment and course of papillary thyroid carcinoma. J Clin Endocrinol Metab 71:414–424
11. Maxon HR, Smith HS (1990) Radioiodine-131 in the diagnosis and treatment of well differentiated thyroid cancer. Endocrinol Metab Clin North Am 19:685–718
12. Riccabona G (1998) Differentiated thyroid carcinoma. In: Murray IPC, Ell PJ (eds) Nuclear medicine in clinical diagnosis and therapy. Churchill and Livingstone, Edinburgh, pp 941–957

13. Goldman JM, Line BR, Aamodt RL et al (1980) Influence of triiodothyronine withdrawal time on 131-I uptake postthyroidectomy for thyroid cancer. J Endocrinol Metab 50:734–739
14. Clark OH, Duh QY (1990) Thyroid cancer. In: Green MA (ed) The thyroid gland. Raven, New York, pp 537–572
15. Sweeney D, Johnston G (2000) Radioiodine treatment of thyroid cancer-II. Maximizing therapeutic and diagnostic 131I uptake. In: Wartofsky L (ed) Thyroid cancer. a comprehensive guide to clinical management. Humana Press, Totowa, NJ, pp 239–250
16. Ladenson PW (2000) Recombinant thyrotropin versus thyroid hormone withdrawal in evaluating patients with thyroid carcinoma. Semin Nucl Med 30:98–106
17. Haugen BR, Pacini F, Reiners C et al (1999) A comparison of recombinant human thyrotropin and thyroid hormone withdrawal for the detection of thyroid remnant or cancer. J Clin Endocrinol Metab 84:3877–3885
18. Harness JK, Fund L, Thompson NW, Burney RE, McLeod MK (1986) Total thyroidectomy: complications and technique. World J Surg 10:781–786
19. Clark OH, Elmhed J (1995) Thyroid surgery-past, present and future. Thyroid Today 38:1–9
20. Lennquist S (1986) Surgical strategy in thyroid carcinoma; a clinical review. Acta Chir Scand 152:321–338
21. Massin JP, Savoie JC, Garnier H, Guiaraudon G, Leger FA, Bacourt P (1984) Pulmonary metastases in differentiated thyroid cacinoma,. Study of 58 cases with implications for the primary tumor treatment. Cancer 53:982–992
22. Freitas JE, Gross MD, Ripley SD, Shapiro B (1986) Radionuclide diagnosis and therapy of thyroid cancer: current status report. In: Freeman LM (ed) Freeman and JohnsonÆs clinical radionuclide imaging. Grune and Stratton, Orlando, FL, pp 1994–2027
23. Shapiro B, Ruffini V, Jarwan A et al (2000) Artifacts, anatomical and physiological variants, and unrelated diseases that might cause false-positive whole body scans in patients with thyroid cancer. Semin Nucl Med 30:115–132
24. Jeevanram RK, Shah DH, Sharma SM, Ganatra RD (1986) Influence of initial large dose on subsequent uptake of therapeutic radioiodine in thyroid cancer patients. Nucl Med Biol 13:277–279
25. Park H (1992) Stunned thyroid after high-dose I-131 imaging. Clin Nucl Med 17:501–502
26. Dadparvars S, Chevres A, Tulchinsky M, Krishna-Badrinath L, Khan AS, Slizofski WJ (1995) Clinical utility of technetium-99m methoxyisobutylisonitrite imaging in Differentiated thyroid carcinoma: comparison with thallium-201 and iodine-131 Na Scintigraphy and thyroglobulin quantitation. Eur J Nucl Med 22:1330–1338
27. Kosuda S, Yokoyama H, Katayama M, Yokokawa T, Kusano S, Yamamoto O (1995) Technetium-99m tetrofosmin and technetium-99m sestamibi imaging of multiple metastases from differentiated thyroid carcinoma. Eur J Nucl Med 22:1218–1220
28. Brendel AJ, Guyot M, Jeandot R, Lefolt G, Manicet G (1998) Thallium-201 imaging in the Follow-up of differentiated thyroid carcinoma. J Nucl Med 29:1515–1520
29. Szakall S, Esik O, Bajzik G, Repa I, Dabasi G, Sinkovacs I, Agoston P, Tron L (2002) 18F-FDG PET detection of lymph node metastases in medullary thyroid carcinoma. J Nucl Med 43:66–71
30. Chin B, Patel P, Cohade C, Ewertz M, Wahl R, Ladenson P (2004) Recombinant human-thyrotropin stimulation of fluoro-D-glucose positron emission tomography uptake in well-differentiated thyroid carcinoma. J Clin Endocrinol Metab 89:91–95
31. Kang KW, Kim S-K, Kang H-S et al (2003) Prevalence and risk of cancer of focal thyroidincidentaloma identified by 18F-fluorodeoxyglucose positron emission tomography for metastasis evaluation and cancer screening in healthy subjects. J Clin Endocrinol Metab 88:4100–4104
32. Baudin E, Schlumberger M, Lumbrosa J et al (1996) Octreotide scintigraphy in patients with Differentiated thyroid carcinoma: contribution for patients with negative radioiodine scans. J Clin Endocrinol Metab 81:2451–2544

33. Burch HB (2000) Papillary thyroid cancer. Follow up. In: Wartofsky L (ed) Thyroid cancer. a comprehensiveguide to clinical management. Humana Press, Totowa, NJ, pp 229–237
34. Fatourechi V, Hay ID (2000) Treating the patient with differentiated thyroid cancer with thyroglobulin-positive iodine-131diagnostic scan-negative metastases: including comments on the role of serum thyroglobulin monitoring in tumor surveillance. Semin Nucl Med 30:107–114
35. Cailleux AF, Baudin E, Travagli JP, Ricard M, Schlumberger M (2000) Is diagnostic iodine-131 scanning useful after total thyroid ablation for differentiated thyroid cancer? J Clin Endocrinol Metab 85:175–178
36. Van de Velde CJH, Hamming JF, Goslings BM, Schelfhout LJDM, Clark OH, Smets S et al (1988) Report of the consensus development conference on the management of differentiated thyroid cancer in the Netherlands. Eur J Cancer Clin Oncol 24:287–292
37. Beierwaltes WH, Rabbini R, Dmuchowski C, Lloyd RV, Eyre P, Mallette S (1984) An analysis of ablation of thyroid remnants with ^{131}I in 511 patients from 1947–1984. J Nucl Med 25:1287–1293
38. Johnston G, Sweeney D (2000) Radioiodine therapy of thyroid cancer. General considerations. I. In: Wartofsky L (ed) Thyroid cancer. A comprehensive guide to clinical management. Humana Press, Totowa, NJ, pp 147–153
39. Grigsby PW, Baglan K, Siegel BA (1999) Surveillance of patients to detect recurrent thyroid carcinoma. Cancer 85:945–951
40. Burman KD (1995) How serious are the risks of thyroid hormone over-replacement? Thyroid Today 18:1–9
41. Burmeister LA, Goumaz MO, Mariassh CN, Oppenheimer JH (1992) Levothyroxine dose requirements for thyrotropin suppression in the treatment of differentiated thyroid cancer. J Clin Endocrinol Metab 75:344–350
42. Ozata M, Suzuki S, Miyamoto T, Liu RT, Fierro-Renoy F, DeGroot LJ (1994) Serum thyrotropin in the follow-up of patients with treated differentiated thyroid cancer. J Clin Endocrinol Metab 79:98–105
43. Samaan NA, Schultz PN. Hickey RC, Haynie TP, Johnston DA, Ordonez NG (1992) Well-differentiated thyroid carcinoma and the results of various modalities of treatment. A retrospective review of 1,599 patients. J Clin Endocrinol Metab 75:714–720
44. Benua RS, Cicale NR, Sonenberg M (1962) The relation of radioiodine dosimetry to results and complications in the treatment of metastatic thyroid cancer. AJR 87:171–182
45. Hurley RJ, Becker DV (1983) The use of radioiodine in the management of thyroid cancer. In: Freeman LM, Weissman HS (eds) Nuclear medicine annual. Raven, New York, pp 348–349
46. Wartofsky L (2000) An approach ot the management of patients with scan negative, thyroglobulin positive, differentiated thyroid carcinoma. In: Wartofsky L (ed) Thyroid cancer. A comprehensive guide to clinical management. Humana Press, Totowa, NJ, pp 251–261
47. Deihl M, Risse JH, Brandt-Mainz K, Dietlein M, Bohuslavizki KH, Matheja P, Lange H, Bredow J, Korber C, Grunwald F (2001) Fluorine-18 fluorodeoxyglucose positron emission tomography in medullary thyroid cancer: results of a multicenter study. Eur J Nucl Med 28:1671–1676
48. Lowe V, Mullan BP, Hay ID, McIver B, Kasperbauer JL (2003) 18F-FDG PET of patients with Hurthle cell carcinoma. J Nucl Med 44:1402–1406
49. Tallroth E, Lundell G, Tennvall J, Wallin G (1990) Chemotherapy and multimodality treatment in thyroid carcinoma: disorders of the thyroid and parathyroid. II. Otolaryngol Clin North Am 32:523–527
50. White RL (2000) Management of papillary thyroid carcinoma. In: Wartofsky L (ed) Thyroid cancer. A comprehensive guide to clinical management. Humana Press, Totowa, NJ, pp 225–228

51. Eng C, Clayton D, Schuffenecker I et al (1996) The relationship between specific RET protooncogene mutations and diseased phenotype in multiple endocrine neoplasia type 2: international RET mutation consortium analysis. JAMA 276:1575–1579
52. Ball DW (2000) Medullary thyroid carcinoma. In: Wartofsky L (ed) Thyroid cancer. A comprehensive guide to clinical management. Humana Press, Totowa, NJ, pp 365–381
53. Sisson JC (1989) Medical treatment of benign and malignant thyroid tumors. Endocrinol Metab Clin North Am 18:359–387
54. Kwekkeboom DJ, Reubi JC, Lamberts SWJ et al (1993) In vivo somatostatin-receptor imaging in medullary thyroid carcinoma. J Clin Endocrinol Metab 76:1413–1417
55. Clarke SEM, Lazarus CR, Wraight P, Sampson C, Maisey MN (1988) Pentavalent [99m-Tc] DMSA, [131-I] MIBG, and [99m-Tc] MDP: an evaluation of three imaging techniques in patients with medullary carcinoma of the thyroid. J Nucl Med 29:33–38
56. O'Byrne KJ, Hamilton D, Robinson I, Sweeney E, Freyne PG, Cullen MJ (1992) Imaging of medullary carcinoma of the thyroid using 111-In labeled anti-CEA monoclonal antibody fragments. Nucl Med Commun 13:142–148
57. Clarke SEM, Lazarus CR, Edwards S et al (1987) Scintigraphy and treatment of medullary carcinoma of the thyroid with iodine-131 metaiodobenzylguanidine. J Nucl Med 28:1820–1825
58. Virgolini I, Traub T, Novotny C, Leimer M, Fuger B et al (2001) New trends in peptidereceptor radioligands. Q J Nucl Med 45:153–159
59. Hooft L, Hoekstra OS, Deville W, Lips P, Teule GJJ, Boers M, van Tulder MW (2001) Diagnostic accuracy of 18F-fluorodeoxyglucose positron emission tomography in the follow up of papillary or follicular cancer. J Clin Endocrinol Metab 86:3779–3786
60. Frilling A, Tecklenborg K, Gorges R, Weber F, Clausen M, Broelsch EC (2001) Preoperative diagnostic value of [18-F] Fluorodeoxyglucose positron emission tomography in patients with radio-iodine negative recurrent well-differentiated thyroid carcinoma. Ann Surg 234:804–811
61. Helal BO, Merlet P, Toubert M-E, Franc B, Schvartz C, Gauthier-Koelesnikov H, Prigent A, Syrota A (2001) Clinical impact of ^{18}F-FDG PET in thyroid carcinoma patients with elevated thyroglobulin levels and negative ^{131}I scanning results. J Nucl Med 42:1464–1496
62. Wang W, Larson SM, Tuttle RM, Kalaigian H, Kolbert K, Sonenberg M, Robbins RJ (2001) Resistance of [^{18}F]-fluorodeoxyglucose-avid metastatic thyroid cancer lesions to treatment with high-dose radioactive iodine. Thyroid 11:1169–1175
63. Clark OH, Hoelting T (1994) Management of patients with differentiated thyroid cancer who have positive serum thyroglobulin levels and negative radioiodine scans. Thyroid 4:501–505
64. Pineda JD, Lee T, Ain K, Reynolds JC, Robbins J (1995) Iodine-131 therapy for thyroid cancer patients with elevated thyroglobulin and negative diagnostic scan. J Clin Endocrinol Metab 80:1488–1492
65. Maxon HR III (1993) The role of I-131 in the treatment of thyroid cancer. Thyroid Today XVI:1–9
66. Schlumberger M, Arcangioli O, Pickarski JD, Tubiana M, Parmentier C (1988) Detection and treatment of lung metastases of differentiated thyroid carcinoma in patients with normal chest X-rays. J Nucl Med 29:1790–1794
67. Beierwaltes WH (1978) The treatment of thyroid carcinoma with radioactive iodine. Semin Nucl Med 8:79–94
68. Schlumberger MJ (1999) Diagnostic follow-up of well-differentiated thyroid carcinoma: historical perspective and current status. J Endocrinol Invest 22:3–7
69. Pacini F, Agate L et al (2001) Outcome of differentiated thyroid cancer with detectable serum Tg and negative diagnostic I-131 whole body scan: comparison of patients treated with high I-131 activities versus untreated patients. J Clin Endocrinol Metab 86:4092–4097

CHAPTER 13

Thyroglobulin as Specific Tumor Marker in Differentiated Thyroid Cancer

13

R. GÖRGES and A. BOCKISCH

13.1 Introduction

Thyroglobulin (Tg) is an iodoglycoprotein with a molecular mass of 660 kDa which is exclusively produced in thyrocytes or tumor cells of thyrocyte origin and which is necessary for the synthesis and storage of thyroid hormones. For a long time it was assumed that no secretion or leakage from the healthy thyroid occurs. In the 1960s, more-sensitive detection tools were developed: the specific hemagglutination-inhibition tests [34] and especially radioimmunoassays [65, 81]. Using these new tests, the detection sensitivity was sufficient to prove the presence of Tg also in the blood of healthy subjects. The reference range (95-percentile of the healthy population) extends to about 50 ng/ml, with quite a high interindividual variance. Some thyroid diseases release considerable amounts of Tg into the blood, particularly differentiated, follicular cell-derived thyroid cancer (DTC). However, also benign thyroid diseases may be associated with (highly) increased serum Tg levels (e.g., thyroid enlargement, thyroid nodules, hyperthyroidism, thyroiditis), and there is a very wide overlap between the serum Tg levels in benign or malignant disease. In Hashimoto's thyroiditis, for example, Tg values up to 22,000 ng/ml have been reported [52].

Like the glandular secretion, tumoral Tg secretion mostly displays a TSH dependency, because follicular-cell derived tumor tissue mostly preserves TSH receptors [72]. Consequently, Tg values measured under maximum TSH stimulation, obtained 3–4 weeks after levothyroxine or 2 weeks after triiodothyronine withdrawal ("off-Tg"), exceed Tg values under TSH suppression ("on-Tg") by one order of magnitude (in poorly differentiated tumors, less than factor 3, and in highly differentiated tumors, factor 10 and more [29, 30, 54, 57, 70, 75]). In an unpublished study of 356 patients in our department, a median stimulation factor of 8 was determined. In less-differentiated carcinomas, when TSH receptors are reduced, the stimulation factor can be much lower or absent.

Even in healthy subjects without thyroid disease, circulating Tg displays a molecular heterogeneity, e.g., in respect of iodine content, which obviously depends on iodine alimentary support. Furthermore, structural distinctions between the predominant Tg forms in benign thyroid diseases and DTC have been detected, which are in part due to the process of release from the thyroid cell [17]. However, assays relying on those structural differences, which measure exclusively or at least preferably "malignant" Tg, are not available yet or in the foreseeable future.

Thus, Tg can be used as a tumor marker only after total thyroidectomy – apart from a few exceptions. In the case of a carcinoma of unknown origin and proven distant metastases which might be thyroid cancer, the level of serum Tg may be a useful indicator. A high Tg value suggests thyroid cancer; a value in normal range nearly excludes at least a well-differentiated carcinoma derived from follicular cells [18]. Furthermore, Spencer et al. [75] proposed the measurement of serum Tg levels in all patients with DTC prior to surgery (in the presence of the primary tumor) in order to achieve information about the Tg secretion activity of the tumor.

The specificity of Tg measurement in the follow-up of thyroid cancer is highest after thyroidectomy and adjuvant radioiodine ablation of the thyroid remnants. Corresponding to the serum half-life, on average 65 h [35], during the first days and weeks after thyroidectomy, still measurable but decreasing Tg values are expected. Thus, depending on the initial level of serum Tg, the full specificity and accuracy is established only several weeks after radioiodine ablation of the thyroid remnants [21]. Assuming the pretherapeutic serum Tg level to be 100 ng/ml arising from the benign thyroid or thyroid carcinoma, Tg might be measurable for approximately 4 weeks even after complete cure.

In thyroid cancer patients with subtotal or "total" thyroidectomy but no radioiodine ablation, Van Wyngaarden and McDougall [82] detected persistent, measurable Tg values in 38% of the patients being judged tumor free, even under TSH-suppressive medication. The proportion of Tg-positive patients necessarily increases with the sensitivity of the Tg test used. In a group of 33 patients who were only thyroidectomized but had no radioiodine ablation, we found measurable serum Tg values under TSH suppression in 50% of the subjects using a test with a lower detection limit of 0.5 ng/ml and even in 100% using a test with a functional sensitivity of 0.03 ng/ml [31].

Nowadays, immunometric assays (IMAs; with isotope or nonisotope technique) are most frequently used for Tg measurement in Europe. Many of the commercialized kits offer a functional sensitivity of about 0.5 ng/ml. However, this lower limit is only a technical threshold and would lead to a high rate of false-positive findings if a single Tg value were to be assessed underlying such low value as cutoff. Therefore, arbitrary cutoff values are introduced intending to find an optimal compromise between diagnostic sensitivity and specificity. Often an arbitrary threshold of about 2 ng/ml is proposed [21, 29, 42, 84]. According to our experience, a significantly lower value can be used for the assessment of *serial* Tg measurement in the individual patient, if the performance of the Tg test is under permanent control. If the test is working perfectly, a newly detected measurable Tg value in the follow-up suggests recurrence.

In their recent meta-analysis concerning the diagnostic value of serum Tg measurements in the follow-up of DTC, Eustatia-Rutten et al. [21] reported for IMAs an average diagnostic sensitivity of 0.778 ± 0.023 (mean ± SE), a specificity of 0.977 ± 0.005, and an accuracy of 0.933 ± 0.007 for on-Tg in patients with thyroid ablation (9 underlying series, with a total of 1,613 patients, median cutoff 2 ng/ml). The respective values for off-Tg were 0.961 ± 0.013, 0.947 ± 0.007, and 0.952 ± 0.006 (12 underlying series, with a total of 1,602 patients, median cutoff 3 ng/ml)

13.2 Thyroglobulin Measurement: Methodology and Problems

Tg measurement – aiming for high sensitivity and keeping up high specificity – is challenging for several reasons that are explained in this section, and encumbered with more serious consequences as compared to many other analytes. High laboratory standards are essential, including the definition of the functional sensitivity, based on a 20% interassay coefficient of variation during an application period of the assay over at least 6 months [73], duplicate measurement of the serum samples, restoring frozen sera for future validation, quality controls, and methods for recognizing interfering/disturbing factors and a high-dose hook effect.

The actual serum Tg level is influenced by various factors, including the amount of active tumor tissue, the histological tumor type (in papillary carcinoma mostly lower than in follicular carcinoma [16, 55, 77]), the grade of tumor differentiation (which may change during the course), the stimulation of tumoral TSH receptors (e.g., through TSH or TSH receptor antibodies), the acute attack of Tg-releasing processes (e.g., irradiation), and the serum clearance rate of Tg. Thus – except for analytical interferences and problems – a false-negative Tg finding could be caused by a deficient release of Tg from the tumor, by a very small amount of tumor tissue, or by a lack of sensitivity of the Tg assay. Bachelot et al. [2] report a ratio of 0.5–1 ng/ml serum Tg concentration per gram of neoplastic tissue. However, the serum Tg concentration largely depends on the abovementioned biological parameters.

For these reasons, not only high laboratory standards are necessary, but the reporting physician must also be aware of interfering factors and needs detailed knowledge of the patient, such as mass of thyroid remnant, possible stimulation factors for Tg secretion, previous and actual therapeutic measures (kind of surgery, radioiodine therapy, external radiation, and other interventions), time interval to therapeutic measures, tumor biology, and the course of follow-up.

The most frequent analytical problems in Tg measurement are due to interfering factors in patient's sera (especially anti-Tg autoantibodies; far less frequently, heterophilic antibodies), also to the high-dose hook effect, and in rare cases to the presence of an abnormal Tg not recognized by the assay antibodies [68, 73]. In the majority of one-step immunoradiometric assays (IRMAs), the high-dose hook effect results in false-low values in cases of excessive high serum Tg levels (depending on the Tg test used, typically for serum Tg exceeding the upper detection limit of the test more than 100-fold), as all binding-sites of the first (e.g., solid-phase) assay antibody are saturated. In consequence, a meaningful proportion of the second, signal antibody binds to unbound Tg in the supernatant and is decanted prior to measurement, resulting in a decreased measurement signal. The high-dose hook effect is uncovered by the recovery test: the recovery is remarkably diminished in such cases. In some modern two-step assays, the high-dose hook effect has been overcome by additional wash procedures [51, 87].

Heterophilic antibodies (e.g., human anti-mouse antibodies, HAMA) in the patient's serum may disturb the measurement (e.g., as the assay employs murine antibodies). In times of in vivo diagnostics and therapy with monoclonal murine antibodies, Tg measurements compromised in that way may actually occur more frequently. In this case, using the IMA methodology, the measured Tg values as a rule overestimate the real serum concentration [61]. Meanwhile, the assays of most manufacturers contain blocking agents to prevent this phenomenon, but the efficacy of these measures is not guaranteed in each case.

Modern Tg assays rely on monoclonal antibodies that are highly epitope-specific. Therefore, there is at least a theoretical risk that "atypical" Tg might not be recognized, as it might not express the tested epitope. That is why there is discussion about whether the use of polyclonal or polyvalent antibodies, or the combination of different antibodies might be advantageous. However, up till now, the proof of clinical relevance of this aspect is missing.

Tg-TgAb interference is a definitely more relevant challenge, and numerous efforts have been undertaken to overcome this problem:

A. The development of assays which employ monoclonal capture antibodies with specificities for Tg epitopes not involved in the autoimmune response [60]
B. Adding a Tg fragment which neutralizes the presence of autoantibodies [39]
C. The use of various polyclonal and monoclonal antibodies to increase the number of epitopes on the Tg molecule that are recognized and possibly not affected by Tg-TgAb interference [19]
D. The use of assay antibodies which bind with markedly higher affinity to the Tg epitopes than the autoantibodies. Thus Tg is stripped from interfering human TgAb and bound to the assay antibodies [4].

Nevertheless, the problem of Tg-TgAb interference could not be eliminated through these modifications, but merely somewhat diminished [44, 67, 86].

TgAb interference can produce either under- or overestimation of serum Tg depending on the assay architecture and therefore can cause discordant results between IMAs and RIAs. Tg IMAs typically underestimate serum Tg when sera contain Tg antibodies (TgAbs), presumably because the endogenous Tg complexed with TgAbs cannot interact with the assay antibodies, whereas RIAs can under- or overestimate Tg depending on the characteristics of the respective assay antibodies [74, 86]. In contrast, Mariotti et al. [44] postulated that low Tg values observed in some patients who also have TgAbs could also be due to an accelerated metabolic clearance rate of the Tg-TgAb complexes from the blood via the reticuloendothelial system. Consequently, very low or negative Tg values in the presence of circulating TgAbs should be interpreted carefully. Some authors recommend serial TgAb measurement in such cases as surrogate tumor marker test, but there is controversy over the clinical relevance [11, 62].

On the other hand, circulating TgAbs – even in high serum concentrations – must not necessarily interfere with the Tg measurement [74], and moreover not only TgAb interference, but other factors, too, may also cause unreliable Tg values. Finally, not only Tg assays, but also TgAb assays can produce unreliable results, e.g., because of interfering high Tg concentrations [24] or epitope incompatibility between TgAbs and the radioligand (Tg) on the one hand and radioligand and assay antibodies on the other hand [6]. Thus, estimation of TgAbs is no ideal tool to authenticate Tg measurements.

In the light of this background, Tg recovery tests have been introduced, allowing control over whether a defined amount of Tg added to the patient's serum sample could be measured adequately. However, there exists no consent about the usefulness of those recovery tests and their validity for recognizing Tg-TgAb interferences. Some authors [74, 86] stress that recovery tests – at least in the usually performed manner concerning the amount and origin of added Tg and the incubation time – cannot be used to validate a Tg measurement in serum containing TgAbs. Particularly, they postulate that the epitopes on the exogenous Tg molecules (glandular origin) may differ from the epitopes of endogenous tumor Tg in the patient's serum. In contrast, other authors emphasize the importance of recovery tests instead of TgAb measurements [10, 41].

If TgAbs were measured in order to authenticate Tg values, one should use a highly sensitive assay and even report very low TgAb values, as there is no established correlation between the TgAb titers and the influence of Tg-TgAb interference on the measured serum Tg level [74]. In their cross-sectional study, Spencer et al. [74] found TgAbs in approximately 25% of the DTC patients as compared to 10% in the general population by using this sensitive assay. Tg-TgAb interference could not be excluded for measurable TgAb within the normal range for subjects without thyroid disease at all, and even TgAb concentrations below the lower detection limits of common assays may result in significant interferences. Spencer et al. [74] also proposed a RIA/IMA discordance test to uncover interfering TgAbs. Other authors recommend performing recovery tests and TgAb measurements in parallel [88], since recovery tests additionally allow the detection of otherwise disturbing factors in Tg measurement, e.g., a possible high-dose hook effect.

If recovery tests are performed, they should not be normalized to the expected concentration of added Tg (e.g., 50 ng/ml), but one should take the actually measured Tg results into consideration in order to diminish possible (e.g., pipetting) errors, using the formula:

$$\frac{Tg_{(\text{patient's serum + recovery buffer})} - Tg_{(\text{patient's serum})}}{Tg_{(\text{Tg-free serum + recovery buffer})}} \times 100\% = \text{recovery}$$

(as a rule, a recovery 70–130% is defined as undisturbed).

In our laboratory, in each assay run, at least half of the patients show up with negative serum Tg levels and a long-term, established complete remission. All the recovery values are finally normalized to the average of those values, resulting in a narrower distribution of the recovery tests, which enables us to reduce the normal interval to 80–120% and to compensate for day by day fluctuations. Because also economical aspects are of increasing importance in our health care system, further data may be helpful on which a pragmatic approach concerning the authentication of Tg values could be based (e.g., low-dose recovery tests; recovery tests using special Tg forms; "cold" preincubation to reach equilibration between TgAbs, assay antibodies, serum Tg and recovery Tg; only initially performed TgAb measurement, and restriction on further controls in cases of initially elevated TgAbs values).

For a long time, the results from different Tg assays and different laboratories could not be compared numerically, as no valid international standard was available [23]. In 1996 the European reference preparation CRM 457 was introduced in order to overcome this drawback [25, 26], and recent assays are calibrated on this preparation. However, the comparability was increased but still is not perfect as, for example, the antibodies of different assays are directed against different epitopes, and the variation between the different assays may still be up to factor 1.5 despite the calibration on the same standard preparation [53].

From a statistical point of view, the abovementioned analytical difficulties cause problems of only minor relevance in the clinical routine of our department, which takes care of far more than 2,000 DTC patients per year, and it has to be emphasized that Tg measurement – performed with assays now available under high laboratory standards – is a highly reliable diagnostic tool in the follow-up of DTC. Nevertheless, one should be aware of the possibility of the above-outlined problems, since they may cause fatal health consequences in some patients, mainly due to unnecessary or delayed diagnostic and therapeutic measures.

13.3 Diagnostic Value of Thyroglobulin in the Spectrum of Follow-Up Methods

Since recurrences in DTC may occur even after decades and the chance for a curative therapy commonly increases with the earliness of the detection of a relapse, most expert organizations recommend a lifelong follow-up. Diagnostic radioiodine whole-body scintigraphy (dWBS), Tg measurement, and neck ultrasonography are the most important tools of the thyroid cancer aftercare found in numerous procedure guidelines (e.g., National Cancer Centre Network [45], German Cancer Society [38], American Associations of Clinical Endocrinology and of Endocrine Surgeons [78]). Subsequent to the ablation of thyroid remnants, both dWBS and Tg measurement have a high specificity regarding the detection of tumor tissue, because the ability to secrete Tg and to concentrate iodine are characteristic features of differentiated carcinomas. However, both features may not always be associated [16] and, in cases of dedifferentiation, the capacity of iodine concentration is more often lost than the Tg secretion.

Data from the literature concerning the sensitivity and specificity for the detection of tumor tissue of dWBS with ^{131}I as compared to Tg measurement under TSH-suppressive thyroid hormone supplementation ("on-Tg") are given in Table 13.1 (studies which only examine the prediction of a positive dWBS as "gold standard" by a positive on-Tg were excluded). The data are highly dependent on the sensitivity of the applied Tg assay and the performance of dWBS;

moreover, the question of the ideal "gold standard" is a point of discussion. In the majority of cases, on-Tg measurement is superior to dWBS, but some authors favor a combination of Tg measurement and routinely performed dWBS in order to maximize the sensitivity, especially concerning patients with interfering TgAbs. Of course, the additional opportunity to measure off-Tg should always be used when thyroid hormones are withdrawn in preparation to dWBS.

It has to be underlined that values for diagnostic sensitivity of dWBS and on-Tg from the literature mostly derive from patients with active tumor disease in general. Diagnostic sensitivity of these two tools concerning early detection of recurrences in patients thought to be in complete remission is a distinctly different situation. Focusing on these patients, significantly lower values for diagnostic sensitivity have been reported, e.g., virtually 0% [79], 14% [36], 27% [46], and 41% [63] for dWBS. Apart from the limited sensitivity for detection of still small amounts of relapsing tumor tissue after diagnostic doses of ^{131}I in general, this could be explained by less radioiodine accumulation in late recurrences, the proportion of which ranges from one-half to two-thirds of all cases [63]. In a comparative study of 44 DTC patients who were in complete remission after primary therapy, we found a diagnostic sensitivity for early detection of recurrences for on-Tg of 27% (RIA with a lower detection limit of 6 ng/ml) and 58% (IRMA with a lower detection limit of 1 ng/ml), respectively, and for dWBS of 2.7% [50].

Schlumberger and Pacini performed a meta-analysis of various studies (with underlying assay sensitivities or cutoff values between 1 and 3 ng/ml) and reported that 20% of the local metastases and 2–5% of the distant metastases were Tg-negative under TSH-suppressive conditions [69]. Under maximum TSH stimulation, the respective rates were 5% and 0%. Thus, particularly local and regional recurrences to a certain extent are missed by on-Tg measurements.

Focusing on detection of neck recurrences, Frasoldati et al. [27] reported a significant superiority of high-resolution ultrasonography (sensitivity 94%) relative to Tg measurement, even when performed under TSH stimulation (sensitivity 57% for an underlying cutoff of 2 ng/ml; 67% for 0.25 ng/ml) and dWBS (sensitivity 45%). The important additional role of ultrasonography is confirmed by the results of other recent studies [14, 80]. In a recent publication [32], we introduced rules for judging the dignity of cervical lesions in thyroid cancer patients using a logistic regression model based on dichotomized B-mode and color flow Doppler criteria. Performing high-end ultrasonography and applying these rules, a diagnostic sensitivity of 90% (95%-CI: 76–97%) and specificity of 82% (95%-CI: 57–96%) could be reached.

13.4 Tg Measurement Under Exogenous TSH Stimulation

Approval for the use of recombinant human TSH (rhTSH) for diagnostic purposes in DTC was granted in 1998 in the USA and in 2001 in Europe. If injected i.m. following the established application scheme (each 0.9 mg rhTSH at days 0 and 1) the median serum TSH-peak (>150 ng/ml) is reached at days 2 and 3, followed by a quite rapid decline. The maximum median serum Tg concentration is

Table 13.1. Data from the literature concerning the diagnostic value of on-Tg compared with diagnostic ^{131}I whole body scintigraphy (WBS) for the detection of follicular cell-derived thyroid cancer (DTC) tumor tissue

Authors	Patients	On-Tg			Diagnostic ^{131}I WBS			On-Tg + WBS
		Lower detection limit or cutoff, respectively	Diagnostic sensitivity	Diagnostic specificity	Dose of ^{131}I	Diagnostic sensitivity	Diagnostic specificity	Diagnostic sensitivity
Ashcraft and van Herle 1981 [1]	Overall 36 (18 with active tumor disease)	1 ng/ml	100%	29%	185 MBq	58%	100%	Not reported
Colacchio et al. 1982 [12]	Overall 67 (37 with recurrences)	15 ng/ml	78%	100%	74 MBq	84%	100%	Not reported
Hüfner et al. 1983 [36]	28 with recurrences	10 ng/ml	71%	Not reported	74 MBq	14%	Not reported	78%
Reiners et al. 1984 [63]	55 with active tumor disease	5 ng/ml	89%	Not reported	74 MBq	58%	Not reported	Not reported
	22 with late recurrences		86%	Not reported		41%	Not reported	Not reported
Sulman et al. 1984 [76]	Overall 115 (23 with active tumor disease)	6.25 ng/ml	83%	95%	37 MBq	35%	100%	83%
Müller-Gärtner et al. 1988 [55]	Overall 374 (30 with active tumor disease)	3 ng/ml	50%	99%	370–740 MBq	57%	Not reported	Not reported
Ronga et al. 1990 [66]	Overall 61 (30 with active tumor disease)	5 ng/ml	83%	58%	74–148 MBq	77%	100%	96%

Table 13.1. *Continued*

Authors	Patients	On-Tg			Diagnostic ^{131}I WBS			On-Tg + WBS
		Lower detection limit or cutoff, respectively	Diagnostic sensitivity	Diagnostic specificity	Dose of ^{131}I	Diagnostic sensitivity	Diagnostic specificity	Diagnostic sensitivity
Berding et al. 1992 [7]	Overall 70 (9 with recurrence)	5 ng/ml	67%	91%	370 MBq	56%	Not reported	78%
		10 ng/ml	56%	94%	370 MBq	56%	Not reported	78%
Lubin et al. 1994 [43]	Overall 261 (59 with active tumor disease)	10 ng/ml	88%	Not reported	185 MBq	55%	Not reported	88%

observed later, with a peak at day 4 [58, 59]. Tg is stimulated by rTSH on average by a factor of 10–20 compared with the "on-Tg" value [75]. Thus, on the average, a similar sensitivity and specificity to endogenously stimulated Tg ("off-Tg") is reached [21]. The advantage of rTSH stimulation is the absence of hypothyroid symptoms induced by thyroid hormone withdrawal, especially the reduction of health-related quality of life [15, 33, 40].

Some authors [3, 56, 85] propose in recent papers the application of rTSH solely to increase the sensitivity of the Tg determination (without dWBS) using assays with a functional sensitivity of about 0.5 ng/ml or cutoff values of 2.0 ng/ml. Based on the results of previous studies, a group of thyroid experts in the United States [47] and in Europe [71] recently proposed a revised follow-up protocol for low-risk DTC patients without interfering TgAbs, where Tg measurement under rhTSH stimulation in combination with neck ultrasonography is routinely performed 6–12 months after primary therapy in all patients without evidence of disease, whereas the routine use of dWBS in the majority of those patients should be abandoned.

However, this proposed follow-up regime was criticized by other thyroid cancer experts for several reasons, including the functional sensitivity of the applied Tg assays and the cutoff values for Tg, the definition of low-risk patients, and the questionable cost-efficiency and impact on the clinical outcome of this paradigm [22, 49]. Yet, there exists no international consent about the routine use of rhTSH-stimulated Tg measurement in DTC aftercare. The broad application of rTSH stimulation (costs: about 900 US dollars) solely in order to increase sensitivity of Tg detection needs a critical discussion, especially if significantly more sensitive Tg assays become available. Already today an increase in the assay sensitivity by a factor of 10 is feasible. This increase in sensitivity is about equivalent to the stimulation effect. In addition, the increased assay sensitivity is of high value for (less differentiated) tumors which do not or only insufficiently react on TSH stimulation due to missing TSH receptors [75].

Moreover, the extent of the Tg increase after TSH stimulation does not correlate with the dignity of the Tg source. The response does not reliably allow differentiation between thyroid remnant and recurrence in each case. In a representative sample of our DTC patients, we found no significant difference of the extent of the Tg response to maximum TSH stimulation: factor 0.6–25.7 in tumor-free patients and 3.2–33.8 in patients with active tumor. In their authors' response to the controversial comments on the abovementioned revised follow-up protocol, Mazzaferri et al. [48] conceded that in the future the availability of Tg assays even more sensitive than used in their studies may "render TSH stimulation unnecessary to identify patients with persistent tumor."

13.5 Ultrasensitive Thyroglobulin Measurement

Meanwhile, Tg assays are commercially available whose sensitivity is one order of magnitude higher than the present assay generation still with a satisfying intra- and interassay precision [31, 37, 51, 87]. Iervasi et al. [37] examined the diagnostic performance of a fully automated, chemiluminescent immunoassay and found the analytical sensitivity to be 0.01 ng/ml and the functional sensitivity (at 20% coefficient of variation) to be 0.1 ng/ml. The ILMA evaluated by Morgenthaler et al. [51] had a lower detection limit of 0.02 ng/ml and a functional sensitivity of 0.06 ng/ml. Wunderlich et al. [87] evaluated an immunoenzymometric assay (IEMA) in a cross-sectional study and found the functional sensitivity to reach as low as 0.03 ng/ml (calibrated on the European Tg-reference preparation CRM 457).

The diagnostic value of such sensitive assays is no longer based on a single measurement (the rate of Tg-positive but tumor-free patients becomes quite high – even after radioiodine ablation), but relies on an early suspicion of recurrence, which is proven by the Tg course in the follow-up. The high clinical value of serial Tg measurements under TSH suppression has already been stressed by various authors at times using less sensitive Tg assays [8, 9, 73, 75]. DTC usually grow quite slowly. By analyzing the Tg course of 20 patients with established metastases which for various reasons did not get any kind of treatment (with the exception of suppressive thyroxine medication), we calculated the median time for doubling the serum Tg concentration to be 6 months (range 1–42 months).

Applying the same ultrasensitive IEMA which was already reported by Wunderlich et al. [87] in a longitudinal study, we could demonstrate that the scale of this "metabolic tumor doubling-time" is also applicable to the very low range of Tg (<1 ng/ml), corresponding to very early development of tumor recurrences. We used the deep-frozen sera of seven patients collected over 5 years in our serum bank and calculated the potential time profit by using the highly sensitive Tg assay, which naturally depends on the growth characteristics of the tumor and the follow-up intervals. A gain of 5–15 months for the detection of the recurrence could be calculated compared with the established assay generation [31]. Zöphel et al. [89] found a similar range using the same IEMA: 6–12 months.

The validity and reliability of the results of this ultrasensitive IEMA are also proven by the fact that TSH stimulation increases the Tg values in the lowest range by the same factor established for higher values. In addition, an excellent intraindividual reproducibility of the lowest values in clinically stable patients (including those who are likely to be in full remission) was found, as well as a continuous and smooth increase in Tg values with progressive disease [31].

The availability of assays with increasing sensitivity which are clinically applicable (stable intra- and interassay precision at very low Tg levels) will enhance the importance of the documentation of the change in Tg levels in serial measurements under TSH suppression for the early detection of recurrence. The often-proposed arbitrary cutoff value of 2 ng/ml (which today is not adequate) definitely needs to be abandoned in the face of high functional sensitivity. However, the reasonably lower normal Tg level needs to be defined in larger prospective studies; the same holds for the threshold of the respective Tg value, or dynamic pattern of consecutive Tg values, which requires further diagnostics or therapeutic interventions (e.g., continuous Tg increase at three consecutive examinations or doubling of the previous value), dependent on the tumor type and individual risk profile.

13.6 Thyroglobulin messenger RNA as Alternative Tumor Marker

In 1996 Ditkoff et al. [13] described for the first time the qualitative detection of circulating thyroid cells in peripheral blood, applying reverse transcription polymerase chain reaction (RT-PCR). As molecular genetic methods become more common in medical diagnostics, this finding has increasing meaning also for thyroid cancer patients. An increased independence from the extent of TSH stimulation and no interference from circulating TgAbs are expected by the molecular genetic approach, displaying potential advantages over Tg measurement.

In the past 8 years, numerous papers have been published, concerning both the qualitative [5, 28] and the quantitative [20, 64] detection of circulating thyroglobulin messenger RNA (mRNA). The results of the different laboratories and therefore their attitude towards clinical usefulness are at least controversial. One reason might be the lack of standardization. Due to an unfavorable "signal to noise ratio," the average specificity is significantly inferior to that of state-of-the-art Tg assays (e.g., "thyroid-specific" mRNAs – even when the applied primer does not recognize splice variants for Tg – are less specific as initially assumed). In a recent review, Verburg et al. [83] concluded that at present Tg-mRNA detection is not a useful tool in the follow-up of DTC, but that the concept of using RT-PCR measurements during follow-up still warrants further research.

References

1. Ashcraft MW, Herle AJ van (1981) The comparative value of serum thyroglobulin measurements and iodine 131 total body scans in the follow-up study of patients with treated differentiated thyroid cancer. Am J Med 71:806–814
2. Bachelot A, Cailleux AF, Klain M, Baudin E, Ricard M, Bellon N, Caillou B, Travagli JP, Schlumberger M (2002) Relationship between tumor burden and serum thyroglobulin level in patients with papillary and follicular thyroid carcinoma. Thyroid 12:707–711
3. Baskin HJ, Atwood TM, Holcomb LP (2000) Recombinant and human thyrotropin stimulation in the follow-up of patients with stage I or II differentiated thyroid carcinoma. Endocr Pract 6:430–434
4. Bayer MF, Kriss JP (1979) Immunoradiometric assay for serum thyroglobulin: semiquantitative measurement of thyroglobulin in antithyroglobulin-positive sera. J Clin Endocrinol Metab 49:557–564
5. Bellantone R, Lombardi CP, Bossola M, Ferrante A, Princi P, Boscherini M, Maussier L, Salvatori M, Rufini V, Reale F, Romano L, Tallini G, Zelano G, Pontecorvi A (2001) Validity of thyroglobulin mRNA assay in peripheral blood of postoperative thyroid carcinoma patients in predicting tumor recurrences varies according to the histologic type: results of a prospective study. Cancer 92:2273–2279
6. Benvenga S, Burek CL, Talor M, Rose NR, Trimarchi F (2002) Heterogeneity of the thyroglobulin epitopes associated with circulating thyroid hormone autoantibodies in Hashimoto's thyroiditis and non-autoimmune thyroid diseases. J Endocrinol Invest 25:977–982
7. Berding G, Hüfner M, Georgi P (1992) Thyroglobulin, ^{131}I whole body scintigraphy and risk factors in the follow-up of differentiated thyroid cancer. Nuklearmedizin 31:32–37

8. Black EG, Sheppard MC, Hoffenberg R (1987) Serial serum thyroglobulin measurements in the management of differentiated thyroid carcinoma. Clin Endocrinol (Oxf) 27:115–120
9. Botsch H, Glatz J, Schulz E, Wenzel KW (1983) Long-term follow-up using serial serum thyroglobulin determinations in patients with differentiated thyroid carcinoma. Cancer 52:1856–1859
10. Bourrel F, Hoff M, Regis H, Courriere P, Caron P (1998) Immunoradiometric assay of thyroglobulin in patients with differentiated thyroid carcinomas: need for thyroglobulin recovery tests. Clin Chem Lab Med 36:725–730
11. Chung JK, Park YJ, Kim TY, So Y, Kim SK, Park DJ, Lee DS, Lee MC, Cho BY (2002) Clinical significance of elevated level of serum antithyroglobulin antibody in patients with differentiated thyroid cancer after thyroid ablation. Clin Endocrinol (Oxf) 57:215–221
12. Colacchio TA, LoGerfo P, Colacchio DA, Feind C (1982) Radioiodine total body scan versus serum thyroglobulin levels in follow-up of patients with thyroid cancer. Surgery 91:42–45
13. Ditkoff BA, Marvin MR, Yemul S, Shi YJ, Chabot J, Feind C, Lo Gerfo PL (1996) Detection of circulating thyroid cells in peripheral blood. Surgery 120:959–964
14. Do Rosario PW, Fagundes TA, Maia FF, Franco AC, Figueiredo MB, Purisch S (2004) Sonography in the diagnosis of cervical recurrence in patients with differentiated thyroid carcinoma. J Ultrasound Med 23:915–920
15. Dow KH, Ferrell BR, Anello C (1997 Quality-of-life changes in patients with thyroid cancer after withdrawal of thyroid hormone therapy. Thyroid 7:613–619
16. Dralle H, Schwarzrock R, Lang W, Bocker W, Ziegler H, Schroder S, Geerlings H (1985) Comparison of histology and immunohistochemistry with thyroglobulin serum levels and radioiodine uptake in recurrences and metastases of differentiated thyroid carcinomas. Acta Endocrinol (Copenh) 108:504–510
17. Druetta L, Croizet K, Bornet H, Rousset B (1998) Analyses of the molecular forms of serum thyroglobulin from patients with Graves' disease, subacute thyroiditis or differentiated thyroid cancer by velocity sedimentation on sucrose gradient and western blot. Eur J Endocrinol 139:498–507
18. Edmonds CJ, Willis CL (1988) Serum thyroglobulin in the investigation of patients presenting with metastases. Br J Radiol 61:317–319
19. Erali M, Bigelow RB, Meikle AW (1996) ELISA for thyroglobulin in serum: recovery studies to evaluate autoantibody interference and reliability of thyroglobulin values. Clin Chem 42:766–770
20. Eszlinger M, Neumann S, Otto L, Paschke R (2002) Thyroglobulin mRNA quantification in the peripheral blood is not a reliable marker for the follow-up of patients with differentiated thyroid cancer. Eur J Endocrinol 147:575–582
21. Eustatia-Rutten CF, Smit JW, Romijn JA, Kleij-Corssmit EP van der, Pereira AM, Stokkel MP, Kievit J (2004) Diagnostic value of serum thyroglobulin measurements in the follow-up of differentiated thyroid carcinoma, a structured meta-analysis. Clin Endocrinol (Oxf) 61:61–74
22. Fatemi S, LoPresti JS (2003) A consensus report of the role of serum thyroglobulin as a monitoring method for low-risk patients with papillary thyroid carcinoma. J Clin Endocrinol Metab 88:4507–4508
23. Feldt-Rasmussen U, Schlumberger M (1988) European interlaboratory comparison of serum thyroglobulin measurement. J Endocrinol Invest 11:175–181
24. Feldt-Rasmussen U, Hoier-Madsen M, Hansen HS, Blichert-Toft M (1986) Comparison between homogeneous phase radioassay and enzyme-linked immunosorbent assay for measurement of antithyroglobulin antibody content in serum. Relation to presence of thyroglobulin. Acta Pathol Microbiol Immunol Scand [C] 94:33–38
25. Feldt-Rasmussen U, Profilis C, Colinet E et al (1996a) Human thyroglobulin reference material (CRM 457). 1. Assessment of homogeneity, stability and immunoreactivity. Ann Biol Clin (Paris) 54:337–342

26. Feldt-Rasmussen U, Profilis C, Colinet E et al (1996b) A human thyroglobulin reference material (CRM 457). 2. Physicochemical characterization and certification. Ann Biol Clin (Paris) 54:343–348
27. Frasoldati A, Pesenti M, Gallo M, Caroggio A, Salvo D, Valcavi R (2003) Diagnosis of neck recurrences in patients with differentiated thyroid carcinoma. Cancer 97:90–96
28. Fugazzola L, Mihalich A, Persani L, Cerutti N, Reina M, Bonomi M, Ponti E, Mannavola D, Giammona E, Vannucchi G, di Blasio AM, Beck-Peccoz P (2002) Highly sensitive serum thyroglobulin and circulating thyroglobulin mRNA evaluations in the management of patients with differentiated thyroid cancer in apparent remission. J Clin Endocrinol Metab 87:3201–3208
29. Girelli ME, Busnardo B, Amerio R, Scotton G, Casara D, Betterle C, Piccolo M, Pelizzo MR (1985) Serum thyroglobulin levels in patients with well-differentiated thyroid cancer during suppression therapy: study on 429 patients. Eur J Nucl Med 10:252–254
30. Girelli ME, Busnardo B, Amerio R, Casara D, Betterle C, Piccolo M (1986) Critical evaluation of serum thyroglobulin (Tg) levels during thyroid hormone suppression therapy versus Tg levels after hormone withdrawal and total body scan: results in 291 patients with thyroid cancer. Eur J Nucl Med 11:333–335
31. Görges R, Brandt-Mainz K, Freudenberg L, Frilling A, Grimm W, Bockisch A (2003a) Kontinuierliche Sensitivitätssteigerung in der Schilddrüsenkarzinom-Nachsorge im Verlauf dreier Thyreoglobulin-IMA-Generationen. Nuklearmedizin 42:157–166
32. Görges R, Eising EG, Fotescu D, Renzing-Köhler K, Frilling A, Schmid KW, Bockisch A, Dirsch O (2003b) Diagnostic value of high-resolution B-mode and power-mode sonography in the follow-up of thyroid cancer. Eur J Ultrasound 16:191–206
33. Görges R, Tagay S, Matyssek K, Freudenberg L, Bockisch A, Langkafel M (2004) Einfluss der Schilddrüsenstoffwechsellage auf den psychosomatischen Status bei Schilddrüsenkarzinom-Patienten. In: Dietlein M, Schicha H (eds) Schilddrüse 2003: Zufallsbefund Schilddrüsenknoten – latente Schilddrüsenfunktionsstörungen. De Gruyter, Berlin, pp 374–80
34. Hjort T (1961 Determination of serum-thyroglobulin by a haemagglutination-inhibition test. Lancet 1:1262–1264
35. Hocevar M, Auersperg M, Stanovnik L (1997) The dynamics of serum thyroglobulin elimination from the body after thyroid surgery. Eur J Surg Oncol 23:208–210
36. Hüfner M, Stumpf HP, Grussendorf M, Hermann HJ, Kimmig B (1983) A comparison of the effectiveness of 131I whole body scans and plasma Tg determinations in the diagnosis of metastatic differentiated carcinoma of the thyroid: a retrospective study. Acta Endocrinol (Copenh) 104:327–332
37. Iervasi A, Iervasi G, Bottoni A, Boni G, Annicchiarico C, Cecco P di, Zucchelli GC (2004) Diagnostic performance of a new highly sensitive thyroglobulin immunoassay. J Endocrinol 182:287–294
38. Informationszentrum für Standards in der Onkologie (ISTO) (2001) Maligne Schilddrüsentumoren. Interdisziplinäre Leitlinie der Deutschen Krebsgesellschaft und der Deutschen Gesellschaft für Chirurgie, 3rd edn. http://www.uni-duesseldorf.de/WWW/AWMF/11/ (accessed 14 February 2005)
39. Kato R, Maruyama M, Sekino T, Kasuga Y (2000) A new assay for thyroglobulin concentration in serum using monoclonal antibodies against synthetic peptides. Clin Chim Acta 298:69–84
40. Langkafel M, Tagay S, Schöpper N, Bockisch A, Senf W, Görges R (2004) Befindlichkeitsstörungen und Lebensqualität bei Schilddrüsenfunktionsstörungen – insbesondere bei Hypothyreose und Schilddrüsenkarzinom. In: Dietlein M, Schicha H (eds) Schilddrüse 2003: Zufallsbefund Schilddrüsenknoten – latente Schilddrüsenfunktionsstörungen. De Gruyter, Berlin, pp 357–362
41. Ligabue A, Poggioli MC, Zacchini A (1993) Interference of specific autoantibodies in the assessment of serum thyroglobulin. J Nucl Biol Med 37:273–279

42. Lima N, Cavaliere H, Tomimori E, Knobel M, Medeiros-Neto G (2002) Prognostic value of serial serum thyroglobulin determinations after total thyroidectomy for differentiated thyroid cancer. J Endocrinol Invest 25:110–115
43. Lubin E, Mechlis-Frish S, Zatz S, Shimoni A, Segal K, Avraham A, Levy R, Feinmesser R (1994) Serum thyroglobulin and iodine-131 whole-body scan in the diagnosis and assessment of treatment for metastatic differentiated thyroid carcinoma. J Nucl Med 35:257–262
44. Mariotti S, Barbesino G, Caturegli P, Marino M, Manetti L, Pacini F, Centoni R, Pinchera A (1995) Assay of thyroglobulin in serum with thyroglobulin autoantibodies: an unobtainable goal? J Clin Endocrinol Metab 80:468–472
45. Mazzaferri EL (1999) An overview of the management of papillary and follicular thyroid carcinoma. Thyroid 9:421–427
46. Mazzaferri EL, Kloos RT (2002) Is diagnostic iodine-131 scanning with recombinant human TSH useful in the follow-up of differentiated thyroid cancer after thyroid ablation? J Clin Endocrinol Metab 87:1490–1498
47. Mazzaferri EL, Robbins RJ, Spencer CA, Braverman LE, Pacini F, Wartofsky L, Haugen BR, Sherman SI, Cooper DS, Braunstein GD, Lee S, Davies TF, Arafah BM, Ladenson PW, Pinchera A (2003a) A consensus report of the role of serum thyroglobulin as a monitoring method for low-risk patients with papillary thyroid carcinoma. J Clin Endocrinol Metab 88:1433–1441
48. Mazzaferri EL, Robbins RJ, Braverman LE, Pacini F, Haugen BR, Wartofsky L, Braunstein GD, Ladenson PW, Pinchera A (2003b) Authors‘ response: a consensus report of the role of serum thyroglobulin as a monitoring method for low-risk patients with papillary thyroid carcinoma. J Clin Endocrinol Metab 88:4508–4510
49. Menzel C, Grünwald F, Biersack HJ (2003) Monitoring of low-risk patients with papillary thyroid carcinoma. J Clin Endocrinol Metab 88:4507
50. Mommert C, Görges R, Brandt-Mainz K, Hüsing J, Mergner J, Bockisch A (2000) Outcome of 1,017 patients with differentiated thyroid carcinoma and detection of recurrences. Eur J Nucl Med 27:1156 (abstract PS581)
51. Morgenthaler NG, Froehlich J, Rendl J, Willnich M, Alonso C, Bergmann A, Reiners C (2002) Technical evaluation of a new immunoradiometric and a new immunoluminometric assay for thyroglobulin. Clin Chem 48:1077–1083
52. Moriyama K, Akamizu T, Umemoto M, Miura M, Saijo M, Taniguchi K, Nakao K (1999) A case of Hashimoto‘s thyroiditis with markedly elevated serum thyroglobulin and evidence of its influence on the measurement of anti-thyroglobulin antibody by highly sensitive assays. Endocr J 46:687–693
53. Morris LF, Waxman AD, Braunstein GD (2002) Interlaboratory comparison of thyroglobulin measurements for patients with recurrent or metastatic differentiated thyroid cancer. Clin Chem 48:1371–1372
54. Müller-Gärtner HW, Schneider C, Tempel MT (1986) Serum-Thyreoglobulin in der Metastasendiagnostik des differenzierten Schilddrüsenkarzinoms. Nuklearmedizin 25:194–200
55. Müller-Gärtner HW, Schneider C (1988) Clinical evaluation of tumor characteristics predisposing serum thyroglobulin to be undetectable in patients with differentiated thyroid cancer. Cancer 61:976–981
56. Pacini F, Lippi F (1999) Clinical experience with recombinant human thyroid-stimulating hormone (rhTSH): serum thyroglobulin measurement. J Endocrinol Invest 22 [Suppl 11]:25–29
57. Pacini F, Lari R, Mazzeo S, Grasso L, Taddei D, Pinchera A (1985) Diagnostic value of a single serum thyroglobulin determination on and off thyroid suppressive therapy in the follow-up of patients with differentiated thyroid cancer. Clin Endocrinol (Oxf) 23:405–411
58. Pellegriti G, Scollo C, Regalbuto C, Attard M, Marozzi P, Vermiglio F, Violi MA, Cianci M, Vigneri R, Pezzino V, Squatrito S (2003) The diagnostic use of the rhTSH/thyroglobulin

test in differentiated thyroid cancer patients with persistent disease and low thyroglobulin levels. Clin Endocrinol (Oxf) 58:556–561

59. Petrich T, Börner AR, Weckesser E, Soudah B, Otto D, Widjaja A, Hofmann M, Kreipe HH, Knapp WH (2001) Nachsorge des differenzierten Schilddrüsenkarzinoms unter Verwendung von rhTSH – vorläufige Ergebnisse. Nuklearmedizin 40:7–14
60. Piechaczyk M, Baldet L, Pau B, Bastide JM (1989) Novel immunoradiometric assay of thyroglobulin in serum with use of monoclonal antibodies selected for lack of cross-reactivity with autoantibodies. Clin Chem 35:422–424
61. Preissner CM, O'Kane DJ, Singh RJ, Morris JC, Grebe SK (2003) Phantoms in the assay tube: heterophile antibody interferences in serum thyroglobulin assays. J Clin Endocrinol Metab 88:3069–3074
62. Quevedo I, Campino C, Rodriguez Portales JA, Arteaga E, Lopez JM, Campusano C, Gonzalez G, Fardella C, Slater J, Valdivia L, Poggi H, Foradori A, Velasco S (2002) Anti thyroglobulin antibodies in the follow-up of patients with differentiated thyroid cancer: residual or relapsing disease markers? Rev Med Chil 130:167–172
63. Reiners C, Reimann J, Schaffer R, Baum K, Becker W, Eilles C, Gerhards W, Schick F, Spiegel W, Wiedemann W et al (1984) Metastatic differentiated thyroid cancer. Diagnostic accuracy of thyroglobulin-RIA in comparison with ^{131}I-whole body scintigraphy. Röfo 141:306–313
64. Ringel MD, Balducci-Silano PL, Anderson JS, Spencer CA, Silverman J, Sparling YH, Francis GL, Burman KD, Wartofsky L, Ladenson PW, Levine MA, Tuttle RM (1999) Quantitative reverse transcription-polymerase chain reaction of circulating thyroglobulin messenger ribonucleic acid for monitoring patients with thyroid carcinoma. J Clin Endocrinol Metab 84:4037–4042
65. Roitt IM, Torrigiani G (1967) Identification and estimation of undegraded thyroglobulin in human serum. Endocrinology 81:421–429
66. Ronga G, Fiorentino A, Paserio E, Signore A, Todino V, Tummarello MA, Filasi M, Baschieri I (1990) Can iodine-131 whole-body scan be replaced by thyroglobulin measurement in the post-surgical follow-up of differentiated thyroid carcinoma? J Nucl Med 31:1766–1771
67. Sapin R, Gasser F, Chambron J (1992) Recovery determination in 600 sera analyzed for thyroglobulin with a recently commercialized IRMA kit. Clin Chem 38:1920–1921
68. Schaadt B, Feldt-Rasmussen U, Rasmusson B, Torring H, Foder B, Jorgensen K, Hansen HS (1995) Assessment of the influence of thyroglobulin (Tg) autoantibodies and other interfering factors on the use of serum Tg as tumor marker in differentiated thyroid carcinoma. Thyroid 5:165–170
69. Schlumberger M, Pacini F (eds) (1999) Thyroid tumors. Serum thyroglobulin measurement, Chap 7.2.3. Éditions Nucléon, Paris, pp 136–140
70. Schlumberger M, Fragu P, Gardet P, Lumbroso J, Violot D, Parmentier C (1991) A new immunoradiometric assay (IRMA) system for thyroglobulin measurement in the follow-up of thyroid cancer patients. Eur J Nucl Med 18:153–157
71. Schlumberger M, Berg G, Cohen O, Duntas L, Jamar F, Jarzab B, Limbert E, Lind P, Pacini F, Reiners C, Sanchez Franco F, Toft A, Wiersinga WM (2004) Follow-up of low-risk patients with differentiated thyroid carcinoma: a European perspective. Eur J Endocrinol 150:105–112
72. Sheils OM, Sweeney EC (1999) TSH receptor status of thyroid neoplasms – TaqMan RT-PCR analysis of archival material. J Pathol 188:87–92
73. Spencer CA, Takeuchi M, Kazarosyan M (1996; Current status and performance goals for serum thyroglobulin assays. Clin Chem 42:164–173
74. Spencer CA, Takeuchi M, Kazarosyan M, Wang CC, Guttler RB, Singer PA, Fatemi S, LoPresti JS, Nicoloff JT (1998) Serum thyroglobulin autoantibodies: prevalence, influence on serum thyroglobulin measurement, and prognostic significance in patients with differentiated thyroid carcinoma. J Clin Endocrinol Metab 83:1121–1127

75. Spencer CA, LoPresti JS, Fatemi S, Nicoloff JT (1999) Detection of residual and recurrent differentiated thyroid carcinoma by serum thyroglobulin measurement. Thyroid 9:435–441
76. Sulman C, Gosselin P, Carpentier P, Lemaire B (1984) Value of the estimation of thyroglobulin levels in the surveillance of treated differentiated thyroid carcinoma. J Clin Chem Clin Biochem 22:215–218
77. Szanto J, Vincze B, Sinkovics I, Karika Z, Daubner K, Peter I, Kazatsay I, Eckhardt S (1989) Postoperative thyroglobulin level determination to follow up patients with highly differentiated thyroid cancer. Oncology 46:99–104
78. Thyroid Carcinoma Task Force (2001) CE/AAES medical/surgical guidelines for clinical practice: management of thyroid carcinoma. American Association of Clinical Endocrinologists. American College of Endocrinology. Endocr Pract 7:202–220
79. Torlontano M, Crocetti U, D'Aloiso L, Bonfitto N, Di Giorgio A, Modoni S, Valle G, Frusciante V, Bisceglia M, Filetti S, Schlumberger M, Trischitta V (2003) Serum thyroglobulin and ^{131}I whole body scan after recombinant human TSH stimulation in the follow-up of low-risk patients with differentiated thyroid cancer. Eur J Endocrinol 148:19–24
80. Torlontano M, Attard M, Crocetti U, Tumino S, Bruno R, Costante G, D'Azzo G, Meringolo D, Ferretti E, Sacco R, Arturi F, Filetti S (2004) Follow-up of low risk patients with papillary thyroid cancer: role of neck ultrasonography in detecting lymph node metastases. J Clin Endocrinol Metab 89:3402–3407
81. Van Herle AJ, Uller RP, Matthews NI, Brown J (1973) Radioimmunoassay for measurement of thyroglobulin in human serum. J Clin Invest 52:1320–1327
82. Van Wyngaarden K, McDougall IR (1997) Is serum thyroglobulin a useful marker for thyroid cancer in patients who have not had ablation of residual thyroid tissue? Thyroid 7:343–346
83. Verburg FA, Lips CJ, Lentjes EG, Klerk JM de (2004) Detection of circulating Tg-mRNA in the follow-up of papillary and follicular thyroid cancer: how useful is it? Br J Cancer 91:200–204
84. Wang PW, Wang ST, Liu RT, Chien WY, Tung SC, Lu YC, Chen HY, Lee CH (1999) Levothyroxine suppression of thyroglobulin in patients with differentiated thyroid carcinoma. J Clin Endocrinol Metab 84:4549–4553
85. Wartofsky L (2002) Using baseline and recombinant human TSH-stimulated Tg measurements to manage thyroid cancer without diagnostic (131)I scanning. J Clin Endocrinol Metab 87:1486–1489
86. Weightman DR, Mallick UK, Fenwick JD, Perros P (2003) Discordant serum thyroglobulin results generated by two classes of assay in patients with thyroid carcinoma: correlation with clinical outcome after 3 years of follow-up. Cancer 98:41–47
87. Wunderlich G, Zöphel K, Crook L, Smith S, Smith BR, Franke WG (2001) A high-sensitivity enzyme-linked immunosorbent assay for serum thyroglobulin. Thyroid 11:819–824
88. Zöphel K, Wunderlich G, Liepach U, Koch R, Bredow J, Franke WG (2001) Recovery test or immunoradiometric measurement of anti-thyroglobulin autoantibodies for interpretation of thyroglobulin determination in the follow-up of different thyroid carcinoma. Nuklearmedizin 40:155–163
89. Zöphel K, Wunderlich G, Smith BR (2003) Serum thyroglobulin measurements with a high sensitivity enzyme-linked immunosorbent assay: is there a clinical benefit in patients with differentiated thyroid carcinoma? Thyroid 13:861–865

Chapter 14

Functional Imaging of Differentiated Thyroid Cancer

F. Grünwald

14.1 Introduction

Due to their relatively unaggressive biological behavior, most differentiated thyroid carcinomas have a good prognosis [7, 33]. This holds true even for patients with lung metastases, particularly in cases with disseminated metastatic sites that are radioiodine-positive. Therefore, thyroid cancer is overall a rare cause of cancer-associated death. Serum thyroglobulin measurement is the most sensitive method to detect recurrence of differentiated thyroid carcinoma during follow-up [46]. Radioiodine scintigraphy can be used as a highly specific method to visualize tumor tissue. But in many cases, particularly in poorly differentiated cancer and in Hürthle cell carcinoma, radioiodine uptake is decreased or absent, owing to several mechanisms. Particularly DNA changes, encoding the Na^+/I^- symporter, have to be considered. Therefore, the sensitivity of radioiodine scintigraphy is decreased from about 70% to less than 50% during the clinical course [44, 54]. Although therapeutic options are often limited to some extent in patients with radioiodine-negative metastases, correct staging is very important to plan further diagnostic and therapeutic steps. But also in cases with known radioiodine-positive tumor tissue, other functional techniques are clinically useful to prove or exclude additional radioiodine-negative tumor sites, which cannot be influenced by further radioiodine treatments. In some cases, recurrence or metastases are suspected during follow-up, even if no increased thyroglobulin values are observed. The reason might be pathological thyroglobulin recovery values or the existence of very poorly differentiated cell lines which have lost the capability to synthesise Tg. Tumor-specific functional imaging techniques are necessary to evaluate equivocal morphological alterations in these patients.

14.2 Tracers

14.2.1 Thallium Chloride

^{201}Tl was initially used to image myocardial viability and blood flow. Thallium is a monovalent cationic isotope and has a high affinity to the Na^+/K^+ pump, but it does not behave exactly like potassium because the affinity of thallium to the pump is even higher than that of potassium itself and there are two binding sites at the ATPase enzyme system for thallium – in contrast to potassium. ^{201}Tl has been used for tumor imaging for more than 20 years. The uptake of this tracer depends mainly on blood flow and metabolic demand. Several factors can influence the metabolic demand of tumor cells. The most important factors are viability and malignancy grade; the latter correlates with tumor growth. Therefore, ^{201}Tl scintigraphy can be used for tumor detection, therapy control, and in vivo grading of several tumor types. The clinical use of ^{201}Tl for tumor imaging has decreased because of its low gamma energy and the increasing importance of the ^{99m}Tc-labeled tracers hexakis 2-methoxyisobutylisonitrile (MIBI) and 1,2-bis [bis(2-ethoxyethyl)phosphino] ethane (tetrofosmin), as well as the increasing availability of ^{18}F-fluorodeoxyglucose (FDG) positron emission tomography (PET).

14.2.2 MIBI and Other ^{99m}Tc-Labeled Tracers

Like ^{201}Tl, MIBI was initially developed as a myocardial tracer. The uptake of this radiopharmaceutical depends mainly on the mitochondrial potential. More than 90% of the tracer is accumulated in the inner mitochondrial matrix [42]. The mitochondrial content of the tumor and the mitochondrial potential have a major influence on the tracer uptake in malignant tissue. The mitochondrial content does not change during the clinical course in most cases, whereas the potential is influenced by several factors. The most important factor is the metabolic demand, depending on the tumor growth. Hürthle cell tumors (which are frequently radioiodine-negative) are known to have a high mitochondrial content and can be detected with a high sensitivity using MIBI (Fig. 14.1) [3]. Since uptake values of ^{201}Tl and MIBI do not differ significantly in most thyroid tumors [10], MIBI is preferred mainly because of its favorable physical characteristics with respect to imaging [particularly single-photon emission computed tomography (SPECT)] and radiation exposure. Other ^{99m}Tc-labeled cationic complexes such as tetrofosmin or ^{99m}Tc-furifosmin (Q12), which have been developed as myocardial tracers also [4], have been used less frequently for thyroid carcinoma imaging. The specific uptake mechanisms of these substances – particularly in tumor cells – are partly unclear; the uptake of tetrofosmin (like that of MIBI) depends at least partially on the mitochondrial potential.

14.2.3 ^{18}F-Fluorodeoxyglucose

Glucose consumption is known to be increased in tumor cells [54]. Malignant tissue can metabolize glucose by oxidation or to lactic acid, even if saturated with oxygen. In addition to this increased use of glucose, trapped in the tumor cells, changes in glucose transporter systems and hexokinase activity influence glucose uptake [38]. Thus, the overexpression of glucose transporter genes

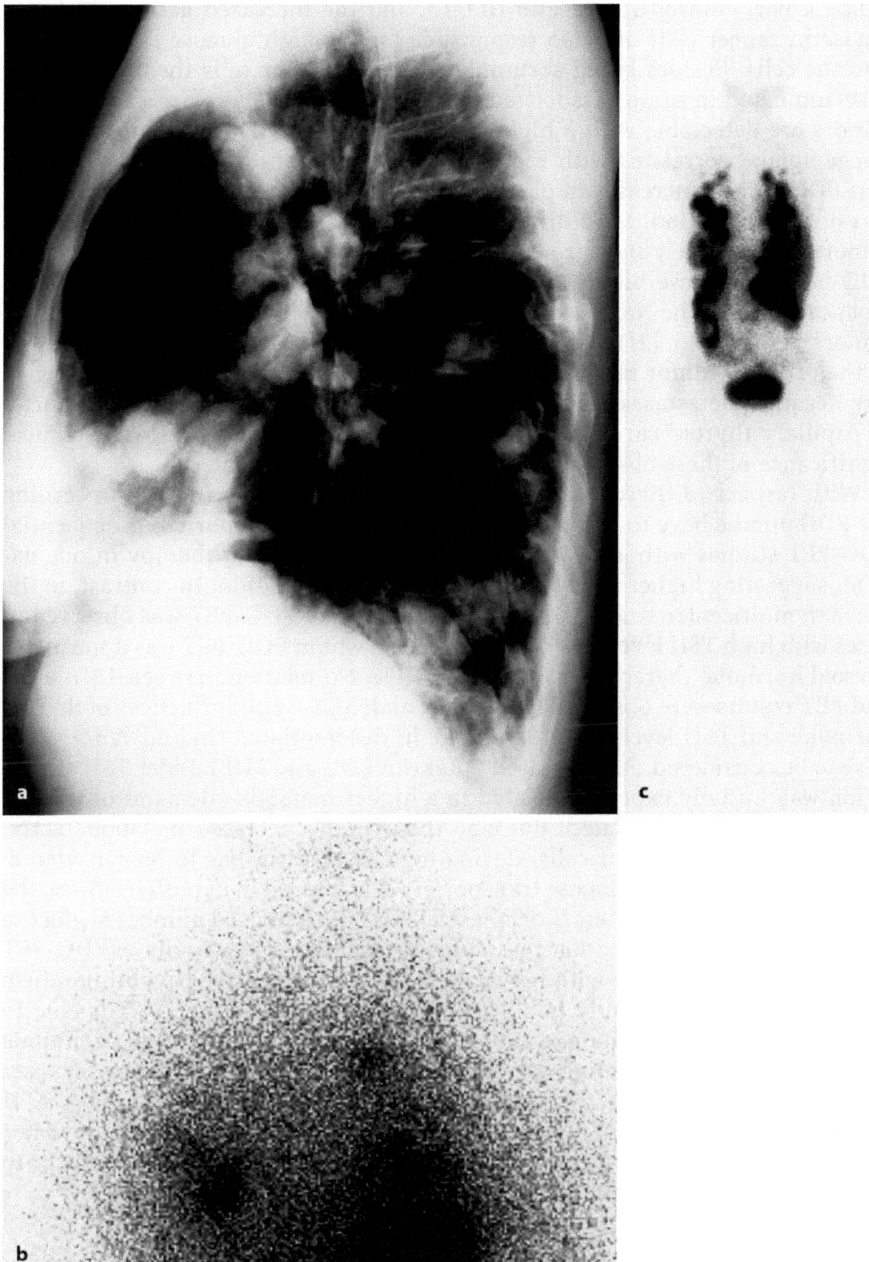

Fig. 14.1 a–d A 71-year-old female patient with Hürthle cell thyroid cancer and multiple lung metastases. The X-ray appearance is shown in **a**. Whole-body scintigraphy with radioiodine (dorsal view) shows faint uptake at one pulmonary site (**b**). Whole-body MIBI scintigraphy (dorsal view) (**c**) and SPECT imaging with MIBI (**d**) show high tracer uptake in the pulmonary metastases

(*GLUT*), particularly *GLUT1* and *GLUT3*, and the increased activity of hexokinase in cancer cells are also responsible for the high glucose transport rate into the cells. Besides being accumulated in the tumor cells themselves, FDG is accumulated in tumor-associated macrophages [31]. Therefore, fast-growing tumors are detectable with a higher sensitivity by FDG-PET. In most tumors, tracer uptake correlates with malignancy grade. Yoshioka et al. [55] showed that FDG uptake increases in pancreatic, gastric, and colonic cancer cells with loss of differentiation. Most differentiated thyroid carcinomas, particularly G1 tumors, are relatively slow growing and are therefore expected to be frequently FDG-negative. These highly differentiated tumors are radioiodine-positive in most cases, since the Na^+/I^- symporter can be expected still to be active in such tumors. Arturi et al. [2] reported a lack of the Na^+/I^- symporter gene expression in the primary tumor in 50% of patients suffering from whole body scintigraphy-negative metastases. In contrast, an increased expression of the symporter in papillary thyroid carcinomas has been described recently [45]. The clinical significance of these observations still remains to be evaluated.

With respect to thyroid carcinoma, some specific mechanisms concerning the FDG uptake have to be considered. Sisson et al. [48] reported on sequential FDG-PET studies with and without thyroxine replacement therapy in one patient, suggesting higher FDG uptake under TSH stimulation. In contrast, in the German multicenter study [26] a lower sensitivity of FDG-PET was observed in cases with high TSH levels (67%). In patients in whom FDG-PET was done under thyroid hormone therapy, sensitivity was 91%. No relation between TSH levels and PET results were observed by Wang et al. [53]. Several influences of thyroid hormone and TSH levels on FDG uptake in differentiated thyroid cancer cells have to be considered. An increased uptake of FDG and MIBI under TSH stimulation was initially expected, related to a higher metabolic demand of thyroid cells, specifically stimulated. But also the overall decreased metabolic activity, which includes tumor cells, during hypothyroidism has to be considered. Whereas the activity of glucose transporters is increased in hypothyroidism, the total number of transporters is decreased [35]. The decreased number of glucose transporters might be another reason for the decreased sensitivity of FDG-PET during thyroid hormone withdrawal, besides the influence of hypothyroidism on tumor growth. Recently published data [13, 41] show that TSH is able to increase FDG uptake in human thyroid cells in vitro and in thyroid carcinoma tissue in vivo. Tumor grading can be expected to affect TSH influence on tracer uptake since well-differentiated cancer cells can be expected to be more TSH dependent. In the German multicenter study on a large patient group, no major differences between tumor types (papillary versus follicular) with respect to sensitivity of any functional imaging technique were observed.

14.2.4 ^{111}In-Octreotide

Somatostatin receptor scintigraphy has predominantly been used for imaging of medullary thyroid cancer, rather than for DTC. Recently, reports on the use of

^{111}In-octreotide in DTC have been published [19, 21, 22, 27, 49, 51]. Somatostatin receptors mediate the antiproliferative effects of somatostatin and are present in normal tissue as well as in a variety of endocrine tumors such as medullary thyroid cancer. In tumor tissue, somatostatin receptor density is usually higher than in nontumoral tissue. In order to visualize somatostatin receptor-containing tumors, a long-acting somatostatin analog was required, because the half-life of native somatostatin in the circulation is extremely short (about 3 min) due to rapid enzymatic degradation [32]. The synthetic peptide (somatostatin analog) octreotide, which was developed by Bauer et al. [5], meets these requirements. However, the labeling procedure for octreotide is not suited for routine use. Therefore, a diethylenetriaminepentaacetic acid (DTPA)-conjugated derivative of octreotide labeled with ^{111}In has been developed for clinical routine use. ^{99m}Tc-labeled octreotide derivatives have been introduced in the clinical routine for some applications [18], with some limitations concerning the abdomen, but can be expected to be comparable in neck and mediastinum.

14.3 Clinical Use of Functional Imaging

14.3.1 Presurgical Evaluation

Several studies have dealt with the clinical significance of ^{201}Tl and MIBI scintigraphy for the evaluation of thyroid nodules. Although no clear-cut differentiation between malignant and benign nodules is possible, particularly MIBI is frequently used for presurgical imaging. The risk that a circumscribed lesion will be malignant seems to be distinctly higher if the lesion is cold on pertechnetate scintigraphy and hot on MIBI scintigraphy [37]. Nevertheless, since thyroid adenomas frequently show increased MIBI uptake, the specificity of MIBI scintigraphy with respect to the detection of malignancy is limited [17, 30, 34]. The specificity of FDG-PET is too low – especially in iodine-deficiency areas with a high incidence of (mostly benign) thyroid nodules – for preoperative use in nodular thyroid diseases. Like MIBI, FDG is taken up by benign adenomas in most cases. In papillary carcinoma, the sensitivity of FDG-PET is lower [29]. Using semiquantitative techniques, Adler and Bloom [1] observed a better differentiation between benign thyroid nodules and thyroid cancer. In summary, the large variety of metabolic rates of malignant and benign thyroid nodules prevents routine clinical use of FDG-PET prior to surgery. Nevertheless, in cases with preoperatively known carcinoma, particularly in medullary thyroid cancer, preoperative scintigraphy with MIBI or FDG-PET can be useful for staging to allow optimized surgical planning. In cases of circumscribed increased FDG uptake in the thyroid gland during a PET study performed for other reasons, particularly malignant melanoma, further evaluation is necessary to exclude malignancy [36]. Scott et al. [47] reported successful preoperative staging of the diffuse sclerosing variant of papillary carcinoma and of cervical lymph node metastases using FDG-PET. But especially in iodine-deficiency areas with a high incidence of nodular goiter and a high rate of surgical procedures concerning the thyroid gland, the definitive diagnosis of DTC is not known before histological evaluation in the majority of cases.

14.3.2 Postsurgical Treatment and Follow-up

It is sometimes difficult to distinguish remnant tissue from local recurrence, particularly during the initial weeks after the first ablative radioiodine therapy, since radiothyroiditis in the remnant tissue can show up with an increase in glucose utilization or MIBI uptake. Therefore it is recommended that FDG-PET and MIBI scintigraphy be used no earlier than 6 weeks after the first radioiodine treatment. Besides problems due to increased tracer uptake in inflammatory remnant tissue, imaging with single-photon emitters cannot be done earlier than about 6 weeks after radioiodine administration since even small amounts of radioiodine can interfere with imaging using ^{99m}Tc or ^{201}Tl owing to the long half-life and the high gamma energy of radioiodine. PET imaging is not affected by single-photon emitters (including radioiodine), although ^{99m}Tc-labeled tracers and ^{201}Tl should not be used on the same day after FDG administration. Exogenic TSH stimulation (rTSH injection) is known to increase PET sensitivity [41], in contrast to TSH stimulation after thyroid hormone withdrawal. The accuracy of ^{201}Tl or tetrofosmin imaging has been described to be independent of thyroid hormone replacement therapy [50]. No data have been published concerning the sensitivity and specificity of MIBI scintigraphy in relation to TSH levels. Morphological techniques such as ultrasonography, computed tomography (CT), or magnetic resonance imaging (MRI) have the disadvantage that the identification of radioiodine-negative tumor masses is often limited because of their inferior specificity, particularly in cases with altered anatomy (e.g., after neck dissection). Therefore, especially in radioiodine-negative cases with recurrence or metastatic disease, additional functional imaging techniques are necessary. The differentiation of scar tissue from local recurrence and of unspecific lymph node enlargement (cervical or mediastinal) from lymph node metastases is often very difficult using CT and MRI. In addition, the use of CT is limited, because this method can only be applied without contrast enhancement in view of further radioiodine administration. Moreover, all morphological imaging techniques lack sensitivity to some extent owing to their limited field of view.

Therapeutic strategies in cases with radioiodine-negative tumor tissue – which is detected by functional imaging – can include surgery, radiation therapy, chemotherapy, or redifferentiation therapy [8, 15, 25, 43]. Radioiodine treatments might be useless if radioiodine-negative tumor sites exist in addition to radioiodine-positive sites because of a variety of less differentiated tumor cell lines, which are more frequently radioiodine-negative.

In radioiodine-negative cases, the sensitivity of FDG-PET is as high as 85% (Fig. 14.2), whereas it is about 75% in the whole group of differentiated thyroid carcinomas [14, 16, 23, 24, 26]. The phenomenon that thyroid tumor cells take up either radioiodine or FDG was called "flip-flop" by Feine et al. [16]. The com-

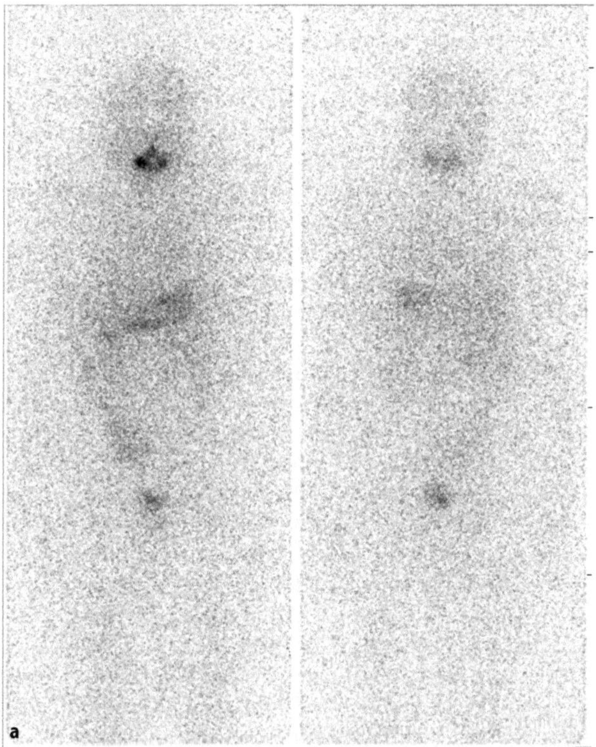

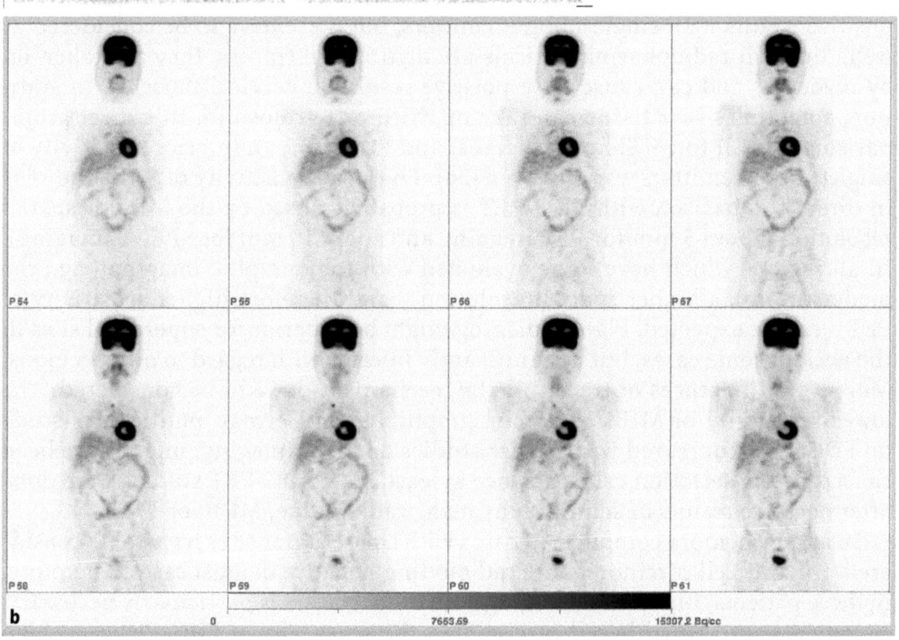

Fig. 14.2 A 30-year-old male patient with papillary thyroid cancer presenting with elevated thyroglobulin values during follow-up. Radioiodine scan (**a**) is completely negative, whereas FDG-PET (**b**) shows a small lymph node metastases behind the right sternoclavicular joint

bination of FDG-PET and posttherapeutic radioiodine scintigraphy gave a sensitivity of 93% in the German multicenter study [26]. In a group of 37 patients with negative radioiodine scan, Wang et al. [53] were able to localize tumor sites in 71% of all cases with elevated thyroglobulin values. The overall specificity of FDG-PET is inferior to that of radioiodine scintigraphy, because increased FDG uptake in nontumor tissue can occur for several reasons. For example in the lung, nontumor-associated FDG uptake can be caused by sarcoidosis, tuberculosis, aspergillosis, or pneumonia [10]. Activation of cervical muscles after tracer injection, which frequently occurs if the patients are not able to relax after tracer injection, can cause significant cervical FDG uptake which can resemble cervical lymph node metastases. In the mediastinum, false-positive results can be due to thymus tissue.

^{201}Tl was used initially for nonradioiodine scintigraphy in thyroid cancer with promising results [28], but its sensitivity is too low for routine clinical use, especially in comparison with MIBI and tetrofosmin, mainly due to inferior physical characteristics of the isotope. Ohnishi et al. [40] reported a false-negative rate of 53%, while MRI was false-negative in only 23% in the same group. In the first years of clinical use, a sensitivity of about 70–90% was reported for MIBI [10, 12, 39]. Recent studies on tetrofosmin [20] have yielded promising results, suggesting this tracer to be comparable with MIBI, as was expected due to comparable tracer uptake mechanisms. Gallowitsch et al. [20] reported sensitivity values up to 100% in small groups, depending on the site of the metastases, but further studies are necessary to confirm these preliminary data. A recently published paper, comparing furifosmin and FDG-PET, gave poor results for this ^{99m}Tc-labeled tracer [9]. Only a few studies have dealt with the causes of false-positive results with single-photon emitters, but these have to be considered as well. Since all radiopharmaceuticals are myocardial tracers, they are taken up by myocytes and can cause false-positive results in cervical muscles. In addition, sometimes scar tissue can take up MIBI or tetrofosmin. In a direct comparison of MIBI (or ^{201}Tl in a few cases) and FDG-PET, an inferior sensitivity of single-photon emitters was observed [26]. The lower sensitivity of MIBI and ^{201}Tl in direct comparison with FDG-PET is probably caused by the inferior spatial resolution (about 5 mm for PET imaging and about 10 mm for SPECT imaging). In all regions which have to be evaluated with tomographic imaging (e.g., the mediastinum), a higher spatial resolution – and therefore higher sensitivity of PET – can be expected. Planar imaging might be superior for superficial sites in the neck in some cases, but is significantly inferior with regard to other regions. Moreover, differences of tracer uptake mechanisms have to be considered. The lower sensitivity of MIBI/^{201}Tl scintigraphy in the German multicenter study on FDG-PET, compared with earlier studies on MIBI imaging, might have been caused by the selection criteria, since at least a few FDG-PET studies were done after negative results of scintigraphy using radioiodine, MIBI, or ^{201}Tl.

In addition, more complicated cases with small tumor sites have to be considered. Hürthle cell carcinomas are radioiodine-negative in most cases. Therefore, in these patients, functional imaging with other tracers is particularly necessary. In patients with Hürthle cell carcinomas, the sensitivity of FDG-PET is as high as 85% [26], whereas it is very low for radioiodine, as might be expected. Since

Hürthle cell carcinomas are known to have a high mitochondria content, they were expected to take up high amounts of all tracers which are accumulated in accordance with the mitochondrial potential and content (MIBI, tetrofosmin). However, the sensitivity of imaging using MIBI in Hürthle cell carcinoma was not observed to be higher than that of FDG-PET.

Somatostatin receptor expression in thyroid tissue (particularly in endemic goiter) was observed by Becker et al. [6]. Recently, somatostatin receptor expression has been described in three patients with Hürthle cell carcinoma using ^{111}In-octreotide [27]. Compared with conventional radiologic procedures, Valli et al. [51] found somatostatin receptor imaging to be inferior with respect to the obtained clinical information. In only one case did somatostatin receptor imaging detect mediastinal lymph node metastases not seen with morphological techniques [51]. Görges et al. [21] reported a good correlation of somatostatin receptor scintigraphy with the autoradiographically measured receptor status. They studied 24 cases of differentiated thyroid cancer and found a higher sensitivity of somatostatin receptor scintigraphy, compared with MIBI and ^{201}Tl. The highest sensitivity was achieved by FDG-PET in this group [21]. As well as for tumor detection, this method can be used to evaluate subsequent therapeutic options with somatostatin analogs. But no correlation between therapeutic effects of cold octreotide and receptor scintigraphy could be proven by Görges et al. [21].

References

1. Adler LP, Bloom AD (1993) Positron emission tomography of thyroid masses. Thyroid 3:195–200
2. Arturi F, Russo D, Schlumberger M, du-Villard JA, Caillou B, Vigneri P, et al. (1998) Iodide symporter gene expression in human thyroid tumors. J Clin Endocrinol Metab 83:2493–2496
3. Balone HR, Fing-Bennett D, Stoffer SS (1992) ^{99m}Tc-sestamibi uptake by recurrent Hürthle cell carcinoma of the thyroid. J Nucl Med 33:1393–1395
4. Bangard M, Bender H, Grünwald F, et al. (1999) Myocardial uptake of technetium-99m-furifosmin (Q12) versus technetium-99m-sestamibi (MIBI). Nuklearmedizin 38: 189–191
5. Bauer W, Briner U, Doepfner W (1982) SMS-201–995: a very potent and selective octapeptide analogue of somatostatin with prolonged action. Life Sci 31:1133–1140
6. Becker W, Schrell U, Buchfelder M, Hensen J, Wendler J, Gramatzki M, et al. (1995) Somatostatin receptor expression in the thyroid demonstrated with ^{111}In-octreotide scintigraphy. Nuklearmedizin 34:100–103
7. Biersack HJ, Hotze A (1991) The clinician and the thyroid. Eur J Nucl Med 18: 761–778
8. Börner AR, Petrich T, Weckesser E, Fricke H, Hofmann H, Otto D, Weckesser M, Langen KJ, Knapp WH (2002) Monitoring isotretinoin therapy in thyroid cancer using ^{18}F-FDG PET. Eur J Nucl Med Mol Imaging 29:231–236
9. Brandt-Mainz K, Müller SP, Sonnenschein W, Bockisch A (1998) Technetium-99m-furifosmin in the follow-up of differentiated thyroid carcinoma. J Nucl Med 39:1536–1541
10. Briele B, Hotze AL, Kropp J, Bockisch A, Overbeck B, Grünwald F, et al. (1991) A comparison of ^{201}Tl and ^{99m}Tc-MIBI in the follow-up of differentiated thyroid carcinoma. Nuklearmedizin 30:115–124

11. Briele B, Willkomm P, Grünwald F, Ruhlmann J, Biersack HJ (1999) Imaging of secondary pulmonary changes in central bronchial carcinomas by F-18-FDG-PET. Nuklearmedizin 38:323–327
12. Dadparvar S, Chevres A, Tulchinsky M, Krishna-Badrinath L, Khan AS, Slizofski WJ (1995) Clinical utility of technetium-99m methoxisobutylisonitrile imaging in differentiated thyroid carcinoma: comparison with thallium-201 and iodine-131 Na scintigraphy, and serum thyroglobulin quantitation. Eur J Nucl Med 22:1330–1338.
13. Deichen JT, Schmidt C, Prante O, Maschauer S, Papadopoulos T, Kuwert T ((2004) Influence of TSH on uptake of [(18)F]fluorodeoxyglucose in human thyroid cells in vitro. Eur J Nucl Med Mol Imaging 31:507–512
14. Dietlein M, Scheidhauer K, Voth E, Theissen P, Schicha H (1997) Fluorine-18 fluorodeoxyglucose positron emission tomography and iodine-131 whole-body scintigraphy in the follow-up of differentiated thyroid cancer. Eur J Nucl Med 24:1342–1348
15. Farahati J, Reiners C, Stuschke M, Müller SP, Stüben G, Sauerwein W, et al. (1996) Differentiated thyroid cancer. Impact of adjuvant external radiotherapy in patients with perithyroidal tumor infiltration (stage pT4). Cancer 77:172–180
16. Feine U, Lietzenmayer R, Hanke JP, Held J, Wöhrle H, Müller-Schauenburg W (1996) Fluorine-18-FDG and iodine-131-Iodide uptake in thyroid cancer. J Nucl Med 37: 1468–1472
17. Foldes I, Levay A, Stotz G (1993) Comparative scanning of thyroid nodules with technetium-99m pertechnetate and technetium-99m methoxyisobutylisonitrile. Eur J Nucl Med 20:330–333
18. Gabriel M, Moncayo R et al (2004) ^{99m}Tc-EDDA/HYNIC-TOC and ^{18}F-FDG in thyroid cancer patients with negative ^{131}I whole-body scans. Eur J Nucl Med Mol Imaging 31:330–341
19. Giammarile F, Borson-Chazot F et al (2004) Diagnostic management of suspected metastatic thyroid carcinoma: clinical value of octreotide scintigraphy in patients with negative high-dose radioiodine scans. Eur J Endocrinol 150:277–283
20. Gallowitsch HJ, Mikosch P, Kresnik E, Unterweger O, Gomez I, Lind P (1998) Thyroglobulin and low-dose iodine-131 and technetium-99m-tetrofosmin whole-body scintigraphy in differentiated thyroid carcinoma. J Nucl Med 39:870–875
21. Görges R, Kahaly G, Müller-Brand J, et al. (1999) Examination of the somatostatin receptor status in non-medullary thyroid cancer. Nuklearmedizin 38:15–23
22. Görges R, Kahaly G, Müller-Brand J, Mäcke H, Roser HW, Bockisch A (2001) Radionuclide-labeled somatostatin analogues for diagnostic and therapeutic purposes in nonmedullary thyroid cancer. Thyroid 11:647-659
23. Grünwald F, Schomburg A, Bender H, Klemm E, Menzel C, Bultmann T, et al. (1996) Fluorine-18 fluorodeoxyglucose positron emission tomography in the follow-up of differentiated thyroid cancer. Eur J Nucl Med 23:312–319
24. Grünwald F, Menzel C, Bender H, Palmedo H, Willkomm P, Ruhlmann J, et al. (1997) Comparison of ^{18}FDG-PET with ^{131}iodine and ^{99m}Tc-sestamibi scintigraphy in differentiated thyroid cancer. Thyroid 7:327–335
25. Grünwald F, Menzel C, Bender H, Palmedo H, Otte R, Fimmers R, et al. (1998) Redifferentiation therapy-induced radioiodine uptake in thyroid cancer. J Nucl Med 39: 1903–1906
26. Grünwald F, Kälicke T, Feine U, et al. (1999) Fluorine-18 fluorodeoxyglucose positron emission tomography in thyroid cancer: results of a multicentre study. Eur J Nucl Med 26:1547–1552
27. Gulec SA, Serafini AN, Sridhar KS, Peker KR, Gupta A, Goodwin WJ, et al. (1998) Somatostatin receptor expression in Hürthle cell cancer of the thyroid. J Nucl Med 39:243–245
28. Hoefnagel CA, Delprat CC, Marcuse HR, deVijlder JJ (1986) Role of thallium-201 total-body scintigraphy in follow-up of thyroid carcinoma. J Nucl Med 27:1854–1857
29. Joensuu H, Ahonen A, Klemi PJ (1988) ^{18}F-fluorodeoxyglucose imaging in preoperative diagnosis of thyroid malignancy. Eur J Nucl Med 13:502–506

30. Koizumi M, Taguchi H, Goto M, Nomura T, Watari T (1993) Thallium-201 scintigraphy in the evaluation of thyroid nodules. A retrospective study of 246 cases. Ann Nucl Med 7:147–152
31. Kubota R, Kubota K, Yamada S, Tada M, Ido T, Tamahashi N (1994) Microautoradiographic study for the differentiation of intratumoral macrophages, granulation tissues and cancer cells by the dynamics of fluorine-18-fluorodeoxyglucose uptake. J Nucl Med 35:104–112
32. Lamberts SW, Koper JW, Reubi JC (1987) Potential role of somatostatin analogues in the treatment of cancer. Eur J Clin Invest 17:281–287
33. Lerch H, Schober O, Kuwert T, Saur HB (1997) Survival of differentiated thyroid carcinoma studied in 500 patients. J Clin Oncol 15:2067–2075
34. Lind P (1999) Multi-tracer imaging of thyroid nodules: is there a role in the preoperative assessment of nodular goiter? Eur J Nucl Med 26:795–797
35. Matthaei S, Trost B, Hamann A, Kausch C, Benecke H, Greten H, et al. (1995) Effect of in vivo thyroid hormone status on insulin signalling and GLUT1 and GLUT4 glucose transport systems in rat adipocytes. J Endocrinol 144:347–357
36. Menzel C, Risse JH, Biersack HJ, Grünwald F (2001) Primary diagnosis of papillary thyroid carcinoma in the framework of staging of malignant melanoma with F-18 deoxyglucose using PET. Nuklearmedizin 40:23–24
37. Mezosi E, Bajnok L, Gyory F, Varga J, Sztojka I, Szabo J, Galuska L, Leovey A, Kakuk G, Nagy E (1999) The role of technetium-99m methoxyisobutylisonitrile scintigraphy in the differential diagnosis of cold thyroid nodules. Eur J Nucl Med 26:798–803
38. Mueckler M (1994) Facilitative glucose transporters. Eur J Biochem 219:713–725
39. Nemec J, Nyvltova O, Blazek T, Vlcek P, Racek P, Novak Z, et al. (1996) Positive thyroid cancer scintigraphy using technetium-99m methoxyisobutylisonitrile. Eur J Nucl Med 1996; 23:69–71
40. Ohnishi T, Noguchi S, Murakami N, Jinnouchi S, Hoshi H, Futami S et al. (1993) Detection of recurrent thyroid cancer: MR versus thallium-201 scintigraphy. AJNR Am J Neuroradiol 14:1051–1057
41. Petrich T, Börner AR, Otto D, Hofmann M, Knapp WH (2002) Influence of rhTSH on [(18)F] fluorodeoxyglucose uptake by differentiated thyroid carcinoma. Eur J Nucl Med Mol Imaging 29:641–647
42. Piwinica-Worms D, Kronauge JF, Chiu ML (1990) Uptake and retention of hexakis (2-methoxyisobutyl isonitrile) technetium (I) in cultured chick myocardial cells, mitochondrial and plasma membrane potential dependence. Circulation 82:1826–1838
43. Raue F (1997) Chemotherapie bei Schilddrüsenkarzinomen: Indikation und Ergebnisse. Onkologe 3:55–58
44. Reiners C, Reimann J, Schaffer R, Baum K, Becker W, Eilles C, et al. (1984) Metastatic differentiated thyroid cancer. Diagnostic accuracy of thyroglobulin-RIA in comparison with I-131-whole-body scintigraphy. RÖFO Fortschr Geb Röntgenstr Nuklearmed 141:306–313
45. Saito T, Endo T, Kawaguchi A, Ikeda M, Katoh R, Kawaoi A, et al. (1998) Increased expression of the sodium/iodide symporter in papillary thyroid carcinomas. J Clin Invest 101:1296–1300
46. Schlumberger M, Fragu P, Gardet P, Lumbroso J, Vilot D, Parmentier C (1991) A new immunoradiometric assay (IRMA) system for thyroglobulin measurement in the follow-up of thyroid cancer patients. Eur J Nucl Med 18:153–157
47. Scott GC, Meier DA, Dickinson CZ (1995) Cervical lymph node metastasis of thyroid papillary carcinoma imaged with fluorine-18-FDG, technetium-99m-pertechnetate and iodine-131-sodium iodide. J Nucl Med 36:1843–1845
48. Sisson JC, Ackermann RJ, Meyer MA (1993) Uptake of 18-fluoro-2-deoxy-d-glucose by thyroid cancer: implications for diagnosis and therapy. J Clin Endocrin Metabol 77:1090–1094

49. Stokkel MP, Verkooijen RB, Smit JW (2004) Indium-111 octreotide scintigraphy for the detection of non-functioning metastases from differentiated thyroid cancer: diagnostic and prognostic value. Eur J Nucl Med Mol Imaging 26
50. Ünal S, Menda Y, Adalet I, Boztepe H, Özbey N, Alagöl F, et al. (1998) Thallium-201, technetium-99-tetrofosmin, and iodine-131 in detecting differentiated thyroid carcinoma metastases. J Nucl Med 39:1897–1902
51. Valli N, Catargi B, Ronci N, et al. (1999) Evaluation of indium-111 pentetreotide somatostatin receptor scintigraphy to detect recurrent thyroid carcinoma in patients with negative radioiodine scintigraphy. Thyroid 9:583–589
52. VanSorge-vanBoxtel RAJ, VanEck-Smit BLF, Goslings BM (1993) Comparison of serum thyroglobulin, I-131 and Tl-201 scintigraphy in the postoperative follow-up of differentiated thyroid cancer. Nucl Med Commun 14:365–372
53. Wang W, Macapinlac H, Larson SM, et al. (1999) [18F]-2-Fluoro-2-deoxy-D-glucose positron emission tomography localizes residual thyroid cancer in patients with negative diagnostic (131)I whole body scans and elevated serum thyroglobulin levels. J Clin Endocrinol Metab 84:2291–2302
54. Warburg O (1956) On the origin of cancer cells. Science 123:309–314
55. Yoshioka T, Takahashi H, Oikawa H, Maeda S, Wakui A, Watanabe T, et al. (1994) Accumulation of 2-deoxy-2[^{18}F]fluoro-D-glucose in human cancer heterotransplanted in nude mice: comparison between histology and glycolytic status. J Nucl Med 35:97–103

Chapter 15

Magnetic Resonance Imaging 15

J.H. Risse

15.1 Introduction

Magnetic resonance imaging (MRI) combines excellent soft tissue contrast with multiplanar capabilities and the lack of ionising radiation. This has lent wings to a still-growing scientific community exploring the imaging possibilities of this medico-technical treasure. To date, vast amounts of MRI literature about almost every body region exist, and we observe continuously increasing knowledge in new applications such as MR angiography (MRA), echoplanar MR imaging (EPI) or functional MRI (fMRI).

In contrast, there is relatively little MRI literature about the thyroid. Early MR investigators expressed optimism that this technique would be capable of distinguishing different pathological thyroid tissues [1–14], but this wish remained unfulfilled [15–18]. Even the most recent efforts to examine thyroid function by EPI remain at the trials stage [19]. Consequently, the use of MRI for assessing the thyroid has developed less rapidly than for other body areas and the literature in this field is not expanding as fast as for other parts of the body. Generally, the role of cross-sectional imaging in this area has been reduced in recent years because the functional nature of nuclear medicine is more useful for this endocrine organ. For morphological questions, the small organ in superficial anatomical localisation is predestined for high-frequency sonography, so usually there is no need for CT or MRI – a condition which the thyroid shares with the testes, for example. Additionally, cost-effectiveness analyses increasingly dominate the health care systems in most countries and suppress MRI of the "usual" thyroid disease. Since the late 1980s, three exceptions have been accepted: the morphological assessment of extent and anatomical relationships of intrathoracic goitre, cancer, and recurrent cancer. The past years have shown that in clinical practice MRI is rarely recommended preoperatively for the former two; occasionally, invasion of neighbouring structures by thyroid carcinoma may be of interest [20]; for initial staging purposes, a recent study showed ultrasound to be superior to MRI [21]. For the latter, MRI remains a useful tool. Therefore, this chapter focuses on the role of MRI in the follow-up of thyroid cancer patients based on our experience in more than 200 examinations.

15.2 Principles of MRI

Readers who are familiar with the technical aspects of MRI can skip this section; for those who are not, the necessary basics are explained as briefly as possible.

15.2.1 Physical and Technical Basis of MRI

The physical basis of MRI comprises the basis of nuclear physics, spin and magnetisation principles, signal production and image reconstruction, and the methods to generate image contrast by different imaging sequences. The technical components are the hardware of a MRI system, including the main field magnet, the gradient systems, the high-frequency system and the computer system. These basic components are complex and their detailed presentation would require too much room here; for more detail, the reader is referred to the References section (e.g. [22]). However, for a better understanding of the sequences used at our institution, some basics and terms of image contrast are explained briefly here.

15.2.1.1 Magnetic Signal

MRI is based on two simple facts: One, every atom with an odd number of protons has got a spin, inducing a magnetic field with a magnetic vector, and a defined resonance frequency. The strongest resonance effect comes from hydrogen nuclei with only one proton – and this is also the most frequent element in the human body.

In a strong, continuous magnetic field, such as is given by a MR system, all spins are organised to paralleled magnetic vectors. An additional short, high-frequency electromagnetic impulse with the resonance frequency will stimulate the spins and thereby change their magnetic vector. This changed vector has got an energy surplus and will immediately begin to switch back into its former orientation, which is called "relaxation" and is combined with the delivery of energy in the form of an electromagnetic signal. This MR "answer signal" is modulated by additional weak gradient fields in all planes and then processed to the MR image; most of the signal is shown as brightness, and some signal becomes dark.

The MR signal is weak: compared with the high-frequency stimulation impulse with a power of up to 20 kW, the MR signal is approximately several microwatts. That means a bad signal-to-noise ratio, which may be overcome by surface coils. They are arranged as near as possible to the body region of interest and render a much better signal than the body coil (the body coil is the same coil used for the stimulation impulse).

15.2.1.2
Image Generation: What are TR and TE? What are T1 and T2?

In biological tissues, liquids yield more signal than solid bodies, so that the MR technique recognises predominantly signals coming from water and lipid protons. Three parameters determine the brightness in a MR image and therefore its contrast: proton density, T1-time and T2-time. The *proton density* equals the number of stimulatable spins per volume. This number determines the possible signal maximum that may be emitted by the given tissue. The proton density becomes accentuated when the two other parameters (T1 and T2) are reduced as far as possible – the resulting image is called "proton-" or "density-weighted". The *T1-time* is required for the longitudinal relaxation, the *T2-time* for the transversal relaxation of the changed magnetic vector. Images that are dominated by T1 are called "T1-weighted" and are analogous with T2. Proton density, T1 and T2 are specific tissue characteristics and different biological tissues show strong differences in these parameters. Dependent on which parameter is accentuated in a MR sequence, images with different contrasts will be generated. This is explained below.

For the build-up of a MR image, any slice must be stimulated repeatedly. The time between these repetitions is called "repetition time" (TR) and is, for the so-called spin-echo (SE) sequences, usually between 0.4 and 3 s. A short TR yields much information about T1 differences in the different tissues, i.e. a sequence with short TR is strongly T1-weighted. Tissues with a short T1 appear bright on a T1-weighted image (e.g. fat, hyaline cartilage).

The time between the stimulating impulse and the MR "answer signal" delivered by the relaxing magnetic vector is called "echo time" (TE; usually 15–200 µs). A long TE yields more information about T2 differences between the tissues, and what follows is (reciprocal) analogous to TR and T1: A sequence with long TE is strongly T2-weighted, and tissues with a long TE appear bright on a T2-weighted image (e.g. water). Tissues with a high content of water-bound protons, such as oedema, tumour or inflammation, demonstrate a signal behaviour near to water.

Blood flow usually shows no signal in spin-echo sequences due to the "outflow effect": The stimulated blood spins have moved elsewhere in the vessel when the MR answer signal is to be recognised by the system; and in the location where the system would expect signal to come from, there is "fresh" blood now, coming from elsewhere, which has not been stimulated. This effect is also called "flow void".

The connections between TR, TE and the resulting image contrast are summarised in Table 15.1. Table 15.2 shows the signal intensity of the most important tissues.

The superior soft tissue contrast is only one reason for the advantages of MRI over other morphological imaging techniques in most instances. Compared with sonography, anatomical relationships and slice planes are not dependent on the investigator's actions, but reproducible, "objective"; and compared with X-ray computed tomography (CT), there is no exposure to ionising radiation, freedom from beam-hardening artefacts, and unlimited multiplanar image

	TR short	TR long
TE short	T1-weighted	Proton weighted (not T1, not T2)
TE long	(T1- and T2-weighted, no clinical use)	T2-weighted

Table 15.1 Relations between TR and TE and the resulting image contrast

Table 15.2. Signal intensity of some important tissues in T1- and T2-weighted images, roughly divided into dark and bright

Tissue	T1-weighted	T2-weighted
Fat	Bright	Bright
Water	Dark	Bright
Oedema	Dark	Bright
Tumour	Dark	Bright
Inflammation	Dark	Bright
Lymph node	Dark	Bright
Muscle	Dark	Dark
Thyroid	Dark	Dark
Cartilage, hyaline	Bright	Bright
Cartilage, fibrous	Dark	Dark
Connecting tissues	Dark	Dark
Compact bone	Nearly no signal	Nearly no signal
Air	No signal	No signal
Blood flow	No signal due to outflow effect ("flow void")	No signal due to outflow effect ("flow void")
Haematoma, acute	Dark	Dark
Haematoma, subacute	Bright	Bright

acquisition capabilities. Of course, the MRI technique has got its own pitfalls and artefacts, such as movement or flow artefacts, phase wrapping, fat shift and susceptibility artefacts. These will not be explained further in this chapter. Movement artefacts arising from the heartbeat, the great intrathoracic vessels or breathing may be overcome by ECG- and breath-triggering. Further developments have led to faster MR image acquisition techniques such as "turbo-spin-echo" (TSE), gradient echo (GE) sequences, combinations of these and others (e.g. EPI); of these, only TSE proved useful for our study.

15.2.1.3
Further Contrast Modifications: Fat Saturation and Contrast Media

Additional techniques have been developed to further improve the contrast behaviour in some constellations. Two of these techniques are used for the sequences presented in this chapter: the use of fat saturation (or fat suppression) techniques and contrast media.

15.2.1.3.1
Fat saturation

When the tissues of interest are surrounded by fat and show a signal behaviour resembling fat, they are not clearly distinguishable. For example, for our purposes, this sometimes may become true for lymph nodes in a T2-(T)SE sequence, or in a T1 sequence after the application of contrast media. The solution of this problem is fat saturation, i.e. lowering the fat signal such that fat appears dark to enhance the signal difference, which provides contrast to the tissue under investigation. Two different techniques are important.

SPIR. One fat-suppression technique is called "spectral presaturation with inversion recovery" (SPIR). It requires high magnetic fields to differentiate the spectral resonance lines of water bound from lipid-bound protons. A special pre-pulse of exact fat resonance frequency saturates the lipid-bound protons before the actual sequence. The lipids then do no more contribute signal to the following normal sequence: the fat is suppressed (i.e. dark), whereas non fatty tissues remain unchanged. This pre-pulse may be combined with any sequence type (T1, T2, TSE etc.) and does not affect contrast studies (see below). The main disadvantage is the necessity of very high homogeneity of the static magnetic field; even small inhomogeneities disturb the image quality and may lead to dramatic signal loss at the image periphery.

STIR. The other technique – "short tau inversion recovery" (STIR) – is quite different. Instead of using the different spectral resonance lines of water versus lipid-bound protons such as in SPIR, STIR takes advantage of the different relaxation times of the tissues. Electromagnetic impulses force the fat-bound protons to go with their relaxation through a zone of "zero signal", during which the image is acquired – only water-bound protons yield a signal. Of course, this procedure takes much more time, so that the main drawback of this sequence type is the long examination time. Additionally, the usefulness of contrast media is restricted, because the signal of enhancing organs may be reduced also. On the other hand, this sequence is independent of the strength of the magnetic field, i.e. it may be run on MR systems with lower magnetic fields. The main advantage, however, is the stable homogeneity of the signal throughout the image, compared with T2-SPIR. The image impression for the rest is quite similar: the contrasts are reduced to dark and bright with virtually no greyscale between.

Such sequences may serve as "quick-finders": water, and thus most pathological changes, appear bright, whereas most normal tissues are dark. The resulting high-contrast image may be read almost like a "hot spot" image as known in nuclear medicine – with the great difference that 25 different images (each slice with a different anatomy!) are to be analysed. The high sensitivity is coupled with the drawback of low specificity and many false-positive findings; these occur particularly in veins with a slower blood flow, when the blood flow is too slow for the flow-void effect. Then the blood increasingly adopts a water signal behaviour and becomes more or less bright, resembling lymph nodes, for instance. Additionally, since most normal tissues are dark, anatomical differentiation is difficult.

15.2.1.3.2 Contrast media

Many MR contrast media types have been developed for different indications. The most important is gadolinium diethylene triamine pentaacetic acid (Gd-DTPA). Gadolinium is an element with a high number of seven unpaired electrons causing a strong paramagnetic effect. This leads mainly to a shortening of the T1 relaxation time, i.e. a signal increase in a T1-weighted sequence. This is called "contrast enhancement" and means a brighter appearance in a T1-weighted image. Since isolated paramagnetic substances are toxic metal ions, they have to be bound in a complex such as DTPA. Gd-DTPA is applied in a dose of 0.2 ml/kg (0.1 mmol/kg) intravenously. Data acquisition should begin immediately with the end of the injection, because the substance shows quick diffusion and redistribution within some minutes. The sequence should be started no later than 5–10 min post-injection. Usually, it is sufficient to do one T1-weighted SE sequence before and after contrast media application ("static contrast study"). Alternatively, a "dynamic contrast study" with multiple fast p.i. T1-weighted GE sequences may be performed; but the best anatomical resolution is achieved by the former. The image software usually provides the option of image subtraction. Provided the patient does not move, only enhancing tissues appear bright (depending on the enhancing amount), whereas non-enhancing tissues become dark; but in practice even the smallest movements of the patient during or between the acquisitions result in multiple subtraction artefacts. Reading such an image subtraction product may be more difficult than comparing a pre- and post-contrast image, which is particularly true for the complex and fine-structured anatomy of the neck.

Enhancing tissues such as lymph nodes or vital thyroid tissue often are no longer distinguishable from surrounding fat in a T1-weighted image. In this case, a post-contrast sequence may be combined with a fat-suppression technique (T1-SPIR SE; see above): the enhancing tissues still appear bright (versus dark in the pre-contrast image), whereas the formerly bright fat darkens. The image impression with the contrasts reduced to dark and bright again resembles a STIR/T2-SPIR or a post-contrast T1 subtraction image; but in each of these, different structures or functions are shown bright, with only a small overlap.

The most promising development for lymph node contrast media are ultrasmall, superparamagnetic iron oxide particles (USPIO; <20 nm). They may be applied intravenously and concentrate in normal lymph nodes within 24 h. Due to their superparamagnetism, they induce a strong shortening of the T2 relaxation time and therefore a signal loss in T2-weighted GE sequences: the normal lymph node, bright before application, becomes dark. A lymph node with metastatic infiltration will not take up the particles and therefore remains bright [23–25].

15.2.2 Safety

15.2.2.1 Safety in the magnetic field

The static magnetic fields of MR systems may be up to 4 T, which is about 100,000-fold the natural magnetic field of the Earth (0.02–0.07 mT). Of course, a lot of effects are imaginable in such a magnetic environment. The most important are biophysical effects in the tissue and, on the other hand, dangers from metallic foreign bodies in or outside the body.

Biophysical effects. Multiple biophysical effects have been found in animals, volunteers and patients in static and gradient magnetic fields; however, a listing is not necessary here, because no noxious effects have been observed under normal circumstances. The scientific discussion concerning the upper limit for whole body exposition in static magnetic fields continues. Finally, the high-frequency impulse is a non-ionising radiation (the energy is much too low for ionisation), but it leads to thermal effects, i.e. a temperature increase (as in a microwave oven, but, of course, to a much lesser degree). The energy deposit in biological tissue is "specific absorption rate" (SAR) and is measured in watts per kilogram. For the whole body, the recommended upper SAR limit is 1.5 W/kg; however, under medical supervision, a maximum of 4 W/kg is allowed. All together, the questions of whether there is no negative effect on the organism or whether the body is able to compensate an effect (e.g., thermoregulation) cannot be answered yet.

Dangers from metallic foreign bodies. Any ferromagnetic material in the body – as incorporated by operation, accident or war injury – may become dangerous in a strong magnetic environment. First, such materials might move and cause local tissue damage. An old aneurysm clip on cerebral arteries, for example, might lead to subarachnoid bleeding; metallic foreign bodies in the eye may lead to blindness. Heart valve prostheses with metallic components such as the Starr-Edwards type are a contraindication, too. Second, metallic materials can serve as receivers for the high-frequency impulses and become hot, so local burning is possible. Particularly patients with cardiac pacemakers are at multiple risk: first, the pacemakers have got a magnetic on/off switch which causes a function stop in a strong magnetic field (the recommended upper limit for cardiac pacemakers is 0.5 mT). The pacemaker electrode is an ideal receiving aerial for the high-frequency impulse, causing rhythm disturbances; and there is the risk of local burning. Similar risks are relevant for neurostimulators, cochlea implants and implanted infusion pumps.

With increasing power of the static magnetic field, any isolated ferromagnetic material near to the tomograph becomes a projectile and a danger to every person (including the staff!) on its way to the gantry. Additionally, even small ferromagnetic masses in the gantry, such as coins or paperclips, or in the body cause massive image artefacts which may make a diagnosis impossible. The patient therefore has got to remove all potentially ferromagnetic materials (don't forget the brassiere clips!). Joint prostheses and amalgam fillings usually are not ferromagnetic, i.e. do not yield serious problems besides the artefacts.

No danger but financial damage is likely when the MR room is entered by a person wearing a watch (which will stop) or carrying a credit card (data will be erased).

15.2.2.2
Safety of contrast media

Gd-DTPA was used in more than ten million cases world-wide until 1994. Besides local sensations, systemic side-effects were observed in about 1% of patients. The quality of the side-effects are comparable with those of iodinated, non-ionic X-ray contrast media, but the incidence is two- to threefold lower. The frequency of allergic reactions is about eightfold lower than that of non-ionic X-ray contrast media. Anaphylactic shock is extremely rare, and there have been very few deaths attributable to Gd-DTPA.

The substance shows no or only minimal biochemical effect on organisms; there is no measurable metabolisation, dissociation or retention of the complex in the body. It undergoes renal excretion in unchanged form, with a half-life of 90 min, under normal renal function.

15.2.2.3
Contraindications

Contraindications result predominantly from the abovementioned risks. These and other contraindications include:

- Cardiac pacemakers
- Heart valve prostheses with metallic components, e.g. Starr-Edwards type
- Neurostimulators
- Cochlea implants
- Implanted infusion pumps
- Metallic foreign bodies, particularly in the eyes
- Older ferromagnetic aneurysm clips
- Operation with clip incorporation within the last 6 weeks
- Intubated patients
- Pregnancy in the first 3 months
- Allergic reaction to contrast media
- (Untreatable claustrophobia; rare, since most patients tolerate the examination after sufficient amounts of diazepam)

Modern joint prostheses and amalgam fillings are not contraindicated (see above). To be sure about possible risks and contraindications in connection with metallic materials, the reader is referred to the book *Pocket guide to MR procedures and metallic objects* [26].

Before starting the MR examination, the patient must be fully informed and sign written consent.

15.2.3 Protocol Recommendations for Thyroid Cancer Follow-up

15.2.3.1 Hardware

The stronger the static magnetic field, the better is the signal-to-noise ratio (e.g. 1.5 T is superior to 0.5 T), but, at the same time, artefacts (such as chemical shift in frequency-coded or ghosting in phase-coded direction) become more pronounced, too. Powerful gradient fields enable shorter acquisition times but increase the electric field changes (see above). For high-resolution images of small superficial organs, surface coils are mandatory. Usually, a head-neck coil is sufficient for covering the required anatomical regions; alternatively, a surface ring coil may be applied to the patient's ventral body surface. Wrap-around coils are applied to the patient's neck but do not cover the lower parts of the mediastinum under investigation. Sometimes, no surface coil is suitable, e.g. in very obese patients; then – in systems with at least 1.0 T – the body coil still will render images of high quality but with diminished resolution.

15.2.3.2 Sequences

A MR protocol for thyroid cancer follow-up should include the following sequences:

- T1 SE before and after Gd-DTPA: high anatomical resolution and differentiation of vital pathological tissue versus scars. Optionally with image subtraction
- T2 TSE: high anatomical resolution in a different view from T1. Few artefacts
- Fat suppression: STIR or SPIR-T2 TSE before Gd-DTPA, SPIR-T1 SE after Gd-DTPA: quick search for possible pathological findings with high sensitivity

The slice thickness should be about 5 mm, with a slice gap of 10%.

15.2.3.3
Planes

The most important plane is the axial (transversal) plane, because the complex neck anatomy, with all the muscles, vessels and fascias, is best resolved in this plane; furthermore, the axial plane is comparable with X-ray CT; and last but not least, many surgeons are most familiar with the axial plane due to their longer experience with CT imaging.

However, a second plane should always be included, rendering more insights into the three-dimensional extension and further anatomical relationships of a pathological formation. Moreover, flow artefacts in vessels with slow blood flow are unmasked in another plane. For the paired anatomy of all neck tissues, particularly the thyroid, great vessels, lymph node lanes and salivary glands, the coronal plane is most suitable. Exceptionally, sagittal planes may be useful for an individual pathoanatomical situation. A preoperative MRI for a pathological mass always requires all three planes at least for the post-contrast T1 images.

15.2.3.4
Covered anatomical regions

Anatomical regions to be covered include the neck, the thoracic inlet and the anterior upper mediastinum. The neck is defined as the area between two planes: the cephalad plane, spanned between mandible, mastoid bone and spinous process of the occipital bone; and the caudad plane, connecting the jugular notch and the spinous process of the seventh cervical vertebra. The thoracic inlet represents the connection to the anterior upper mediastinum, which reaches down to the aortic arch. The ideal protocol covers a craniocaudad extension, including the parotid glands down to the aortic arch, all with thin slices; but this is not always possible with a technically limited slice number, depending on the patient's body length. In most instances, the solution of the problem is either to sacrifice some less interesting region or to make the slices thicker. As "ultima ratio", when the anatomical volume of interest exceeds the sequence possibilities by far, sequences must be repeated in another table position – but this doubles the examination time.

15.2.3.5
Our protocol

Our protocol is run on a 1.5-T system with strong gradients. We prefer the head-neck coil whenever suitable; otherwise we use a surface ring coil (or, rarely, the body coil). An automatic injector serves for remote-controlled contrast-medium injection. The protocol includes a defined succession of sequences, all with a slice thickness of 5 mm:

1. STIR axial. This fat suppression sequence is the first sequence in our protocol, because it serves as an initial quick-finder of high sensitivity for patho-

logical changes (see Chap 2.1.3, Fat Saturation). Drawbacks are false-positive findings and difficult differentiation of the complex neck anatomy.
2. T2 TSE axial. This shows exact anatomical relationships in a differentiated greyscale image and helps to identify false-positives in the STIR sequence.
3. T1 SE axial before and after Gd-DTPA. The native T1 SE sequence again shows true anatomical relationships, but with contrasts different from T2, and thus helps to further identify the "what's what" of the complex neck anatomy in the preceding sequences. Vitality of suspect lesions and lymph nodes is checked by contrast enhancement after application of Gd-DTPA.
4. T1-SPIR SE coronal. Enhancing lymph nodes, masked by surrounding fat in the preceding sequence, become clearly unmasked now. The coronal represents the mandatory second plane and nicely shows enhancing lymph node chains in the deep cervical segment.
5. T1 SE coronal (facultatively). If, after the first two sequences, doubt still exists about slow-flow artefacts in vessels versus true pathological changes, this sequence should be inserted after the second: slow-flow artefacts usually disappear in another plane, becoming real flow void now. An anatomical overview of the symmetric long neck structures such as muscles and vessels is shown.

In summary, this sequence succession helps to subdue the complexity of the neck anatomy by rendering prominent pathological changes in the first step. The following steps eliminate false-positives and clarify doubtful findings, until (in an ideal case) only the "truths" remain for making a correct diagnosis.

15.3 Normal MR Anatomy of the Neck, Thyroid, and Upper Mediastinum

In this section, the text focuses on the pertinent anatomical structures; it does not replace a general anatomy book, nor a dedicated MR anatomy book – there are detailed publications, to which the reader is referred (e.g. [27–30]).

15.3.1 Normal Anatomy

15.3.1.1 Neck compartments

The neck is divided into multiple compartments by fascial planes. For the interpretation of transverse images it has proved useful to define three anatomical compartments: visceral, lateral, and posterior.

Visceral compartment. This is the most anterior compartment and contains the thyroid and parathyroid glands as well as structures of the aerodigestive tract, including larynx, trachea and oesophagus (Fig. 15.1). The cranial part of the oesophagus lies in the midline dorsal to the trachea; the descending oesophagus

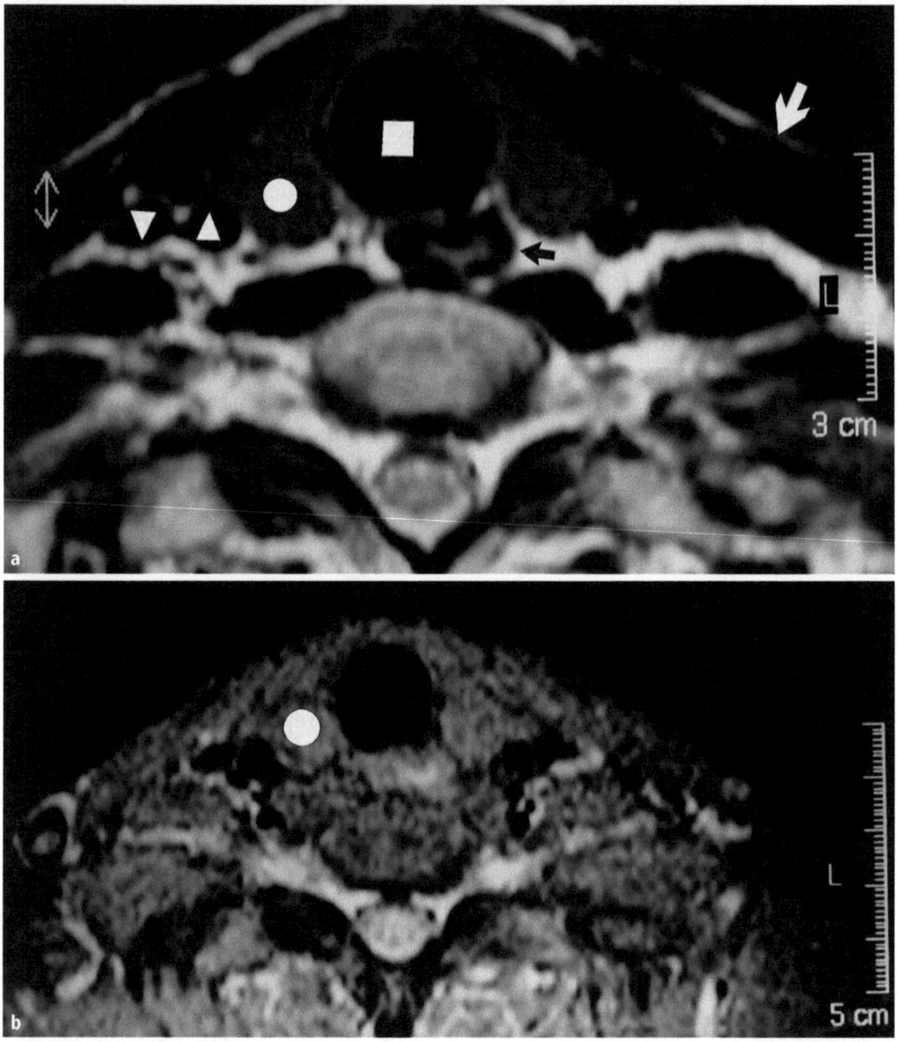

Fig. 15.1a-c Normal anatomy of the neck and mediastinum. **a** A transversal T2 TSE image of the neck at the level of the thyroid isthmus (i.e. thoracic vertebra 1). **b** The corresponding STIR image at the same level. The pertinent anatomical structures are marked. *Circle*, thyroid; *square*, trachea; *filled arrow*, oesophagus; note outer dark muscles and inner bright mucosa. In this slice, the oesophagus is half-way from the midline behind the trachea to the left dorsal paratracheal space; *triangle*, carotid artery, *inverted triangle*, internal jugular vein; *white arrow*, sternocleidomastoid muscle. **c** Transversal T2 TSE image of the upper mediastinum. *Filled arrow*, oesophagus; *triangle*, carotid artery; *circle*, subclavian artery; *inverted triangle*, internal jugular vein; *curved arrow*, lymph node

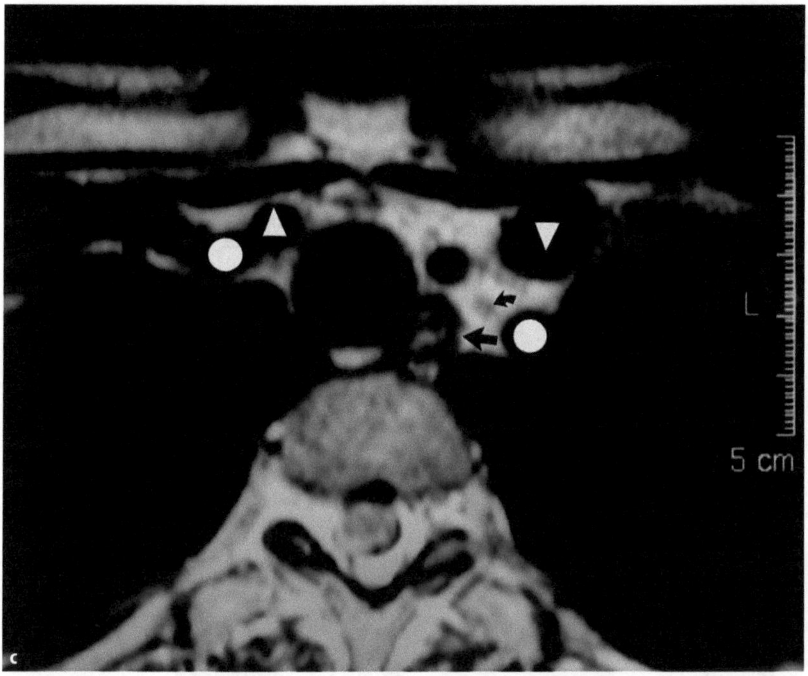

Fig. 15.1c

turns to the left dorsal paratracheal space (Fig. 15.1a, c). The normal laryngeal cartilage appears bright in all sequences used here. The lateral and posterior boundaries of the visceral compartment are formed by the sternocleidomastoid and pharyngeal constrictor muscles.

Lateral compartments. Also called vessel-nerve compartments, they contain the carotid sheaths, with carotid arteries and jugular veins. In the cranial part, the carotid artery (CA) is situated anterior to the internal jugular vein (IJV; Fig. 15.2). In the middle part, the CA lies medially to the IJV (Fig. 15.1a), and in the caudal part, the vessels come apart so that there remains some space between them until the subclavian artery appears at that depth (Fig. 15.1c).

Posterior compartment. This includes cervical vertebrae, posterior extensor muscles and anterior flexor muscles, including the scalene, longus capitis and longus colli muscles (Fig. 15.1a).

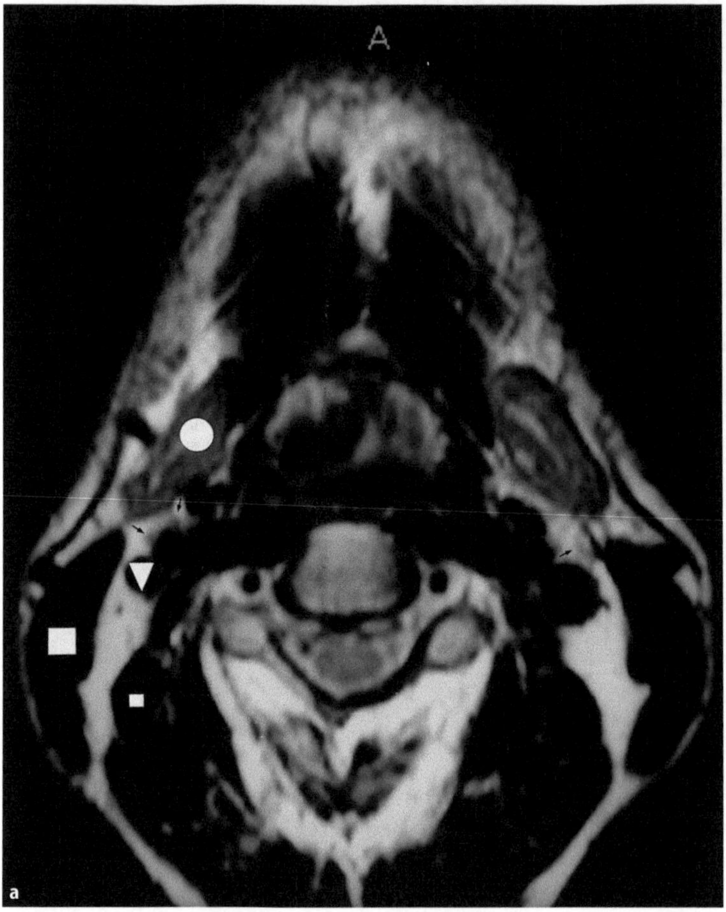

Fig. 15.2a, b Normal anatomy of the cranial neck region at the floor of mouth level. **a** Transversal T2 TSE image; **b** corresponding STIR image. *Circle*, submandibular gland; *triangle*, internal jugular vein; *large square*, sternocleidomastoid muscle; *small square*, levator scapulae muscle. Note small prejugular lymph nodes dorsal to the submandibular glands on both sides in **b** (*arrowheads*): easy to find in the STIR, more difficult in the T2 TSE image (*small arrows*)

15.3.1.2
Thyroid and parathyroid glands

The thyroid in adults extends approximately over 5 cm in craniocaudal distance as a symmetric, homogenous, wedge-shaped structure on either side of the trachea. The average normal volume is up to 18 ml in women and 25 ml in men. The thyroid isthmus usually crosses anterior to the second and third tracheal rings. The normal thyroid can be distinguished from the sternothyroid and sternocleidomastoid muscles by its greater signal intensity in T2-weighted

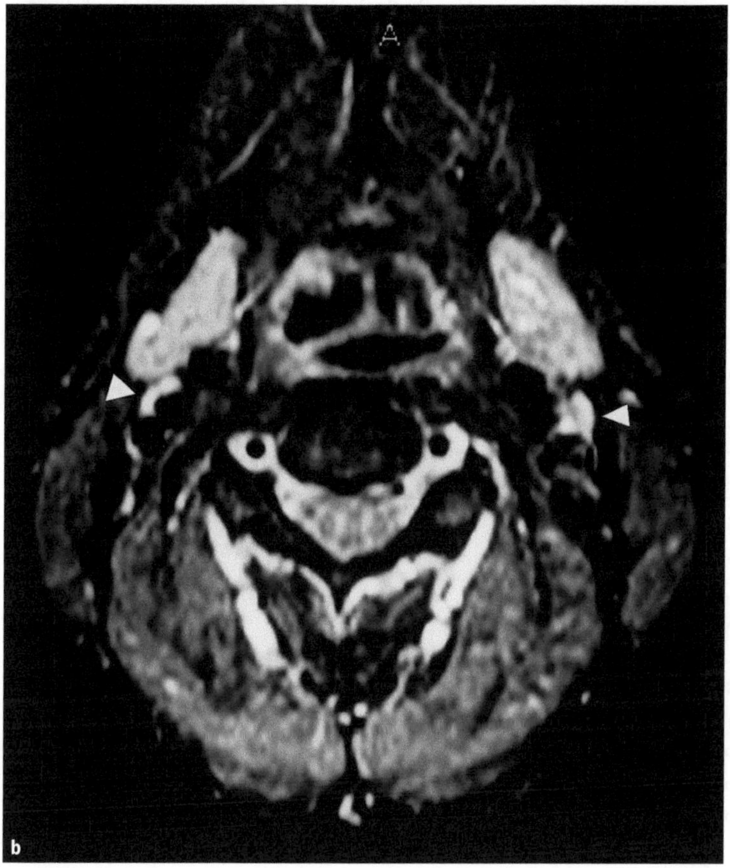

Fig. 15.2b

images (Fig. 15.1a). In T1-weighted images, the gland is isointense to slightly hyperintense to the surrounding muscles; in the STIR, it is isointense (Fig. 15.1b). The normal parathyroid glands are situated dorsally to but not distinguishable from the thyroid.

15.3.1.3 Salivary glands

The major salivary glands of the head are three large, paired glandular structures: the parotid, submandibular and sublingual glands. They consist mainly of mucous- and serous-secreting cells with variable numbers of fat cells. Consequently, the salivary glands are somewhat hyperintense to the thyroid, both

Table 15.3 Lymph node stations of primary lymphatic drainage of the thyroid gland

Lnn cervicales anteriores	Lnn. cervicales laterales profundae
Lnn cervicales ant. superficiales	Lnn. jugulares ant. et lat. craniales
Lnn cervicales anteriores	Lnn. cervicales laterales profundae
Lnn suprasternales	Lnn. jugulares ant. et lat. caudales
Lnn infrahyoidales	Lnn. supraclaviculares
Lnn praelaryngeales	Lnn. jugulodigastricus
Lnn praetracheales	Lnn. juguloomohyoidei
Lnn paratracheales	Lnn. retropharyngeales
Lnn thyroidei	–

Lnn, lymphonoduli

Table 15.4 Neck lymph node levels according to the guidelines of the New American Joint Committee on Cancer (AJCC)

Level	Lymph nodes
I	Submental
	Submandibular
II	Upper deep neck
III	Middle deep neck
IV	Lower deep neck
V	Spinal accessorial
	Transverse neck (supraclavicular)
VI	Pretracheal
	Prelaryngeal
	Paratracheal
VII	Upper mediastinal

in the T1 and T2 image, but pronounced in the STIR image (Fig. 15.2). This becomes important when changes occur after radioiodine therapy.

15.3.1.4
Lymphatic drainage

The head-neck region has many lymph nodes which usually are smaller than in other body regions. The normal lymph node shows a diameter of <10 mm [31, 32], maximal <15 mm [33], and a long oval or spindle form. Submandibular or mandibular angle lymph nodes may be somewhat bigger. Sometimes, and if the normal lymph node is big enough, it shows a fatty central sinus (best seen as a hyperintense centre in the T1-weighted image). Otherwise, lymph nodes appear dark (isointense to muscle) in T1 images, middle-greyscale in T2 images and bright in STIR images. Compared with other bright structures in the STIR, the sequence is (in declining brightness): small, slow-flow veins > lymph nodes > salivary glands > thyroid (Fig. 15.2b). Lymph nodes show strong contrast enhancement. The lymphatic drainage of the thyroid gland, which possesses a highly differentiated lymphatic capillary system, flows into two groups of regional lymph node stations: the anterior and profound lateral cervical lymph nodes. The detailed thyroidal lymph node stations are listed in Table 15.3. The neck lymph node-level classification according to the guidelines of the new American Joint Committee on Cancer (AJCC) is listed in Table 15.4.

15.3.1.5 Upper anterior mediastinum

Between the thoracic inlet and the level of the aortic arch, predominantly there are great vessels, easily distinguishable by mediastinal fat; sometimes, the lower poles of the thyroid reach here and, rarely, thymic remnants may be encountered. Lymph nodes up to 1 cm are frequent (Fig. 15.1c).

Gd-DTPA-enhanced images only show an enhancement of structures rich in vascularity, such as the thyroid, salivary glands, lymphoid tissue, mucosa and the lining of the pharynx. Vessels, fascial planes and muscles typically do not show significant enhancement except slow-flow veins.

15.3.2 Inconspicuous Anatomy After Thyroidectomy

Four to eight weeks after thyroidectomy, postoperative changes such as oedema or haematoma should have disappeared. Small thyroid remnants may be found, but the remaining neck anatomy is unchanged. After successful radioiodine therapy, the thyroid is either no longer visible or the remnants become fibrous. After 12–18 months, developing scars exhibit significant signal loss, i.e. become dark in all sequences used here and no longer show contrast enhancement. Small lymph nodes following the abovementioned normality criteria are a frequent finding. Figure 15.3 shows a normal unsuspected situation after total thyroidectomy followed by two radioiodine therapies.

15.4 Pathological Changes

Compared with normal thyroid tissue, nearly all thyroid abnormalities tend to have prolonged T1 and T2 relaxation times with a large interindividual variability. This is due to mixed composition of colloid, fibrosis, necrosis and haemorrhage. Hyperintense lesions in T1-weighted images usually result from haemorrhage or colloid cyst; in T2-weighted images, almost all pathological changes demonstrate homogeneous or heterogeneous increased intensity [11, 12, 15]. Unfortunately, there are significant similarities and overlaps between

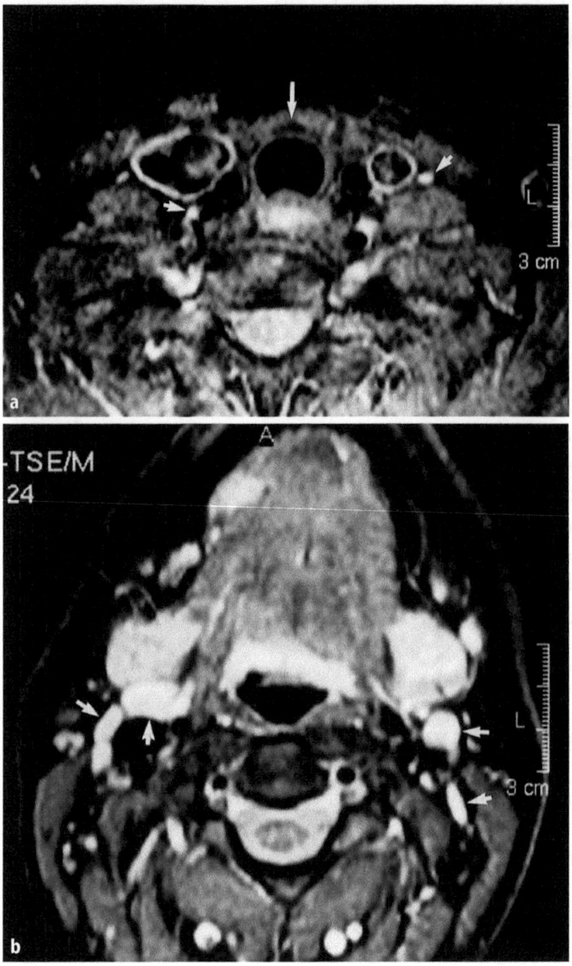

Fig. 15.3a, b Normal unsuspected MR anatomy after total thyroidectomy followed by two radioiodine therapies (transversal STIR). **a** In the thyroid bed, recurrent thyroid cancer or remnants can be ruled out, because there is no hyperintense tissue around the trachea. In the midline ventrally to the trachea, some small scars may be present (small hypointense lesion, *arrow*). Normal bright appearance of the oesophageal mucosa, the outer diameter of the internal jugular veins (flow phenomenon), and some very small perivascular lymph nodes (*short arrows*). **b** At the mandibular level, somewhat larger lymph nodes are encountered that are not considered malignant. All findings were confirmed in the T1 and T2 TSE studies

the MR appearance in various pathological thyroid conditions including cancer. Clinicians are unable to distinguish benign from malignant lesions by T1 and T2 relaxation times, diffusion values or various recent attempts of dynamic contrast studies [34–36]. There are promising preliminary reports on the use of MR spectroscopy for this purpose [37, 38], but unfortunately the ability of MR spectroscopy to truly predict benign follicular lesions has not yet been confirmed by long-term follow-up [36]. However, scars may be clearly distinguished from recurrent thyroid cancer in T2-weighted images, since fibrous tissue is hypointense to muscle [39].

Hyperintense lesions in T2-weighted images appear much more pronounced in STIR images (see Chap 2.1.3). Usual thyroid protocols in the current MRI literature include standard T2- and T1-weighted sequences with or without intravenous contrast studies [34–36, 39–48]. There is only one recent study in

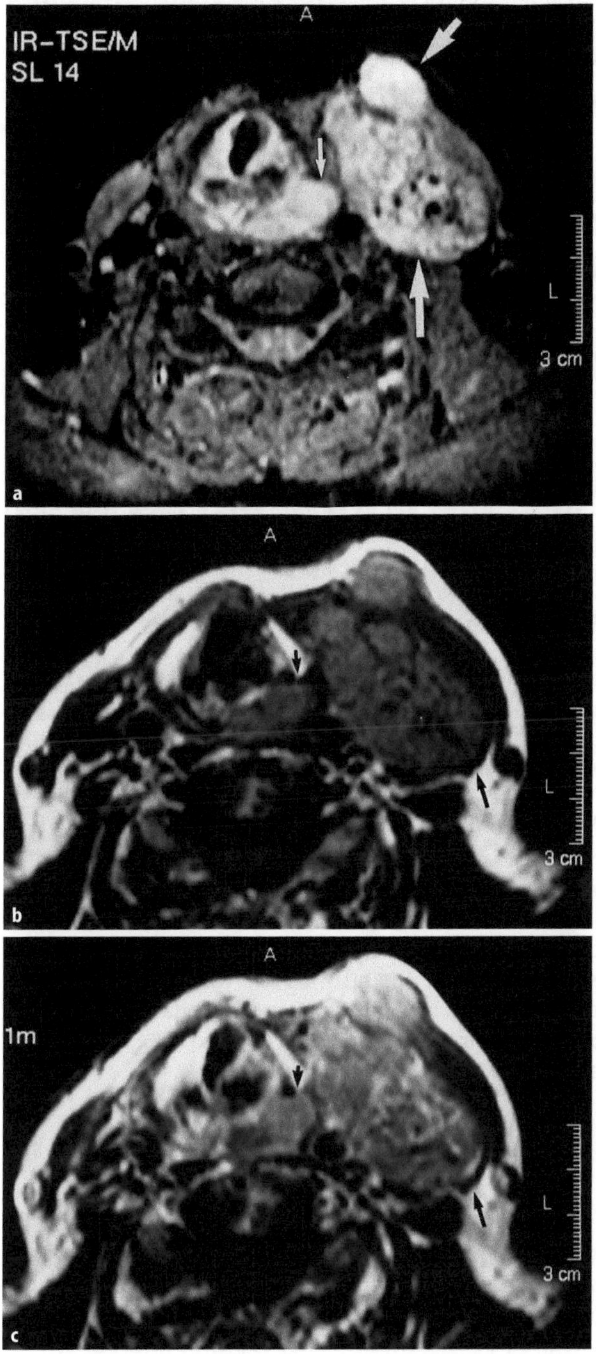

Fig. 15.4a–c Primary left-sided follicular thyroid cancer with secondary dedifferentiation and a cranio-caudad extension of 10 cm. **a** STIR; **b** T1-weighted image; **c** T1-weighted post-Gd image: Inhomogeneous hyperintense mass with complex extensions to the ventral muscles and paralaryngeal space (*arrows*). The tumour tissue reaches the carotid artery with suspected invasion, the internal jugular vein is no longer distinguishable

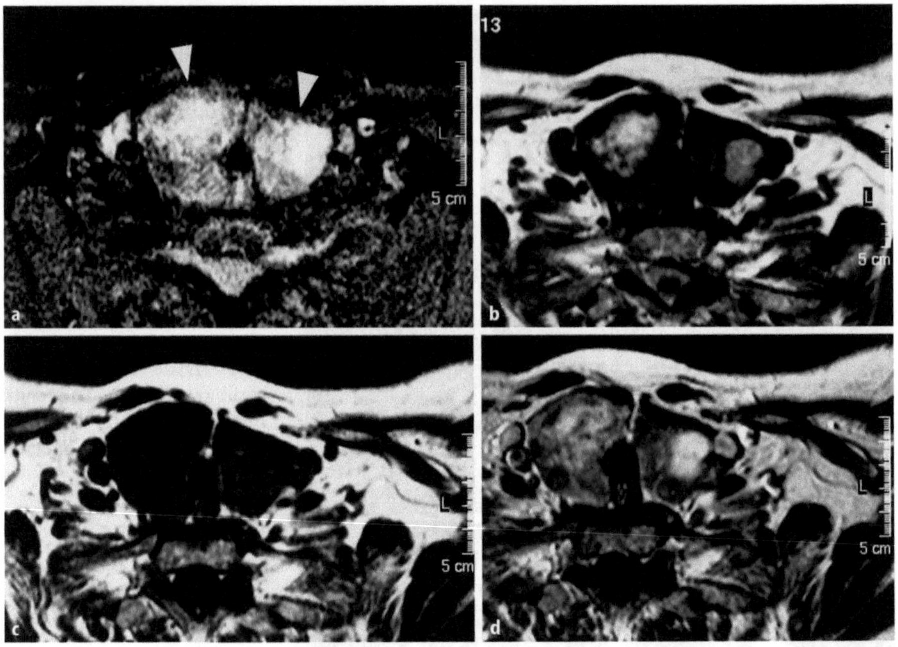

Fig. 15.5a–d Multinodular intrathoracic goitre reaching down to the roof of the aortic arch (thyroid volume approximately 100 ml). The study was performed with the body coil, because the obese patient did not tolerate surface coils. **a** STIR: Inhomogeneous hyperintense enlargement of both thyroid lobes. **b** T2 TSE-weighted image: Multiple nodules of variable hyperintensity. Note: no flow phenomenon, compared with the STIR. **c** T1-weighted native image: Compared with the muscles, slightly hyperintense thyroid with discrete inhomogeneities, but no nodule distinguishable. **d** T1-weighted post-Gd image: multiple nodules with differing enhancement patterns become apparent

which the authors report on the use of a STIR sequence [49]. We have always used an initial fat-suppression sequence (usually STIR) which (a) shows all possible pertinent pathological changes at first sight and (b) enables detection even of very small findings. For this reason, most of the following figures are introduced by STIR images.

15.4.1 Primary Thyroid Cancer

The role of MRI in primary cancer is the morphological assessment of tissue mass extent as well as involvement of surrounding anatomical structures such as vessels or muscles [15, 20, 36, 39, 50–52]. Tumour invasion of adjacent tissue can be ruled out by demonstration of an intermediate, continuous fat line, best seen in native T1-weighted images. However, a fat line is not always present, and it may be difficult to differentiate tumour invasion from adjacent tissue.

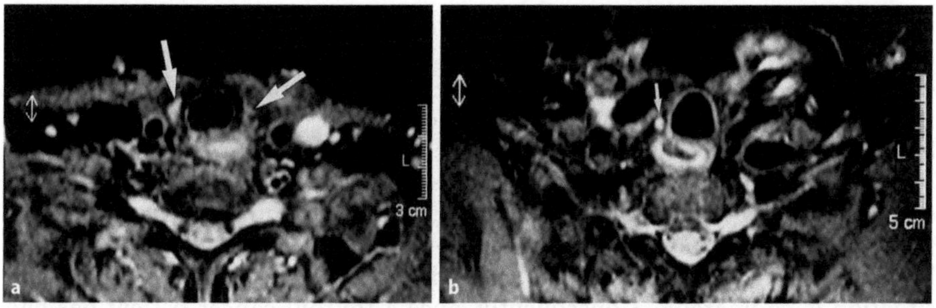

Fig. 15.6a, b Thyroid remnants, transversal STIR images. **a** Typical appearance of thyroid remnants. This patient had had total thyroidectomy and twofold RIT for papillary thyroid cancer with the last therapeutic radioiodine scan negative. Follow-up sonography 4 months later showed equivocal tissue in the right thyroid bed. MRI proved thyroid remnants not only on the right but also on the left side (*arrows*). Note flow phenomenon (high signal) in the left internal jugular vein. **b** Demonstration of the MRI capabilities in delineating even minimal lesions: residual thyroid tissue of about 3 mm right to the trachea (*arrow*). Such small findings are hardly identified by sonography, particularly in this anatomical region (thoracic inlet). Without this STIR image, the lesion would have been much more difficult to identify on T1- and T2-weighted images

Tumour invasion of muscles is best shown as hyperintensity in STIR and in Gd-DTPA-enhanced T1-weighted sequences; normal muscle adjacent to a tumour probably excludes muscle invasion.

An example of primary follicular thyroid cancer is shown in Fig. 15.4. For differential diagnosis, Fig. 15.5 shows a case of benign multinodular goitre: note the intralesional similarities in signal behaviour.

15.4.2 Thyroid Remnants

After thyroidectomy for differentiated thyroid cancer, radioiodine therapy (RIT) usually is performed until no more pathological uptake can be shown. If after multiple RIT cycles there is still some uptake remaining in the thyroid bed, it becomes important to know how much thyroid tissue mass has been persistent and whether a second surgical exploration may become necessary. Thyroid remnants sometimes are difficult to demonstrate by sonography, particularly in obese patients or in the upper mediastinum. In the current MRI literature, thyroid remnants and their appearance are virtually unrecognised; in our experience, they are frequently observed in MRI after one or two RIT cycles and then show up as hyperintense tissue in STIR or T2 TSE-weighted images (Fig. 15.6). In post-Gd T1-weighted sequences, remnants usually show contrast enhancement. This is probably due to inflammatory and oedematous changes, usually following surgery and radiation.

Thyroid remnants become fibrous after successful RIT. Fibrous tissue has a relatively short T2 relaxation time and consequently low intensity on T2-

weighted images [15, 39]. This makes a scar distinguishable from a vital remnant, particularly in STIR sequences. Additionally, scar tissue (stable fibrosis) does not enhance after Gd-DTPA. However, the time frame until a vital tissue finally becomes a scar is uncertain: as known from other body areas (e.g. the breast), healing scars or granulation tissues enhance to a variable degree. Postoperatively, fresh scars enhance for the first 3–6 months; only when more than 6 months have elapsed after surgery do they no longer enhance. After radiation therapy, this time interval can reach 12–18 months [53]. These time courses have not been investigated for the thyroid region yet but, in our opinion, the situation is comparable. Consequently, once a thyroid cancer patient has had surgery and finished RIT, we believe that it may take more than a year until thyroid remnants finally become scars.

15.4.3 Recurrent Thyroid Cancer

There is agreement that MRI is a useful tool for the detection of recurrent thyroid cancer and sometimes superior to other follow-up studies such as scintigraphy with ^{131}I or ^{201}Tl, or sonography [39–42], particularly if serum thyroglobulin (Tg) is negative. The most important differential diagnosis to recurrent cancer is scar. As discussed before, scars are hypointense (dark) in T2-weighted or STIR images, whereas recurrent thyroid carcinoma produces high intensity [15, 39] and enhances after Gd-DTPA. Differential diagnostic difficulties occur when a cancer recurs early, i.e. in the time interval during which remnants become scar-like: both the remnant and the recurring cancer are (a) hyperintense in the T2-weighted or STIR images and (b) enhance after Gd-DTPA. This problem may be overcome by comparison with previous MR examinations: a new lesion in the thyroid bed region which occurs additionally to well-known thyroid remnants, and which seems not to be a typical unsuspicious lymph node is highly suspicious of recurrent cancer (Figs. 15.7 and 15.8).

15.4.4 Pathological Lymph Nodes

Malignant lymph nodes represent a form of metastatic spread or relapse. The MRI appearance of normal lymph nodes in the head-and-neck region has been described in Chap 3.1.4. By definition, criteria of malignant lymph node involvement include [54]:

- A diameter of more than 10 mm
- More than three grouped nodes
- Central necrosis
- Infiltrative growth
- Fixation on surrounding structures

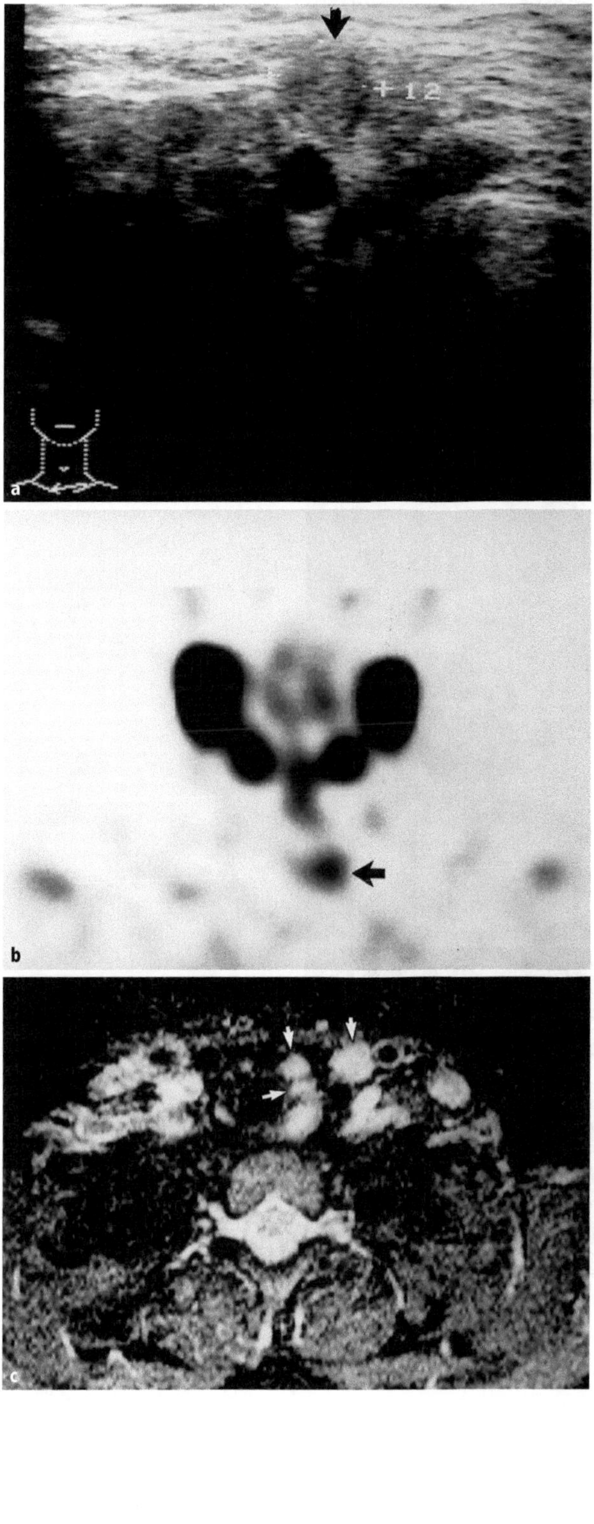

Fig. 15.7a–f Follow-up of a papillary thyroid cancer patient with the last RIT 1 year ago. The RI scan was negative, but sonography showed a hypoechoic lesion with a diameter of 12 mm near to the left carotid artery (**a**). A ^{99m}Tc-sestamibi scan was positive (**b**; coronal SPECT). The MRI demonstrated three lesions between the trachea and the left carotid artery (*arrows*) and some additional small lesions in the right paratracheal space (**c**, STIR; **d**, T2 TSE-weighted sequence; **e**, T1-weighted sequence). The greater lesions on the left side showed significant post-Gd contrast enhancement (**f**)

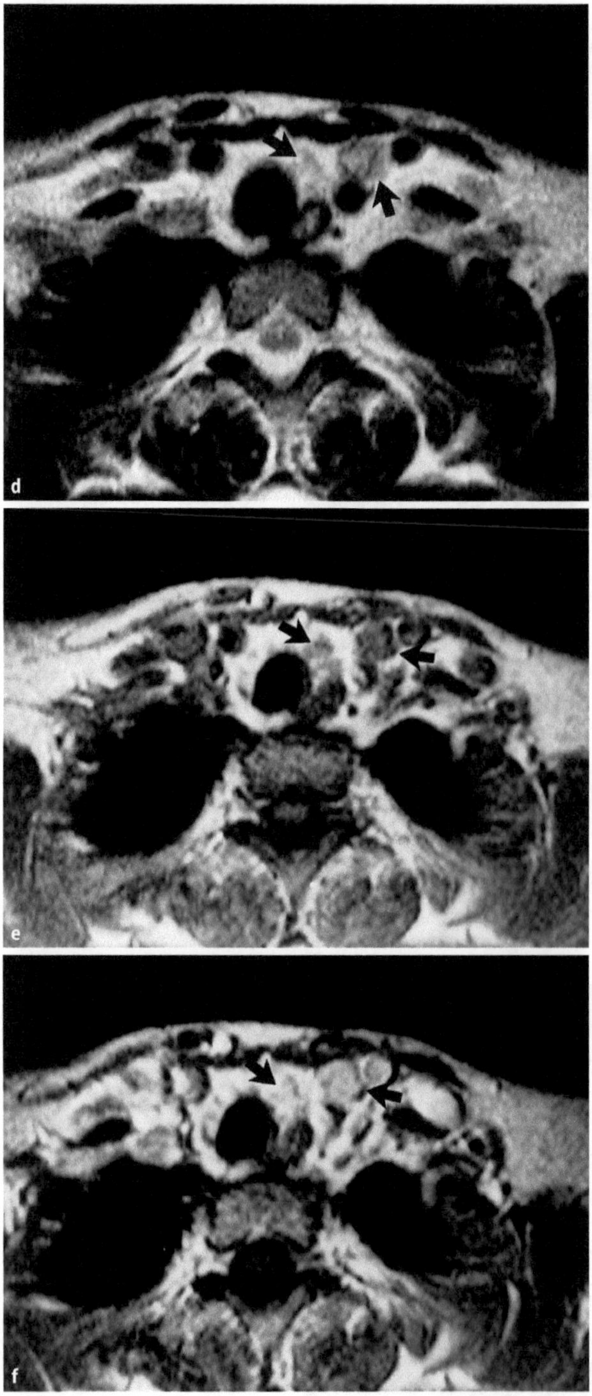

Fig. 15.7a–f

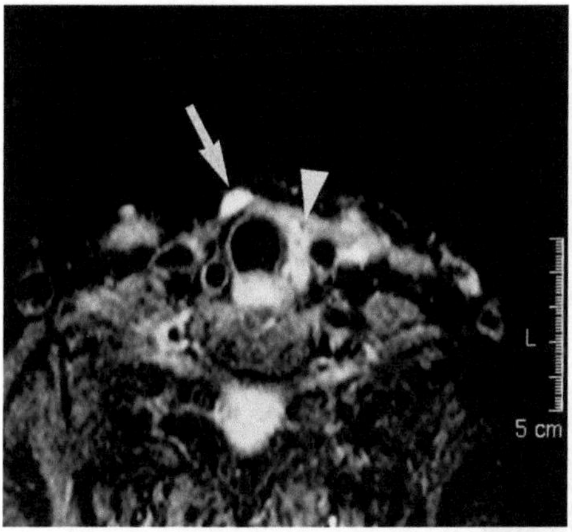

Fig. 15.8 Follow-up of a differentiated thyroid cancer with clear, unsuspicious thyroid remnants. Two years after a sella metastasis was treated by external beam radiation, a palpable mass occurred in the pretracheal region, which was also shown by sonography. In contrast, ^{99m}Tc-sestamibi showed two lesions. MRI demonstrated one larger lesion in the pretracheal midline corresponding to the sonographic finding (not shown) and a smaller one caudally. The STIR image shows the smaller finding (*arrow*) at the same level of some contralateral thyroid remnant (*arrowhead*)

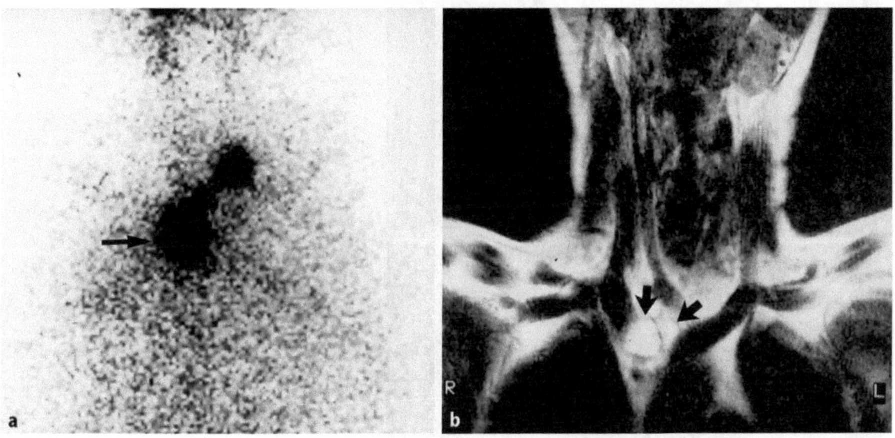

Fig. 15.9a, b Persistent lymph node metastases despite fivefold high-dose RIT following total thyroidectomy for papillary cancer. MRI prior to a second operation for lymph node dissection. **a** Posttherapeutic ventral planar RI scan with three metastases in the lower neck and upper mediastinum. **b** Coronal T2 TSE showing the most caudal finding to be two confluent lymph nodes in the upper mediastinum. All RI scan findings were clearly shown by MRI, successfully removed and proven to be lymph node metastases histopathologically

Two criteria should be added for MRI: (1) not only central necrosis is predictive of a metastasis, but also complete cystic appearance or general inhomogeneity of the lymph node are highly suspicious (Fig. 15.9); (2) a high signal intensity in T1- and T2-weighted images is a sign of either haemorrhage and/or other protein content, here, thyroglobulin, and therefore suspicious [55, 56].

The diameter criterion is unsafe and needs to be discussed. First, there is significant overlap between unspecific and metastatic lymph nodes (Fig. 15.10). One recent study showed that nodes down to 2 mm in transverse diameter were

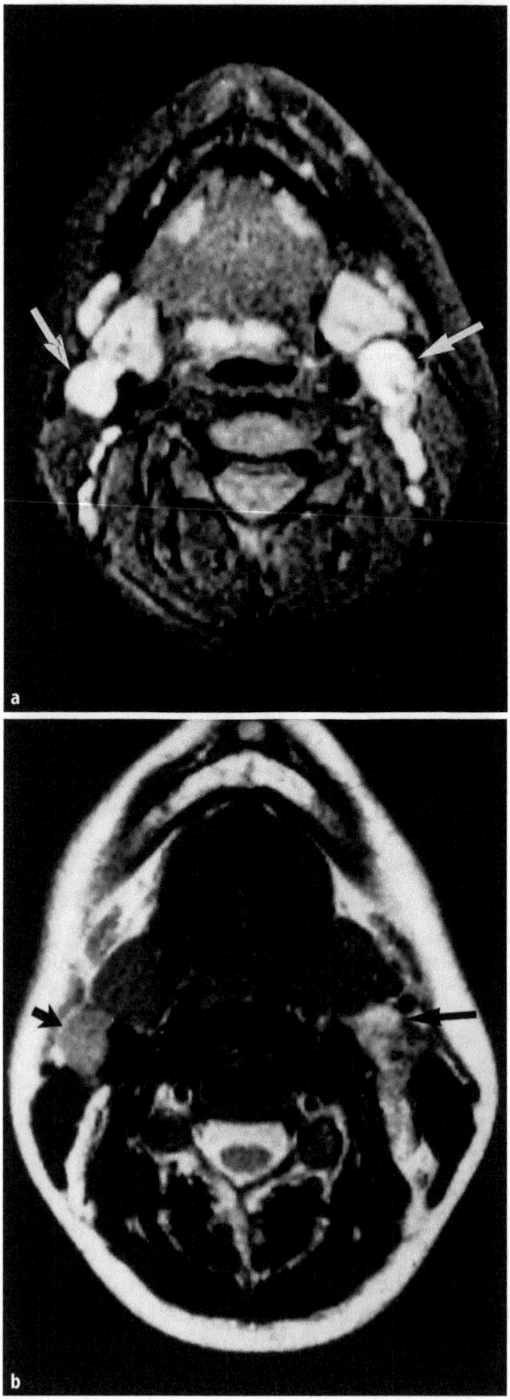

Fig. 15.10a, b **a** STIR, **b** T2 TSE-weighted image. Submandibular lymph nodes of 11 mm (*right*) and 12 mm (*left, arrows*): Both diameters exceed 10 mm. In this case, the left lesion is inhomogeneous hyperintense compared with the right; only the left one was RI-positive and histopathologically malignant

metastatic [56], i.e. even lymph nodes smaller than 5 mm might be considered malignant [56, 57]. Second, lymph nodes may be enlarged due to unspecific, benign inflammatory reaction [33, 43, 49, 58], which is a frequent finding in this anatomical region. Independent of the cause of enlargement, lymph nodes often show similar signal patterns in T1- (isointense to muscle, i.e. hypointense), T2-, proton density-weighted or STIR sequences (hyperintense). Numerous proposals have been made to define maximal diameters for non-malignant changes, either in the transversal or longitudinal plane, and dependent on the specific anatomical site [31–33, 57, 59, 60]; but no real consensus could be found. To increase the accuracy in distinguishing malign from reactive lymph nodes by metric measures, the so-called m/t ratio was transferred from sonography to MRI, i.e. the maximal divided by the corresponding perpendicular transversal diameter [33]. Normal ratio values are 3–5; less than 2 is suggestive of malignancy. Although there remains some overlap, this seems to be the most reliable metric parameter yet.

Following the administration of Gd-DTPA, all enlarged lymph nodes show contrast enhancement. The only reliable (enhancement) sign of a lymph node metastasis is the observation of a central necrosis (hypointensity) with marginal hyperintensity. However, only 50–60% of cervical lymph node metastases demonstrate this enhancement pattern, dependent on their size (mostly >15 mm; for review see [33]). In conclusion, lymph node differentiation remains a problem [61, 62].

In our experience, more than three grouped nodes are not always conclusive of malignancy: there is again some overlap with unspecific reactive hyperplasia. Moreover, lymph node chains are a frequent finding in normal follow-up MR examinations, particularly when they are small (<10 mm).

15.4.5 Distant Metastases

Distant metastases of differentiated thyroid cancer may occur in almost any body region, predominantly the lungs and bones, and can be demonstrated by adequate MRI examination. Data from many metastatic sites are not appropriate for this book, but two examples are shown in Fig. 15.11.

15.4.6 Accidental Pathological Findings

Since MRI demonstrates the complete anatomy of the examined body region, accidental findings are encountered frequently. These may be divided into thyroid cancer-related changes and completely independent lesions. Disease-related findings include postoperative sequelae such as haematoma or recurrent nerve palsies (Fig. 15.12a), and post-RIT sequelae such as salivary gland atrophy (post-RIT fibrosis, sicca syndrome; Fig. 15.12b). Other lesions comprise harmless findings such as pharyngo- or laryngoceles (Fig. 15.13), although a frequent

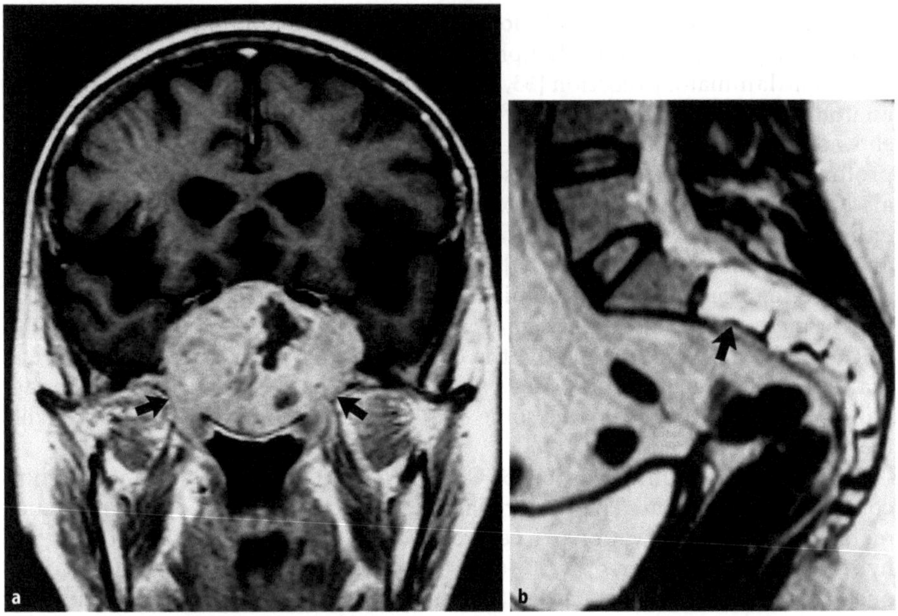

Fig. 15.11a, b **a** Metastasis to the sella region (coronal T1-weighted post-Gd image). RI scan was negative, whereas ^{99m}Tc-sestamibi and ^{18}FDG-PET were positive. The tumour shows inhomogeneous contrast enhancement, destroys the surrounding osseous structures, infiltrates the cavernous sinuses and the carotid arteries, and the optic chiasm is no longer identifiable. **b** Metastases to the sacral bones (except S1; sagittal T2-TSE). RI scan was positive but skeletal scintigram, ^{99m}Tc-sestamibi and ^{18}FDG-PET were negative

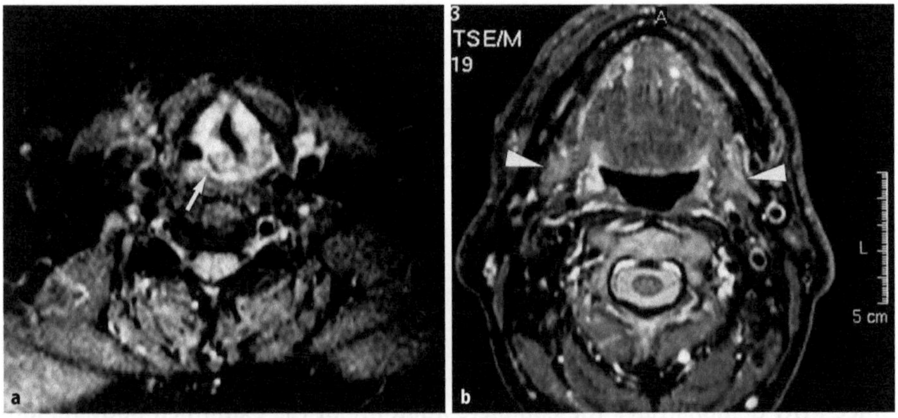

Fig. 15.12a, b **a** The right vocal cords are deformed. This finding is not unusual, if positive only in one or two sequences, due to normal laryngeal motility (breathing, swallowing). A pathological situation may be suspected if the finding is constant in all sequences. In this case, the patient suffered from recurrent nerve palsies due to thyroidectomy (STIR). **b** Repeated RIT with a cumulated applied activity of 1,200 mCi led to progressive sicca symptoms. The STIR shows the submandibular glands much smaller and with less signal than normal (compare with Fig. 15.2)

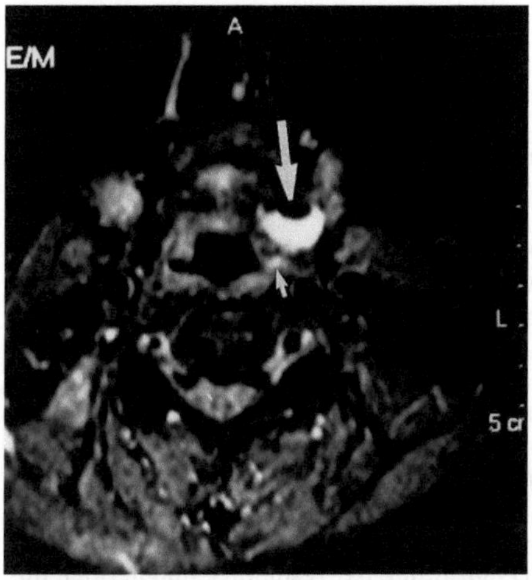

Fig. 15.13 Air- and fluid-filled cavity in the left paralaryngeal space, a typical aspect of a laryngocele (*arrow*; STIR). The connection to the respiratory tract might be a small canaliculus, represented by the hyperintense line (*small arrow*)

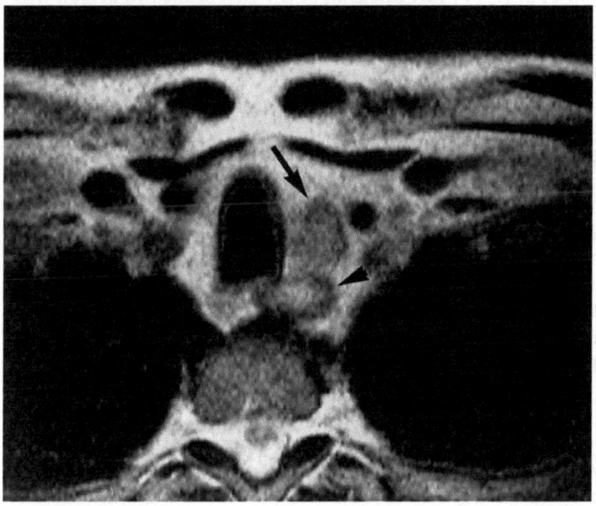

Fig. 15.14 Pathological tissue (*arrow*) in the left paratracheal space after thyroidectomy and two-fold RIT with normal post-therapeutic RI scan and recent negative serum TG. In the T2-TSE sequence, the lesion seems to be distinguishable from the oesophagus (*arrowhead*). ^{99m}Tc-sestamibi was equivocal, but ^{18}FDG-PET was positive. Surgery yielded the diagnosis of oesophageal cancer

coincidence between malignant tumours and tuberculosis is known [54]. Finally, secondary malignancies may be encountered: in one case, we detected an oesophageal cancer in a patient with recently treated papillary thyroid cancer (Fig. 15.14).

References

1. Schara M, Sentjurc M, Auersperg M et al (1974) Characterization of malignant thyroid gland tissue by magnetic resonance methods. Br J Cancer 29:483–486
2. Sinadinovic J, Ratkovic S, Kraincanic M et al (1977) Relationship of biochemical and morphological changes in rat thyroid and proton spin-relaxation of the tissue water. Endokrinologie 69:55–66
3. DeCertaines J, Herry JY, Lancien G et al (1982) Evaluation of human thyroid tumors by proton nuclear magnetic resonance. J Nucl Med 23:48–51
4. Stark DD, Moss AA, Gamsu G et al (1984) Magnetic resonance imaging of the neck. Radiology 150:455–461
5. Stark DD, Clark OH, Moss AA (1984) Magnetic resonance imaging of the thyroid, thymus, and parathyroid glands. Surgery 96:1083–1091
6. Tennvall J, Björklund A, Möller T et al (1984) Studies of NMR-relaxation-times in malignant tumours and normal tissues of the human thyroid gland. Prog Nucl Med 8:142–148
7. Higgins CB, McNamara MT, Fisher MR et al (1986) MR imaging of the thyroid. Am J Roentgenol 147:1255–1261
8. DeCertaines J, Beurton D, Le Jeune JJ et al (1986) Etude par resonance magnetique nucleaire du tissu thyroidien en fonction de son histologie. Ann Endocrinol 47:197–200
9. Mountz JM, Glazer HS, Gan M et al (1987) MR imaging of the thyroid: comparison with scintigraphy in the normal and diseased gland. J Comput Assist Tomogr 11:612–619
10. Sandler MP, Patton JA (1987) Multimodality imaging of the thyroid and parathyroid glands. J Nucl Med 28:122–129
11. Gefter WB, Spritzer CE, Eisenberg B et al (1987) Thyroid imaging with high-field-strength surface coil MR. Radiology 164:483–490
12. Noma S, Nishimura K, Togashi K et al (1987) Thyroid gland: MR imaging. Radiology 164:495–499
13. Tennvall J, Olsson M, Möller T et al (1987) Thyroid tissue characterization by proton magnetic resonance relaxation time determination. Acta Oncol 26:27–32
14. Noma S, Kanaoka M, Minami S et al (1988) Thyroid masses: MR imaging and pathological correlation. Radiology 168:759–764
15. Higgins CB, Auffermann W (1988) MR imaging of thyroid and parathyroid glands: a review of current status. Am J Roentgenol 151:1095–1106
16. James C, Starks M, MacGillivray DC, White J (1999) The use of imaging studies in the diagnosis and management of thyroid cancer and hyperparathyroidism. Surg Oncol Clin North Am 8:145–169
17. Gotway MB, Higgins CB (2000) MR imaging of the thyroid and parathyroid glands. Magn Reson Imaging Clin North Am 8:163–182, ix
18. Weber AL, Randolph G, Aksoy FG (2000) The thyroid and parathyroid glands. CT and MR imaging and correlation with pathology and clinical findings. Radiol Clin North Am 38:1105–1129
19. Tezuka M, Murata Y, Ishida R, Ohashi I, Hirata Y, Shibuya H (2003) MR imaging of the thyroid: correlation between apparent diffusion coefficient and thyroid gland scintigraphy. J Magn Reson Imaging 17:163–169
20. Takashima S, Takayama F, Wang J, Kobayashi S, Kadoya M (2003) Using MR imaging to predict invasion of the recurrent laryngeal nerve by thyroid carcinoma. Am J Roentgenol 180:837–842
21. King AD, Ahuja AT, To EW, Tse GM, Metreweli C (2000) Staging papillary carcinoma of the thyroid: magnetic resonance imaging vs ultrasound of the neck. Clin Radiol 55:222–226
22. Stark DD, Bradley WG (eds) (1999) Magnetic resonance imaging, 3rd edn. Mosby, St Louis

23. Weissleder R, Elizondo G, Wittenberg J et al (1990) Ultrasmall superparamagnetic iron oxide: an intravenous contrast agent for assessing lymph nodes with MR imaging. Radiology 175:494–498
24. Anzai Y, Blackwell KE, Hirschowitz SL et al (1994) Initial clinical experience with dextran-coated superparamagnetic iron oxide for detection of lymph node metastases in patients with head and neck cancer. Radiology 192:709–715
25. Wagner S, Pfefferer D, Ebert W et al (1995) Intravenous MR lymphography with superparamagnetic iron oxide particles: experimental studies in rats and rabbits. Eur Radiol 5:640–646
26. Shellock FG (2003) Reference manual for magnetic resonance safety. Amirsys, Salt Lake City
27. Hansen JT (1990) Surgical anatomy and embryology of the lower neck and superior mediastinum. In: Falk S (ed) Thyroid disease: endocrinology, surgery, nuclear medicine, and radiotherapy. Raven, New York
28. Prescher A, Bohndorf K (1996) Radiologische Anatomie und Topographie des Halses. Thieme, Stuttgart
29. Stone JA, Figueroa RE (2000) Embryology and anatomy of the neck. Neuroimaging Clin North Am 10:55–73
30. Küper K (2001) MR/CT atlas anatomy (Scheringatlas) CD-ROM (Version 5.0). Thieme, Stuttgart
31. Van den Brekel MW, Stel HV, Castelijns JA et al (1990) Cervical lymph node metastasis: assessment of radiologic criteria. Radiology 177:379–384
32. Jabour BA, Lufkin RB, Layfield LJ et al (1990) Magnetic resonance imaging of metastatic cervical adenopathy. Top Magn Reson Imaging 2:69–75
33. Steinkamp HJ, Heim T, Schubeus P et al (1992) The magnetic resonance tomographic differential diagnosis between reactively enlarged lymph nodes and cervical lymph node metastases. Röfo Fortschr Geb Röntgenstr Neuen Bildgeb Verfahr 157:406–413
34. Nakahara H, Noguchi S, Murakami N et al (1997) Gadolinium-enhanced MR imaging of thyroid and parathyroid masses. Radiology 202:765–772
35. Kusunoki T, Murata K, Hosoi H et al (1998) Malignancies of human thyroid tumors and dynamic magnetic resonance imaging (MRI). Auris Nasus Larynx 25:419–424
36. McDermott VG, Spritzer CE (1999) Parathyroid and thyroid glands. In: Stark DD, Bradley WG (eds) Magnetic resonance imaging, 3rd edn. Mosby, St Louis, pp 1807–1820
37. Russell P, Lean CL, Delbridge L et al (1994) Proton magnetic resonance and human thyroid neoplasia. 1. Discrimination between benign and malignant neoplasms. Am J Med 96:383–388
38. Lean CL, Delbridge L, Russell P et al (1995) Diagnosis of follicular thyroid lesions by proton magnetic resonance and fine needle biopsy. J Clin Endocrinol Metab 80:1306–1311
39. Auffermann W, Clark OH, Thurnher S et al (1988) Recurrent thyroid carcinoma: characteristics on MR images. Radiology 168:753–757
40. Dorr U, Wurstlin S, Frank-Raue K, et al (1993) Somatostatin receptor scintigraphy and magnetic resonance imaging in recurrent medullary thyroid carcinoma: a comparative study. Horm Metab Res [Suppl] 27:48–55
41. Ohnishi T, Noguchi S, Murakami N et al (1993) Detection of recurrent thyroid cancer: MR versus thallium-201 scintigraphy. Am J Neuroradiol 14:1051–1057
42. Mallin WH, Elgazzar AH, Maxon HR III (1994) Imaging modalities in the follow-up of non-iodine avid thyroid carcinoma. Am J Otolaryngol 15:417–422
43. Burman KD, Anderson JH, Wartofsky L et al (1990) Management of patients with thyroid carcinoma: application of thallium-201 scintigraphy and magnetic resonance imaging. J Nucl Med 31:1958–1964
44. Funari M, Campos Z, Gooding GA et al (1992) MRI and ultrasound detection of asymptomatic thyroid nodules in hyperparathyroidism. J Comput Assist Tomogr 16:615–619
45. Reading CC, Gorman CA (1993) Thyroid imaging techniques. Clin Lab Med 13:711–724

46. Eisenberg B, Velchick MG, Spritzer C et al (1990) Magnetic resonance imaging and scintigraphic correlation in thyroid disorders. Am J Physiol Imaging 5:8–21
47. Freitas JE, Freitas AE (1994) Thyroid and parathyroid imaging, Semin Nucl Med 24:234–245
48. Yousem DM, Scheff AM (1995) Thyroid and parathyroid gland pathology: role of imaging. Otolaryngol Clin North Am 28:621–649
49. Toubert ME, Cyna-Gorse F, Zagdanski AM et al (1999) Cervicomediastinal magnetic resonance imaging in persistent or recurrent papillary thyroid carcinoma: clinical use and limits. Thyroid 9:591–597
50. Takashima S, Takayama F, Wang Q, Kawakami S, Saito A, Kobayashi S, Sone S (2000) Differentiated thyroid carcinomas. Prediction of tumor invasion with MR imaging. Acta Radiol 41:377–383
51. Wang JC, Takashima S, Takayama F, Kawakami S, Saito A, Matsushita T, Matsuba H, Kobayashi S (2001) Tracheal invasion by thyroid carcinoma: prediction using MR imaging. Am J Roentgenol 177:929–936
52. Takashima S, Matsushita T, Takayama F, Kadoya M, Fujimori M, Kobayashi T (2001) Prognostic significance of magnetic resonance findings in advanced papillary thyroid cancer. Thyroid 11:1153–1159
53. Heywang-Köbrunner SH, Viehweg P (1999) Breasts. In: Stark DD, Bradley WG (eds) Magnetic resonance imaging, 3rd edn. Mosby, St Louis, pp 307–319
54. Vogl TJ, Balzer J, Mack M et al (1998) Radiologische Differentialdiagnostik in der Kopf-Hals-Region. Thieme, Stuttgart
55. Som PM, Brandwein M, Lidov M et al (1994) The varied presentations of papillary thyroid carcinoma cervical nodal disease: CT and MR findings. Am J Neuroradiol 15:1123–1128
56. Takashima S, Sone S, Takayama F et al (1998) Papillary thyroid carcinoma: MR diagnosis of lymph node metastasis. Am J Neuroradiol 19:509–513
57. Van den Brekel MWM, Castelijns JA, Stel HV et al (1991) Occult metastatic neck disease: detection with US and US-guided fine-needle aspiration cytology. Radiology 180:457–461
58. Schlumberger M, Challeton C, Vathaire F de, et al (1996) Radioactive iodine treatment and external radiotherapy for lung and bone metastases from differentiated carcinoma. J Nucl Med 37:598–605
59. Van den Brekel MW, Castelijns JA, Stel HV et al (1990) Detection and characterization of metastatic cervical adenopathy by MR imaging: comparison of different MR techniques. J Comput Assist Tomogr 14:581–589
60. Van den Brekel MW, Castelijns JA, Croll GA et al (1991) Magnetic resonance imaging vs palpation of cervical lymph node metastasis. Arch Otolaryngol Head Neck Surg 117:663–673
61. Van den Brekel MW (2000) Lymph node metastases: CT and MRI. Eur J Radiol 33:230–238
62. Gross ND, Weissman JL, Talbot JM, Andersen PE, Wax MK, Cohen JI (2001) MRI detection of cervical metastasis from differentiated thyroid carcinoma. Laryngoscope 111:1905–1909

Chapter 16

Thyroid Cancer in Chernobyl Children 16

C. Reiners, J. Biko, E.P. Demidchik, and V. Drozd

16.1 Experiences from the Past

It has been well known for 50 years that exposure of the thyroid to ionizing radiation in childhood produces an appreciable cancer risk [7]. The thyroid gland and the bone marrow are considered to be the most radiosensitive cancer sites [25]. Concerning thyroid cancer, many epidemiological studies in populations of children treated with external radiotherapy for benign or malignant lesions in the head and neck region have been published [14, 25, 26, 30, 31]. The diverse indications for treatment have included skin hemangioma, enlarged thymus and tonsils, lymphoid hyperplasia, tuberculous adenitis, acne, and tinea capitis. A pooled analysis [25] using the data of cohort studies in individuals exposed to acute external ionizing radiation before the age of 20 years found an average excess relative risk of 7.7/Gy [95% confidence interval (CI) 4.9–12], while the excess absolute risk was $4.4/10^4$ person-year Gy (95% CI 1.9–10). A linear dose-response function was found to fit the data well; the risk was about 30% lower for fractionated doses than for unfractionated exposure. Almost no thyroid cancers prior to 5 years after irradiation have been reported; the pooled analysis suggested that the excess relative risk per gray was greatest about 15 years after exposure, but was still elevated 40 or more years after irradiation [25].

Unlike studies of external irradiation, where epidemiological data of more than 50,000 exposed children and adolescents are available, only sparse data from childhood exposure to radioiodine (^{131}I) have been published [13, 14, 31]. Cohort studies in approximately 9,000 children exposed to ^{131}I before the age of 20 years suggested no significant increase in thyroid cancer risk for diagnostic or therapeutic use of ^{131}I [13, 14]. A small, but significant increase in thyroid cancer risk has been seen in children and adolescents from the Marshall Islands exposed to fallout from atomic bomb experiments, amounting to an excess relative risk of 0.3 (95% CI 0.1–0.8). However, 80% of this dose originated from short-lived radioiodines and external radiation rather than from ^{131}I [31]. The situation after the atomic bomb explosions of Hiroshima and Nagasaki was similar. However, the data from the Japanese atomic bomb study may be used to estimate age-related excess relative risk coefficients per gray at ages 0–9, 10–19, 20–39, and 40 years, calculated at 9.5, 3.0, 0.3, and –0.2, respectively [1].

These risk coefficients show that the risk for thyroid cancer induction by radiation from atomic bomb explosions is high in children, intermediate in adolescents, and negligible in adults. Epidemiological studies in adults indicating no increased risk for thyroid cancer after external or internal irradiation underline this hypothesis [25, 30]. The publications include comprehensive studies in patients diagnosed or treated with ^{131}I [13, 14]. In general, microdosimetric considerations [2] and/or the low dose rates involved with ^{131}I as compared to external thyroid irradiation with kilovoltage X-rays appear to reduce the carcinogenic potency substantially [30]. External irradiation seems to be 1.5–2 times more dangerous than ^{131}I [18]. Concerning the age-related effects of ^{131}I, it is important to mention that besides the higher cancer risk in children and adolescents whose thyroids are still growing, considerably higher absorbed doses for a given activity of ^{131}I play an important role. The doses to the thyroid (in gray) per ingested activity of ^{131}I (in kilobecquerels) in a newborn and at age 1, 5, 10, 15, and $\geq$20 years amount to 9.6, 3.9, 2.2, 0.9, 0.6, and 0.4 respectively [38].

It has been claimed that malignant thyroid tumors after external irradiation typically present as papillary cancers in approximately 85% of exposed children and adolescents [23, 25, 31, 37]. However, comparing two cohorts of thyroid cancer patients with and without a history of head and neck irradiation as children, Samaan et al. [27] showed that the proportion of papillary cancers in the two cohorts was not significantly different, at 87% and 84% respectively. This indicates that papillary histology per se is typical for thyroid cancer in childhood and adolescence. But Samaan's study revealed with statistical significance that bilateral lobe involvement (51%) and cancer not limited to the thyroid gland (70%) seemed to be characteristic for radiation-induced thyroid cancer [27].

16.2 The Chernobyl Accident

During the night from 25 to 26 April 1986, the most severe reactor accident happened at the nuclear power plant, Chernobyl 30 km south of the border of the Ukraine and Belarus. The reactor core exploded and caught fire, and the fire could not be extinguished until 9 May 1986. Due to the burning graphite, enormous amounts of radioactivity were released during the first 10 days. According to recent calculations, approximately 12×10^{18} Bq ($\cong$ 0.3 billion Ci) of radioactivity was released, including 1.8×10^{18} Bq of ^{131}I. The radioactivity was transported with the prevailing winds from the northern parts of the Ukraine to Belarus and the western parts of Russia and later to Scandinavia and parts of western Europe. Belarus has been most heavily contaminated, with 70% of the released activity. Extremely high contaminations have been found in the regions surrounding the cities of Gomel and Brest [16].

16.3 Thyroid Cancer in Belarus After Chernobyl

The frequency of thyroid cancer in children from Belarus, the Ukraine and the western parts of Russia has been increasing since 1990 [5, 6, 8, 32, 33]. In total,

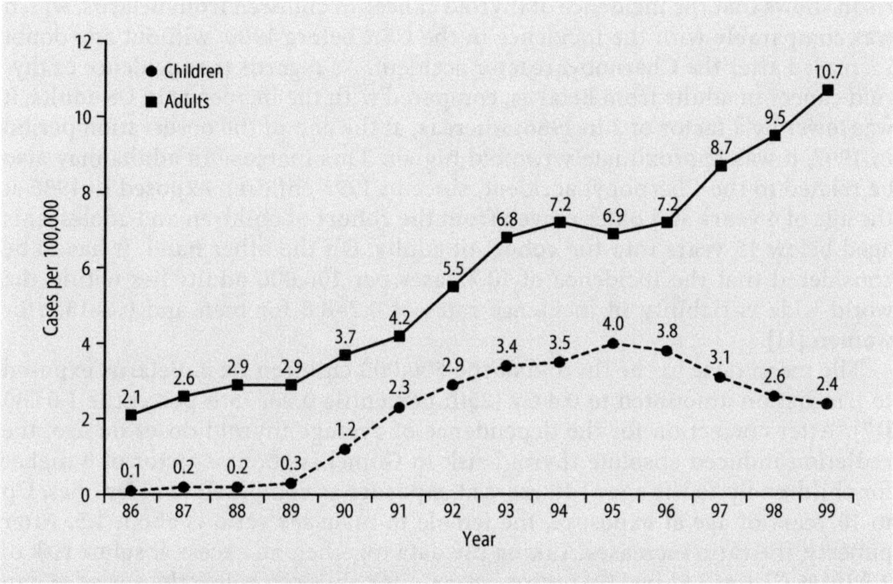

Fig. 16.1 Relative incidence of thyroid cancer in adults and children below the age of 15 years in Belarus between 1986 and 1999

in the three republics afflicted by radioactive fallout from the Chernobyl accident, approximately 1,500 cases of thyroid cancer in children below the age of 15 were diagnosed between 1990 and 1998, as compared to approximately 100 cases between 1968 and 1989 [5, 6, 8, 32, 33].

The most reliable epidemiological data seem to be available from Belarus [5, 6]. The relative incidence of thyroid cancer per 100,000 children below the age of 15, which amounted to 0.1–0.3 between 1986 and 1989, increased to 4.0 in 1995 (Fig. 16.1). In the region of Gomel, which was most heavily contaminated after the Chernobyl accident by radioactive fallout containing ^{131}I and short-lived radioisotopes of iodine, the relative incidence increased to 13.5 in 1995. Since 1996, the relative incidence of thyroid cancer in children has been decreasing (Fig. 16.1).

Figure 16.1 shows that the relative incidence of thyroid cancer in adults from Belarus has also been increasing since 1986. However, whereas the increase in children was approximately 20-fold comparing the year 1995 to the mean of the years 1986–1989, the increase in the relative incidence in adults between 1986 and 1997 was only fivefold. According to data of the Survival Epidemiology and End Results Programme [29] from the USA, the yearly incidence of thyroid cancer between 1990 and 1994 amounted to 4.9 per 100,000 inhabitants (women 6.9, men 2.8 per 100,000). In children and adolescents below the age of 20, the incidence was 0.1 per 100,000 US inhabitants. Between 1950 and 1994, the incidence of thyroid cancer in the USA increased by approximately 22% [29]. This comparison shows that the incidence of thyroid cancer in children from Belarus, which was comparable with the incidence in the USA before 1990, without any doubt increased after the Chernobyl reactor accident. As regards the incidence of thyroid cancer in adults from Belarus, compared with the incidence in US adults, it was lower by a factor of 2 in 1986; whereas, at the end of the observation period in 1997, it was approximately twofold higher. This increase in adults may also be related to the Chernobyl accident, since in 1997 children exposed in 1986 at the age of 4 years and older moved from the cohort of children and adolescents aged below 15 years into the cohort of adults. On the other hand, it has to be considered that the incidence of 10.7 cases per 100,000 adults lies within the world-wide variability in incidence rates of 0.2–8.8 for men and 0.8–18.2 for women [11].

The mean dose to the thyroid of the 500,000 children from Belarus exposed to irradiation amounted to 0.4 Gy (25th percentile 0.08, 75th percentile 1.0 Gy) [17]. After correction for the dependence of average thyroid doses on age, the radiation-induced absolute thyroid risk in Gomel is about a factor of 3 higher for children up to the age of 10 years at exposure as compared to older ones. Up to 10 years of age at exposure, the female to male sex ratio is about 1.5. After puberty, the ratio increases. Taking the data together, an excess absolute risk of 2.3 (95% CI 1.4–3.8) per 10^4 person-year Gy for children below the age of 15 can be calculated [15]. This is a factor of 2 lower than the best estimate derived from the pooled study of thyroid cancer after external exposures [18]. Projecting the age-adjusted average excess risk per unit thyroid dose for the period of 5–50 years following the Chernobyl accident, it has been estimated that about 15,000 cases (95% CI 5,000–45,000) may develop [19].

In total, 673 cases of childhood thyroid cancer were detected and operated on by the Center for Thyroid Tumors in Minsk between 1986 and 1997 [5, 6]. Of these children, 52% lived in the Gomel region. Histologically, 94% of the tumors were classified as papillary thyroid cancer. At the time of surgical intervention in Minsk, 26% of the cases were staged as pT1 (tumors of less than 1 cm in diameter), 28% as pT2 (between 1 and 4 cm in diameter), 1% as pT3 (more than 4 cm in diameter, without invasion of surrounding tissue), and 45% as the most advanced stage pT4 (tumors invading soft tissue surrounding the thyroid gland). In 25% of pT1–2 tumors and 45% of pT4 tumors, cancer growth was classified histologically as multicentric. In 50% of the cases staged pT1–3 and 81% of patients staged pT4, lymph node metastases were observed during surgery. The relative frequency of distant metastases diagnosed in Minsk immediately postoperatively amounted to 5% in tumor stages pT1–3 and 24% in tumor stage pT4.

16.4 Treatment of Thyroid Cancer in Children from Belarus

The German project “Scientists help Chernobyl Children” was established within the framework of bilateral cooperation between two centers in Minsk

Patients	231 children 885 treatment courses
Origin	98 Gomel area 133 other parts of Belarus
Gender	135 girls 96 boys
Age	7–18 years (12.7±2.5)
Histology	229 papillary cancers 2 follicular cancers
Stage	pTx: 2 pT1: 3 pT2: 71 pT3: 4 pT4: 151 pN0: 6 pN1: 225 pM0: 130 pM1: 101 98 lung 2 bone 1 brain
Pretreatment	39 radioiodine therapies in Minsk 6 radioiodine therapies in Italy 19 percutaneous irradiations 6 chemotherapies

Table 16.1. Children with thyroid cancer from Belarus treated with ^{131}I in Germany between 1 April 1993 and 31 March 2000

and the University Clinics for Nuclear Medicine in Essen and later Würzburg. Surgical resection of thyroid tumors and removal of lymph nodes have been performed by the surgical team of the Center for Thyroid Tumors in Minsk. Radioiodine treatment and staging with nuclear medicine procedures has been the task of the Clinics for Nuclear Medicine in Essen and Würzburg. Follow-up has been performed in Minsk by the Center for Thyroid Tumors and the Research and Clinical Institute of Radiation Medicine and Endocrinology in Minsk [24].

16.4.1 Patients

Between 1 April 1993 and 31 March 2003, 231 children from Belarus with the most advanced stages of thyroid cancer were selected for treatment in Germany (Table 16.1). In total, 885 courses of ^{131}I therapy had been applied by 31 March 2003.

Forty-two percent of the children originated from the Gomel region. The mean age of the children at the time of the reactor accident was 2.6±2.2 years (78% of the children were below the age of 5 years). Their age at the time of surgery ranged from 7 to 18 years with a mean age of 12.7±2.5 years. This corresponds to a mean latency time of approximately 10 years; the shortest time interval between exposure and surgery was 3.2 years. Of the children, 58% were female and 42% male. Ninety-nine percent of the cancers were typed histologically as papillary and 1% as follicular carcinomas.

Seventy-two percent of the cases selected for treatment in Germany because of the tumor aggressiveness were classified as stage pT4. In 97% of the cases, lymph node metastases were found, and in 44% distant metastases were detected. With the exception of two cases with secondaries to bone, distant metastases were localized in the lungs (among these cases, one child had metastases to lungs and brain). Nearly all of the cases with lung metastases presented as disseminated miliary spread; only 4% of the children showed single localized nodular lesions. Only 53% of the children with lung metastases detectable by ^{131}I scanning showed positive thoracic X-rays; this proportion was higher (82%) for high-resolution computed tomography (CT). In 39 of the 231 children, radioiodine treatment had been performed with different activities in Minsk previously (mainly low activities up to 1 GBq); 19 of the children had been irradiated percutaneously with mainly low radiation doses (up to 20 Gy). In six children, chemotherapy with different drugs had been performed in Minsk.

16.4.2 Protocol

The diagnostic protocol included ultrasonography and scintigraphy of the neck, thoracic X-ray, computer tests of pulmonary function, and determinations of thyroglobulin, TSH, free T_4, and free T_3 in serum, as well as measurements of calcium, phosphate, and differential blood cell counts. Additionally, X-ray CT, whole body counter measurements of incorporated radionuclides, and biological dosimetry were performed in a subset of children.

For treatment, 50 MBq ^{131}I/kg of body weight was administered to eliminate thyroid remnants. For ablation of metastases, 100 MBq ^{131}I/kg of body weight was given. Simultaneously, antiemetics and emulsions for the protection of the gastric mucosa were given to reduce gastrointestinal side-effects. Two days after treatment, replacement therapy with levothyroxine, which had been withdrawn 4 weeks before treatment, was restarted. The mean dose amounted to 2.5 μg levothyroxine/kg of body weight. For staging, whole body scans were performed 4 days after the administration of radioiodine.

16.4.3 Results of Treatment

In 202 of the 231 children, more than one course of radioiodine treatment has been performed in Germany up to now. In these cases, the results of treatment have been assessed by follow-up with ^{131}I scintigraphy, ultrasonography of the neck, X-ray of the thorax, and determinations of thyroglobulin in serum.

In 168 out of 202 children (83%), complete or stable partial remissions (stable partial remission means negative posttherapeutic scan and TSH-stimulated

Table 16.2 Thyroid cancer in children: data from Belarus in comparison with data from Italy, France, and Germany

Study	Belarus [6]	Italy and France [21]	Germany [9]
No. of children	574	369	114
Mean age	9.9 years	14.6 years	13.2 years
Female:male ratio	1.5:1	2.5:1	2.4:1
Papillary histology	98%	82%	78%
Multicentric growth	33%	–	20%
pT4	45%	25%	29%
pN1	68%	54%	52%
pM1	16%	17%	25%

thyroglobulin <10ng/ml) of thyroid cancer have been achieved up to now. In 16% we were able to recognize partial remissions, defined as decrease in tumor volume, tumor marker serum level, or intensity of radioiodine uptake of at least 50%. Fortunately, in no case has progressive disease been observed. It is important to mention that the results given here are not the final results of treatment since in some cases without complete remission further courses of radioiodine are required.

16.5 Discussion and Conclusions

There is no doubt that exposure to radiation may induce thyroid cancer in children [36]. According to the review of Ron et al., "The thyroid gland in children has one of the highest risk coefficients of any organ and is the only with [sic] convincing evidence for risk at about 0.1 Gy" [25]. Linearity best describes the dose response in children exposed to radiation before the age of 15. Risk decreases significantly with increasing age at exposure, with little risk apparent after the age of 20. The excess relative risk seems to be higher for girls than for boys [25].

Latency times between radiation exposure and development of thyroid cancer range between minimally 3–7 years and maximally 40–50 years. Between 10 and 15 years, a nadir of the statistical distribution may be presumed [30]. The relative incidence of thyroid cancer per 100,000 children below the age of 15 increased in Belarus from 0.1–0.3 cases between 1986 and 1989 to 4.0 cases in 1995. For comparison: According to figures from the USA [12, 20, 29] and data from the German Cancer Registries in Hamburg and the Saarland, the incidence of thyroid cancer in children below the age of 15 is approximately 0.3–0.5 cases per 100,000.

Table 16.2 compares recent multicenter studies on childhood thyroid cancer from Italy, France, and Germany [9, 21] to the statistical material which is available at the Center for Thyroid Tumors in Minsk, Belarus, on 574 cases of childhood cancer diagnosed after the Chernobyl accident between 1986 and 1997 [5, 6]. Table 16.2 proves that a high proportion of papillary histology is typical for thyroid cancer in children and adolescents [27]. But, in children exposed to irradiation from Belarus, the percentage of papillary cancers is extremely high, at 98%, as compared to children from Italy and France (82%) and Germany (78%). In addition, the proportions of tumors with multicentric growth (33% versus 20%) and pT4 stage (45% versus 25% and 29% respectively) are higher in children from Belarus. Lymph node involvement is also more frequent in children from Belarus (68%) as compared to children from Italy and France (54%) or Germany (52%). An unequivocal difference in the frequency of distant metastases is not evident (16% versus 17% and 25% respectively). However, the data available from Belarus may underestimate the frequency of distant metastases, because routine ^{131}I whole body scans have been performed only in a small subgroup of the patients.

To summarize, the characteristics of thyroid cancer in children exposed to Chernobyl fallout seem to be papillary histology and signs of aggressive growth. However, it cannot be ruled out completely that these peculiarities are related to the younger age of Chernobyl children (mean 9.9 years) as compared to the mean ages of children from Italy and France (14.6 years) and Germany (13.2 years) (Table 16.2).

It is well known that papillary thyroid cancers tend to spread via the lymphatic pathway to the lungs [34]. Frequently, this miliary type of disseminated pulmonary metastases may only be detected by whole body scintigraphy and not by thoracic X-ray [28], as was observed in 47% of our children with lung metastases. Of the 98 children from Belarus with secondaries to the lungs treated in Germany, 92 presented with disseminated pulmonary lesions. These could be eradicated completely by ^{131}I therapy in 28% of the children. In the remaining 72% of patients, partial remissions have been observed, with decreasing intensity of radioiodine uptake and reduction of the mostly extremely elevated thyroglobulin levels in serum. However, 8 of 90 children with radioiodine uptake in lung metastases have shown decreases in vital capacity, which has been measured routinely during therapy. Computed tomography proved that pulmonary fibrosis had developed. Lung fibrosis is one of the possible complications of high-dose radioiodine treatment in patients with pulmonary metastases of thyroid cancer. However, five of the eight cases diagnosed in our study had been treated previously with bleomycin, which itself is known to induce pulmonary fibrosis. According to the literature, fibrosis may develop in up to 10% of children with lung metastases [22].

However, generally the prognosis of thyroid cancer in children is reported to be excellent [3, 4, 12, 20, 27, 35]. Children have a better prognosis than adults. Even in cases of scintigraphically persistent pulmonary metastases, prognosis seems to be good [28, 29]. Today, it is generally accepted that treatment guidelines for children and adults have to be identical [3, 4, 12, 20, 27, 35]. Routine treatment has to include thyroidectomy and selective removal of positive lymph nodes, followed by radioiodine treatment. Only in cases staged pT1 are total thyroidectomy and subsequent radioiodine ablation of thyroid remnants not mandatory, because of the excellent prognosis of such tumors. However, it should be taken into consideration that a tumor diameter of 1 cm in a 10-year-old child with a thyroid volume of approximately 10 ml is relatively larger by a factor of 2 than a tumor of the same size in an adult with a thyroid volume of 20 ml [10].

References

1. Akiba S, Lubin J, Ezaki E, Ron E, Ishimaru T, Asona Y, Shimizu Y, Kato H (1991) Thyroid cancer incidence among atomic bomb survivors in Hiroshima and Nagasaki 1958–1979. Technical Report TR 5-91, Radiation Effects Research Foundation, Hiroshima, Japan
2. Brenner DJ (1999) The relative effectiveness of exposure to ^{131}I at low doses. Health Phys 76:180–185
3. Danese D, Gardini A, Farsetti A, Sciacchitano S, Andreoli M, Pontecorvi A (1997) Thyroid carcinoma in children and adolescents. Eur J Pediatr 156:190–194
4. Dottorini ME, Vignati A, Mazzucchelli L, Lomuscio G, Colombo L (1997) Differentiated thyroid carcinoma in children and adolescents: a 37-year experience in 85 patients. J Nucl Med 38:669–675
5. Demidchik EP, Mrochek A, Demidchik Yu, Vorontsova T, Cherstvoy E, Kenigsberg J, Rebeko V, Sugenoya A (1999) Thyroid cancer promoted by radiation in young people of Belarus (clinical and epidemiological features). In: Thomas G, Karaoglou A, Williams ED (eds) Radiation and thyroid cancer. World Scientific, Singapore, pp 51–54
6. Demidchik EP (2000) Personal communication
7. Duffy BJ, Fitzgerald P (1950) Thyroid cancer in childhood and adolescence. Report of 28 cases. J Clin Endocr Metab 10:1296–1308
8. Epsthein OE (2000) Personal communication
9. Farahati J, Parlowsky T, Mäder U, Reiners C, Bucsky P (1998) Differentiated thyroid cancer in children and adolescents. Langenbeck's Arch Surg 383:235–239
10. Farahati J, Reiners C, Demidchik EP (1999) Is the UICC/AJCC classification of primary tumor in childhood thyroid carcinoma valid? J Nucl Med 40:2125
11. Franceschi S, Boyle P, Maisonneuve P, La Vecchia C, Burt AD, Kerr DJ, MacFarlane GJ (1993) The epidemiology of thyroid carcinoma. Crit Rev Oncogenesis 4:25–52
12. Gorlin JB, Sallan SE (1990) Thyroid cancer in childhood. Endocrinol Metab Clin North Am 19:649–662
13. Hall P, Holm LE (1997) Late consequences of radioiodine for diagnosis and therapy in Sweden. Thyroid 7:205–208
14. Hall P, Holm LE (1998) Radiation-associated thyroid cancer – facts and fiction. Acta Oncol 37:325–330
15. Heidenreich WF, Kenigsberg J, Jacob P, Buglova E, Goulko G, Paretzke HG, Demidchik EP, Golovneva A (1999) Time trends of thyroid cancer incidence in Belarus after the Chernobyl accident. Radiat Res 151:617–625
16. International Atomic Energy Agency (1996) One decade after Chernobyl: summing-up the consequences of the accident. IAEA and WHO, Vienna
17. Jacob P (1998) Thyroid cancer risk to children calculated. Nature 392:31–32
18. Jacob P, Kenigsberg Y, Zvonova I, Goulko G, Buglova E, Heidenreich WF, Golovneva A, Bratilova AA, Drozdovitch V, Kruk J, Pochtennaja GT, Balonov M, Demidchik EP, Paretzke HG (1999) Childhood exposure due to the Chernobyl accident and thyroid cancer risk in contaminated areas of Belarus and Russia. Br J Cancer 80:1461–1469
19. Jacob P, Kenigsberg Y, Goulko G, Buglova E, Gering F, Golovneva A, Kruk J, Demidchik EP (2000) Thyroid cancer risk in Belarus after the Chernobyl accident: comparison with external exposures. Radiat Environ Biophys 39:25–31

20. Moir CR, Telander RL (1994) Papillary carcinoma of the thyroid in children. Semin Pediatr Surg 3:182–187
21. Pacini F, Vorontsova T, Demidchik EP, Molinaro E, Agate L, Romei C, Shavrova E, Cherstvoy ED, Ivashkevitch Y, Kuchinskaya E, Schlumberger M, Ronga G, Filesi M, Pinchera A (1997) Post-Chernobyl thyroid carcinoma in Belarus children and adolescents: comparison with naturally occurring thyroid carcinoma in Italy and France. J Clin Endocrinol Metab 82:3563–3569
22. Reiners C, Perret G, Sonnenschein W, John-Mikolajewski V (1994) Radiation reactions to the lung after radioiodine therapy for thyroid cancer. In: Herrmann T, Reiners C, Messerschmidt O (eds) Strahlenschutz in Forschung und Praxis, vol 36. Fischer, Stuttgart, pp 139–146
23. Reiners C, Biko J, Kruglova N, Demidchik EP (1996) Therapy of thyroid carcinoma in children from Belarus after the Chernobyl accident. In: Nauman J, Glinoer D, Braverman LE, Hostalek U (eds) The thyroid and iodine. Merck European Thyroid Symposium, Warsaw, 16–18 May 1996. Schattauer, Stuttgart, pp 89–97
24. Reimers C, Demidchik EP (2003) Differentiated thyroid cancer in childhood: pathology, diagnosis, therapy. Pediatr Endocr Review 1 [Suppl2]:230–236
25. Ron E, Lubin JH, Shore RE, Mabuchi K, Modan B, Pottern LM, Schneider AB, Tucker MA, Boice JD (1995) Thyroid cancer after exposure to external radiation: a pooled analysis of seven studies. Radiat Res 141:259–277
26. Ron E, Schneider AB (1999) External radiation and the thyroid cancer risk in humans. In: Thomas G, Karaoglou A, Williams ED (eds) Radiation and thyroid cancer. World Scientific, Singapore, pp 5–12
27. Samaan NA, Schultz PN, Ordonez NG, Hickey RC, Johnston DA (1987) A comparison of thyroid carcinoma in those who have and have not had head and neck irradiation in childhood. J Clin Endocrinol 64:219–223
28. Samuel AM, Rajashekharrao B, Shah DH (1998) Pulmonary metastases in children and adolescents with well-differentiated thyroid cancer. J Nucl Med 39:1531–1536
29. Surveillance, Epidemiology and End Results (SEER) Program of the USA 1973–1994 (1998) National Cancer Institute, Bethesda
30. Shore RE (1992) Issues and epidemiological evidence regarding radiation-induced thyroid cancer. Radiat Res 131:98–111
31. Shore RE (1996) Human thyroid cancer induction by ionizing radiation: summary of studies based on external irradiation and radioactive iodines. In: Karaoglou A, Desmet G, Kelly GN, Menzel HG (eds) European Commission and the Belarus, Russian and Ukrainian Ministries on Chernobyl Affairs, Emergency Situations and Health: the radiological consequences of the Chernobyl accident. European Commission, Brussels, pp 669–675
32. Tronko M, Bogdanova T, Komisarenko I, Rybakov S, Kovalenko A, Epsthein O, Oliynik V, Tereshchenko V, Likhtarev I, Kairo I, Chepurnoy M (1999) The post-Chernobyl incidence of childhood thyroid cancer in Ukraine. In: Thomas G, Karaoglou A, Williams ED (eds) Radiation and thyroid cancer. World Scientific, Singapore, pp 61–69
33. Tsyb AF, Shakhtarin, Lushnikov EF, Stepanenko VF, Snykov VP, Parshkov EM, Trofimova SF (1999) Development of cancer and non-cancer thyroid diseases in children and adolescents after the Chernobyl accident. In: Thomas G, Karaoglou A, Williams ED (eds) Radiation and thyroid cancer. World Scientific, Singapore, pp 79–87
34. Vassilopoulou-Sellin R, Klein MJ, Smith TH, Samaan NA, Frankenthaler RA, Goepfert H, Cangir A, Haynie TP (1993) Pulmonary metastases in children and young adults with differentiated thyroid cancer. Cancer 71:1348–1352
35. Vassilopoulou-Sellin R, Goepfert H, Raney B, Schultz PN (1998) Differentiated thyroid cancer in children and adolescents: clinical outcome and mortality after long-term follow-up. Head Neck 20:549–555
36. Williams D (1996) Editorial: thyroid cancer and the Chernobyl accident. J Clin Endocrinol Metab 81:6–8

37. Winship T, Rosvoll RV (1970) Thyroid carcinoma in childhood: final report on a 20-year study. Clin Proc Child Hosp (Washington, DC) 26:327–349
38. Zanzonico PB (2000) Age-dependent thyroid absorbed doses for radiobiologically significant radioisotopes of iodine. Health Phys 78:60–67

PART III

Medullary Thyroid Cancer III

Chapter 17

Diagnosis of Medullary Thyroid Cancer

F. Raue and K. Frank-Raue

17.1 Introduction

Medullary thyroid carcinoma (MTC) is a rare calcitonin (CT)-secreting tumor of the parafollicular or C cells of the thyroid. As the C cells originate from the embryonic neural crest, MTC often has the clinical and histological features of neuroendocrine tumors such as carcinoid and islet-cell tumors. It accounts for 8–12% of all thyroid carcinomas and occurs in both sporadic and hereditary forms. The discovery of an MTC in a patient has several diagnostic implications involving a specific strategy: preoperative evaluation of the extent of the disease, classification of MTC as sporadic or hereditary by DNA testing, and screening for associated endocrinopathies in hereditary MTC.

17.2 Classification and Epidemiology

MTC occurs in both sporadic and hereditary forms [20]. The familial variety of MTC is inherited as an autosomal dominant trait with a high degree of penetrance and is associated with multiple endocrine neoplasia (MEN) type 2 syndrome [4, 31]. Three distinct hereditary varieties of MTC are known:

1. The MEN 2A syndrome, characterized by MTC in combination with pheochromocytoma and tumors of the parathyroids; it accounts for more than 90% of all MEN 2 syndromes
2. The MEN 2B syndrome, consisting of MTC, pheochromocytoma, ganglioneuromatosis, and marfanoid habitus [26, 40]
3. Familial MTC (FMTC), without any other endocrinopathies

These four varieties of MTC, three heritable and one nonheritable, are clinically distinct with respect to incidence, genetics, age of onset, association with other diseases, histopathology of the tumor, and prognosis. Many patients with MEN 2B do not have a family history of the disease. Their tumors and characteristic appearance are therefore due to new mutations, which present as sporadic cases of potentially heritable disease. About 30% of MEN 2A and especially FMTC gene carriers never manifest clinically manifest disease. Therefore a family history is often inadequate in establishing familial disease, and more thorough evaluation by genetic and biochemical screening often reveals a family history of MTC in a patient originally thought to have the sporadic form of the disease.

The majority of patients have sporadic MTC (75%), while 25% suffer from hereditary MTC. The sex (male to female) ratio in sporadic MTC is 1:1.3, while both sexes are nearly equally affected in the familial variety [28]. The highest incidence of sporadic disease occurs in the fifth decade of life, while hereditary disease can be diagnosed earlier, depending on the possibility of genetic and biochemical screening.

The mode of discovery of MTC has changed within the last decade, based on the use of specific strategies: CT screening in patients with thyroid nodules and screening with molecular methods for *RET* proto-oncogene mutations in patients with apparently sporadic MTC and family members at risk for MTC. The earlier identification of patients with MTC has altered the presentation from clinical tumors to preclinical disease, resulting in a much better prognosis, with a high cure rate in affected patients.

17.3 Pathology and Biochemical Markers

The histological appearance of MTC is enormously variable with regard to cytoarchitecture (solid, trabecular, or insular) and cell shape (spindle, polyhedral, angular, or round) [37]. MTC is most commonly confused with anaplastic carcinoma, Hürthle cell tumor, or papillary thyroid carcinoma. Characteristic is the presence of stromal amyloid in about 50–80% of MTC patients. This feature was an auxiliary diagnostic criterion for MTC before the use of CT immunocytochemistry.

Hereditary MTC characteristically presents as a multifocal process with C-cell hyperplasia in areas distinct from the primary tumor. Bilateral C-cell hyperplasia is a precursor lesion to hereditary MTC, with a penetrance of nearly 100%. C-cell hyperplasia may also be a precursor lesion to sporadic MTC. It has also been described in 20% of patients with chronic lymphocytic thyroiditis. This type of C-cell hyperplasia can cause elevated CT levels and positive stimulation tests but poses no risk of progression to MTC. The time frame of the progression from C-cell hyperplasia to microscopic carcinoma in hereditary MTC remains unclear but may take years. Metastasis may be found first in central and lateral, cervical and mediastinal lymph nodes in 10% of patients with a micro-MTC operated on after discovery at familial screening, and in up to 90% of patients operated on for clinical MTC. Metastases outside the neck and mediastinum may occur during the course of the disease in the lung, liver, and bone.

The primary secretory product of MTC is CT, a peptide hormone consisting of 32 amino acids and with a molecular mass of 3,400 daltons. CT serves as a tumor marker, and measurement of monomeric CT with two-site assays remains the definitive test for prospective diagnosis of MTC [18]. The test is widely available, accurate, reproducible, and cost-effective. Either basal or stimulated plasma CT levels are elevated in virtually all patients with MTC. Basal CT concentrations usually correlate with tumor mass and are almost always high in patients with palpable tumors [5]. Similarly, elevated plasma CT levels following surgery to remove the tumor are indicative of persistent or recurrent disease. Therefore the preferred biochemical screening method for MTC is provocative stimulation of CT release using pentagastrin. The test is administered by giving 0.5 μg pentagastrin/kg body weight as an intravenous bolus over 5–10 s; CT measurement are made at 2 and 5 min. Abnormal elevation of CT is a reliable predictor of C-cell hyperplasia or MTC [31].

Measurement of serum CT has been part of the routine evaluation of patients with thyroid nodules: up to 3% of patients with thyroid nodules have pathological serum CT concentrations [21, 27, 33, 41]. The prevalence of MTC was found to be 100% when basal CT levels were more than 200 pg/ml, as measured with specific and sensitive two-site assays. This procedure allows early diagnosis and early surgery of MTC, reducing the significant mortality associated with this malignant tumor. It is well known that basal plasma CT can also be elevated during normal childhood and pregnancy in different malignant tumors, Hashimoto's thyroiditis, and chronic renal failure. Patients with these conditions, however, usually have blunted or absent stimulatory responses to CT secretagogues. Provocative CT stimulation tests thus help to sort out these false-negative and false-positive conditions. Therefore routine measurement of serum CT in thyroid nodules is the most informative test for the early diagnosis and treatment of sporadic MTC, resulting in a better outcome than for MTC not detected by serum CT measurement [8].

There are a number of other substances, including carcinoembryonic antigen (CEA), PDN-21 (katacalcin), chromogranin A, neuron-specific enolase, somatostatin, and ACTH, that are produced by MTC and which may help to differentiate it from other tumors.

17.4 Genetic Abnormalities

The MEN 2 gene was localized to centromeric chromosome 10 by genetic linkage analysis in 1987. Point mutations of the *RET* proto-oncogene were identified in 1993 in MEN 2A, MEN 2B, and FMTC in six closely located exons [6, 10, 11, 14]. Analysis of *RET* in families with MEN 2A and FMTC revealed that only affected family members had germline missense mutations. This has brought major advances in our understanding of the molecular genetic basis of MTC and has significantly changed the clinical management of these families with hereditary tumors.

The *RET* proto-oncogene (REarranged during Transfection) has long been known as an oncogene involved in approximately 25% of human papillary thyroid carcinomas. Several studies have demonstrated that *RET* is activated through somatic rearrangements [19]. This may be especially important in radiation-induced thyroid cancers, as in approximately 60% of the papillary thyroid carcinomas found in children from areas contaminated by the Chernobyl accident, somatic rearrangements of the *RET* gene have been demonstrated [15].

Table 17.1 Germline mutations in the RET proto-oncogene according to various hereditary syndromes (September 2004)

Exon RET	Codon	Phenotype Incidence (%)		
		MEN 2A	FMTC	MEN 2B
8	533		<1	
10	609,611	3	8	
10	618,620	9	40	
11	630,631,632		-	
11	<u>634</u>,635,636,649	<u>85</u>	30	
13	768,769,781	1	5	
13	790,791	1	5	
14	804,844		10	
15	891		<1	
15	883		-	2
16	912		<1	
16	<u>918</u>,922			<u>97</u>

The *RET* gene has 21 exons and encodes a receptor tyrosine kinase that appears to transduce growth and differentiation signals in several developing tissues including those derived from the neural crest. It is expressed in cells such as C cells, the precursors of medullary thyroid carcinoma, and in pheochromocytomas (Table. 17.1). The *RET* gene codes for a receptor that has a large extracellular cysteine-rich domain which is thought to be involved in ligand binding, a short transmembrane domain, and a cytoplasmic tyrosine kinase domain, which is activated upon ligand-induced dimerization.

Recent studies have provided evidence for an activating effect of receptor mutations associated with MEN 2/FMTC. It was demonstrated that mutation of the extracellular cysteine at codon 634 causes receptor dimerization, enhanced phosphorylation, and cell transformation [1, 35]. Mutation of the intracellular tyrosine kinase (codon 918) has no effect on receptor dimerization but causes enhanced phosphorylation of a different set of substrate proteins and also results in cellular transformation.

Point mutations in the *RET* proto-oncogene have been identified in 91–100% of MEN 2 and FMTC families [2, 11, 14]. In the majority of these families, germline point mutations are found tightly clustered in five cysteine (TGC) codons in a cysteine-rich region of the extracellular domain of the RET protein. Four of these codons, 609, 611, 618, and 620, are in exon 10, and a fifth, 634, in exon 11. In 87%

of MEN 2A families, cysteine codon 634 is affected, and in particular the most common mutation of this codon, TGC-CGC (Cys-Arg), has been associated with pheochromocytoma and parathyroid gland involvement in MEN 2A families [25]. Therefore individuals with this mutation should be screened annually for these endocrinopathies.

In about 50% of the FMTC families, cysteine codons 618 or 620 in exon 10 and codons 790, 791, 768, 804, 891 in exon 13-15 [12] are mutated. It is of considerable interest to note that identical germline mutations have been reported in families with MEN 2A and FMTC. In 87% of FMTC families the same codons as in MEN 2A are mutated; however, the classic MEN 2A mutation, Cys-634-Arg, in exon 11, was not present in one large series [25]. In the Netherlands, two large families with cysteine codon 618 (exon 10) mutations were investigated. Pheochromocytomas were found in only two of 60 patients in one family and in one of 20 patients in the other [24]. Therefore the authors concluded that FMTC associated with a *RET* gene exon 10 mutation constitutes a subtype of MEN 2A with a low frequency of pheochromocytoma, rather than a separate clinical entity. Initially it was thought that the recently reported mutations in exon 13 (Glu-768-Asp) [10] and in exon 14 (Val-804-Leu) [3] of the *RET* gene were specific for FMTC. However, heterozygous missense mutations were also identified in exon 13 codons 790 and 791 in five families, four with FMTC and one with MTC and pheochromocytoma [2].

In 95% of families with MEN 2B a mutation in codon 918 in exon 16 was found [11]. In each family this mutation resulted in an ATG (methionine) to ACG (threonine) alteration. In the rare families with typical clinical manifestations of MEN 2B but no mutation at codon 918, none of the mutations found in MEN 2A or FMTC were detected, and either unidentified mutations in the *RET* gene or involvement of another gene was suggested. In 1997 a germline mutation of *RET* codon 883 in two cases of de novo MEN 2B were described [39].

Approximately 23–60% of sporadic MTCs have a codon 918 somatic (present in tumor only) mutation identical to the germline mutation found in MEN 2B [43]. In one study, 40% of sporadic MTCs were found to have a codon 768 somatic mutation [10]. Some reports suggest that patients with sporadic MTC with codon 918 somatic mutations have more aggressive tumor growth [36, 44].

The association between disease phenotype and *RET* mutation genotype may have important implications for the clinical management of MEN 2 patients and their families. If the genotype can be correlated with the presence of certain phenotypic features, this information could be used to intensify screening for pheochromocytoma of hyperparathyroidism in mutations associated with a higher risk of disease or to postpone prophylactic thyroidectomy in mutations associated with a mild course of disease [4, 23, 24].

17.5 Clinical Syndrome and Diagnostic Procedure

17.5.1 Sporadic Medullary Thyroid Carcinoma

The most common clinical presentation of sporadic MTC is a single nodule or thyroid mass found incidentally during routine examination [17, 20]. The presentation does not differ from that observed in papillary or follicular thyroid carcinoma. A thyroid nodule identified by physical examination is generally evaluated by ultrasonography and radioisotopic scanning (Fig. 17.1). MTC shows hypoechoic regions, sometimes with calcifications, and a thyroid scan almost always shows no trapping of radioactive iodine or technetium. Cytologic examination of the cold, hypoechoic nodule will lead to strong suspicion or a correct diagnosis in most cases of sporadic MTC. Plain X-ray film of the neck sometimes reveals a characteristic dense, coarse calcification pattern.

A plasma CT measurement can clarify the diagnosis, since preoperative CT levels correlate significantly with tumor size [5] and, in the presence of a palpable MTC, the plasma CT concentration will usually be greater than 100 pg/ml. CEA level will be elevated in most cases with clinically evident tumors. Therefore measurement of plasma CT in patients with thyroid nodules has become a routine procedure [8, 21, 27, 41]. However, as the frequency of MTC is low (0.4%), the cost-benefit ratio should be carefully evaluated before routine CT measurements in all subjects with a thyroid nodule.

Genetic testing for *RET* mutations in patients with elevated CT levels may also be helpful in apparently sporadic cases of MTC, since, if a mutation is found, it will imply that the disease is hereditary and that the family should be screened. The frequency of germline mutations, either inherited or de novo, in a larger series of apparently sporadic MTC patients varied between 1% and 6% [42].

A much higher percentage (approximately 50%) of patients with sporadic MTC have somatic (acquired) mutations in exons 13 and 16, most commonly on codon 918, identical to germline mutation in MEN 2B patients [11, 36]. This 918 mutation has been used for PCR-based genetic analysis in fine-needle aspiration biopsy specimens to identify sporadic MTC before surgery [34]. These mutations are present only in tumor cells and are not detected by standard genetic testing, e.g., using leukocyte DNA.

Metastases to cervical and mediastinal lymph nodes are found in one-half of the patients at the time of initial presentation. Distant metastases to lung, liver, and bone occur late in the course of the disease. Diarrhea is the most prominent of the hormone-mediated clinical features of MTC and is often seen in patients with advanced disease. In addition, occasional tumors secrete ACTH, causing Cushing's syndrome. Given the possibility that any patient with MTC may have MEN 2, preoperative testing must also include a 24-h urinary excretion of catecholamine (to rule out pheochromocytoma) and measurement of calcium (to rule out hyperparathyroidism).

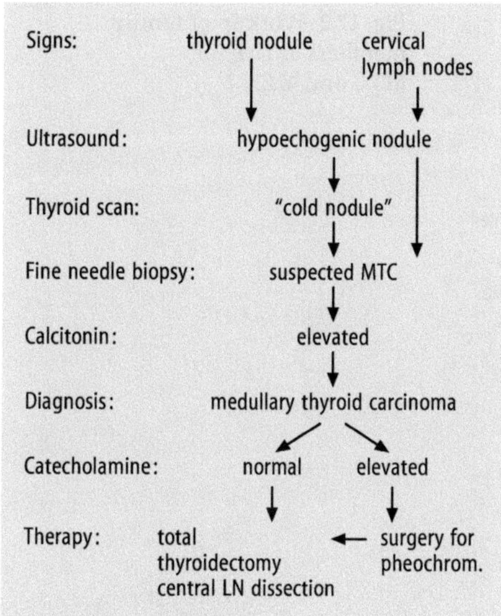

Fig. 17.1 Clinical evaluation of patients at risk for MTC

17.5.2
Hereditary Medullary Thyroid Carcinoma

Only 70% of all genetically determined MEN 2A patients develop clinically apparent MTC by the age of 70 years, but the penetrance of MTC by histological criteria is nearly 100%. The clinical presentation of familial MTC in index cases does not appear to differ from that in patients with sporadic MTC. MTC is often the initial manifestation of MEN 2 syndrome, as the other manifestations, pheochromocytoma and hyperparathyroidism, develop later in the disease with a high inter- and intra-family variabitity [31]. Less common presentations of MTC include recognition during search initiated after an associated disease such as bilateral pheochromocytoma or multiglandular hyperparathyroidism becomes apparent. The diagnosis of familial MTC in index cases is often made postoperatively when histopathological examination may show multifocal bilateral MTC accompanied by diffuse C-cell hyperplasia. MTC/C-cell hyperplasia in other family members is detected at early ages by genetic and biochemical screening and the clinical presentation is silent. The pentagastrin stimulation test may be positive in gene carriers at the age of 6 years; at the age of 30 years nearly 100% of gene carriers show a positive test.

In some MEN 2A families, a skin disorder known as cutaneous lichen amyloidosis is observed. It is characterized by bilateral or unilateral pruritic and lichenoid skin lesions located over the upper portion of the back. It often appears before development of MTC and may be a phenotypic marker of MEN 2A. Skin biopsy specimens show deposition of amyloid at the dermal-epidermal junction [16].

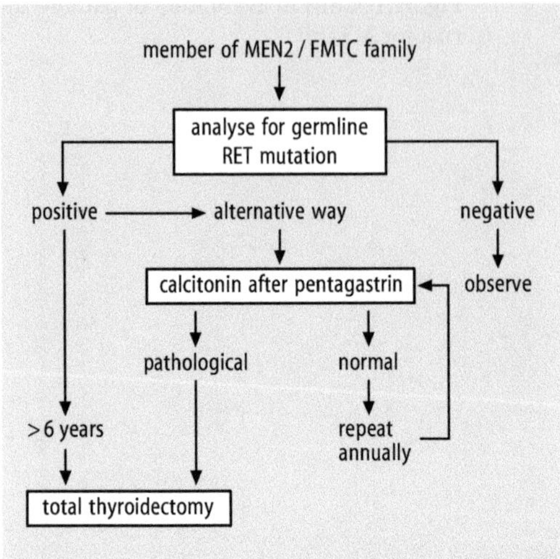

Fig. 17.2 Workup of family members at risk for MTC and MEN 2

FMTC is a variant of MEN 2A in which there is a strong predisposistion to MTC but not to the other clinical manifestations of MEN 2A (or 2B). Distinguishing FMTC from MEN 2A may be difficult in small families. Therefore rigorous criteria for FMTC should be used in order not to miss a pheochromocytoma [4]: more than 10 carriers in the kindred, multiple carriers or affected members over the age of 50 years, and an adequate medical history. A genotype–phenotype correlation has been established, showing clustering of mutations in exon 10 and 11 in classic MEN 2A syndrome, in exon 16 codon 918 in MEN 2B syndrome, and in exon 13–15 in FMTC. A line of evidence suggested that the development and the aggressiveness of MTC in the different cancer syndromes is variable. Patients with codon 790, 791, 804, 891 (exon 13–15) mutations displayed a later onset and a more indolent course than those with codon 634 mutation [4, 12], allowing a more individualized approach to the timing and extent of prophylactic surgery [23].

DNA testing is the optimal test for the early detection of MEN 2. Early diagnosis by genetic screening of "at risk" family members is essential because MTC is a life-threatening disease that can be cured or prevented by early prophylactic thyroidectomy. At present, genetic testing is performed before the age of 6 years in all first-degree relatives. Mutations in the *RET* proto-oncogene can be used to confirm the clinical diagnosis and identify asymptomatic family members with the syndrome (Fig. 17.2). Those who have a negative test can be reassured and require no further biochemical screening. Genetic analysis allows biochemical screening to be focused on those who need it and will reduce the possibility of false-positive interpretations of biochemical tests, for example a "false-positive" pentagastrin test in members of MEN 2 families who have had inappropriate thyroidectomy because of C-cell hyperplasia associated with other disease such as autoimmune thyroid disease. Testing for mutations may also be helpful in apparently "sporadic" cases of MTC, since, if a mutation is found, it will imply that the disease is hereditary and that the family should be screened.

17.5.2.1 Pheochromocytoma

Pheochromocytoma occurs in approximately 20–50% of MEN 2A patients depending on the mutation. As with MTC, the pheochromocytoma of MEN 2 is also multicentric, with diffuse adrenomedullary hyperplasia developing bilateral pheochromocytoma in half of the cases, but often after an interval of several years [14]. Almost all pheochromocytomas are located in an adrenal gland; malignant pheochromocytomas are rare. In index cases, the clinical manifestation of pheochromocytoma associated with MEN 2 is similar to that in sporadic cases, with signs and symptoms such as headache, palpitations, nervousness, tachycardia, and hypertension. However, pheochromocytomas are usually identified early as a result of regular biochemical screening in gene carriers- and clinical manifestations are thus subtle or absent. It is unusual for pheochromocytoma to precede the development of MTC and be the initial manifestation of MEN 2. Annual biochemical screening by measuring 24-h urinary excretion of catecholamines and metanephrines should be performed. Once the biochemical diagnosis is made, imaging studies such as magnetic resonance imaging or metaiodobenzylguanidine scanning are appropriate. The presence of pheochromocytoma must be ruled out prior to any surgical procedure. Patients with MTC should be evaluated for possible pheochromocytoma. A coexisting pheochromocytoma should be removed before thyroidectomy.

17.5.2.2 Primary Hyperparathyroidism

Primary hyperparathyroidism, with hypercalcemia and an elevated serum parathyroid hormone level, occurs in 10–25% of MEN 2 gene carriers. MTC postpones the occurrence of primary hyperparathyroidism often seen in codon 634 mutations, usually after the third decade of life. Hyperparathyroidism develops slowly and is usually mild; clinical features do not differ from those seen in mild sporadic hyperparathyroidism. The diagnosis is established by finding high parathyroid hormone concentrations in the presence of hypercalcemia. Pathological findings show chief cell hyperplasia involving multiple glands. Annual measurement of serum calcium concentration in gene carriers is probably adequate for screening purposes.

17.5.2.3 Multiple Endocrine Neoplasia Type 2B

MEN 2B is clinically characterized by the presence of mucosal neuromas located on the distal tongue and subconjunctival areas, thickened lips, a marfanoid habitus (long, thin extremities, an altered upper-lower body ratio, slipped femoral epiphysis, pectus excavatum), and mucosal neuromas throughout the gastrointestinal tract [26, 40]. The mucosal neuromas are pathognomonic clinical features presenting during childhood which make it possible to diagnose MTC. Other features of the syndrome occurring in childhood include gastrointestinal colic or obstruction and abnormal cramping or diarrhea. Hypertrophy of corneal nerves is frequent and is evaluated by slit-lamp ophthalmic examination. In general, MEN 2B is a more aggressive form of the syndrome, with an earlier clinical presentation of MTC, usually before the age of 10 years. As a result, early diagnosis and prevention are particularly critical. Pheochromocytomas occur as often as in MEN 2A, but primary hyperparathyroidism is absent or rare in MEN 2B.

17.6 Natural History and Prognostic Factors

The natural history of sporadic MTC is variable. The spectrum ranges from years of dormant residual disease after surgery to rapidly progressive disseminated disease and death. The 10-year survival rate for all MTC patients ranges from approximately 61–76% [7, 22, 28, 30, 38]. The overall prognosis is intermediate between that of differentiated papillary and follicular carcinoma of the thyroid and the more aggressive anaplastic thyroid cancer. Early detection and surgical treatment of MTC is likely to be curative. The main factors that influence survival are the stage of disease at the time of diagnosis, the variety of the tumor (sporadic vs familial), and the age and sex of the patient: stage I disease, familial MTC, age less than 40 years, and female gender are favorable prognostic factors. In a multivariate analysis adjusted for tumor stage, the significant difference in survival advantage between patients with sporadic and patients with familial disease disappears. The excellent prognosis associated with identification of MTC at its earliest stage underscores the importance of prospective screening and early diagnosis followed by adequate therapy [23].

References

1. Asai N, Iwashita T, Matsuyama M, Takahashi M (1995) Mechanism of activation of the RET proto-oncogene by multiple endocrine neoplasia 2A mutations. Mol Cell Biol 15:1613–1619
2. Berndt I, Reuter M, Saller B, Frank-Raue K, Groth P, Grußendorf M, Raue F, Ritter MM, Höppner W (1998) A new hotspot for mutations in the RET proto-oncogene causing familial medullary thyroid carcinoma and multiple endocrine neoplasia type 2A. J Clin Endocrinol Metab 83:770–774

3. Bolino A, Schuffenecker I, Luo Y, Seri M, Silengo M, Tocco T, Chabrier G, Houdent C, Murat A, Schlumberger M, Tourniaire J, Lenoir GM, Romeo G (1995) RET mutations in exons 13 and 14 of FMTC patients. Oncogene 10:2415–2419
4. Brandi ML, Gagel R, Angeli A, Bilezikian J, Beck-Peccoz P, Bordi C, Conte-Devolx B, Falchetti A, Gheri R, Libroia A, Lips C, Lombardi G, Manelli M, Pacini F, Ponder B, Raue F, Skogseid B, Tamburrano G, Thakker R, Thompson N, Tomasetti P, Tonelli F, Wells S, Marx S (2001) Guidelines for diagnosis and therapy of MEN type 1 and type 2.J Clin Endocrinol Metab 86:5658–5671
5. Cohen R, Campos JM, Salaün C, Heshmati M, Kraimps JL, Proye C, Sarfati E, Henry JF, Niccoli-Sire P, Modigliani E (2000) Preoperative calcitonin levels are predictive of tumor size and postoperative calcitonin normalization in medullary thyroid carcinoma. J Clin Endocrinol Metab 85:905–918
6. Donis-Keller H, Dou S, Chi D, Carlson KM, Toshima K, Lairmore TC, Howe JR, Moley JF, Goodfellow P, Wells SA (1993) Mutations in the RET proto-oncogene are associated with MEN 2A and FMTC. Hum Mol Genet 2:851–856
7. Dottorini M, Assi A, Sironi M, Sangalli G, Spreafico G, Colombo L (1996) Multivariate analysis of patients with medullary thyroid carcinoma. Cancer 77:1556–1565
8. Elisei R, Bottici V, Luchetti F, Di Coscio G, Romei C, Grasso L, Miccoli P, Iacconi P, Basolo F, Pinchera A, Pacini F (2004) Impact of routine measurement of serum calcitonin on the diagnosis and outcome of medullary thyroid cancer: experience in 10,864 patients with nodular thyroid disorders. J Clin Endocrinol Metab 89:163–168
9. Eng C (1996) The RET proto-oncogene in multiple endocrine neoplasia type 2 and Hirschsprung's disease. N Engl J Med 335:943–951
10. Eng C, Smith DP, Mulligan LM, Healey CS, Zvelebil MJ, Stonehouse TJ, Ponder MA, Jackson CE, Waterfield MD, Ponder BAJ (1995) A novel point mutation in the tyrosine kinase domain of the RET proto-oncogene in sporadic medullary thyroid carcinoma and in a family with FMTC. Oncogene 10:509–513
11. Eng C, Clayton D, Schuffenecker I, Lenoir G, Cote G, Gagel RF, van Amstel H-KP, Lips CJM, Nishisho I, Takai S-I, Marsh DJ, Robinson BG, Frank-Raue K, Raue F, Xu F, Noll WW, Romei C, Pacini F, Fink M, Niederle B, Zendenius J, Nordenskjöld M, Komminoth P, Hendy G, Gharib H, Thibodeau SN, Lacroix A, Frilling A, Ponder BAJ, Mulligan LM (1996) The relationship between specific RET proto-oncogene mutations and disease phenotype in multiple endocrine neoplasia type 2: International RET Mutation Consortium analysis. JAMA 276:1575–1579
12. Frank-Raue K, Heimbach C, Rondot S, Usadel KH, Meng W, Varma C, Fuchs-Hammoser R, Hoppner W, Schulze E, Raue F (2003) Hereditäres medulläres Schilddrüsenkarzinom –Genotyp-Phänotyp Charakterisierung. Dtsch Med Wochenschr.128:1998–2002
13. Frank-Raue K, Höppner W, Frilling A, Kotzerke J, Dralle H, Haase R, Mann K, Seif F, Kirchner R, Rendl J, Deckart HF, Ritter MM, Hampel R, Klempa J, Scholz GH, Raue F, and the German Medullary Thyroid Carcinoma Group (1996) Mutations of the RET proto-oncogene in German multiple endocrine neoplasia families: relation between genotype and phenotype. J Clin Endocrinol Metab 81:1780–1783
14. Frank-Raue K, Kratt T, Höppner W, Buhr H, Ziegler R, Raue F (1996) Diagnosis and management of pheochromocytomas in patients with multiple endocrine neoplasia type 2 – relevance of specific mutations in the RET proto-oncogene. Eur J Endocr 135:222–225
15. Fugazzola L, Pilotti S, Pinchera A, Vorontsova TV, Mondellini P, Bongarzone I, Greco A, Astakhova L, Butti MG, Demidchik EP, Pacini F, Pierotti MA (1995) Oncogenic rearrangements of the RET proto-oncogene in papillary thyroid carcinomas from children exposed to the Chernobyl nuclear accident. Cancer Res 55:5617–5620
16. Gagel RF, Levy ML, Donovan DT, Alford BR, Wheeler T, Tschen JA (1989) Multiple endocrine neoplasia type 2a associated with cutaneous lichen amyloidosis. Ann Intern Med 111:802–806
17. Giuffrida D, Gharib H (1998) Current diagnosis and management of medullary thyroid carcinoma. Ann Oncol 9:695–701

18. Grauer A, Raue F, Ziegler R (1998) Clinical usefulness of a new chemoluminescent two-site immunoassay for human calcitonin. Exp Clin Endocrinol Diabetes 106:353–359
19. Grieco M, Santoro M, Berlingieri MT, Melillo RM, Donghi R, Bongarzone I, Pierotti MA, Della Porta G, Fusco A, Vecchio G (1990) PTC is a novel rearranged form of the RET proto-oncogene and is frequently detected in vivo in human thyroid papillary carcinomas. Cell 60:557–563
20. Heshmati HM, Gharib H, van Heerden JA, Sizemore GW (1997) Advances and controversies in the diagnosis and management of medullary thyroid carcinoma. Am J Med 103:60–69
21. Karges W, Dralle H, Raue F, Mann K, Reiners C, Grussendorf M, Hüfner M, Niederle B, Brabant G (2004) Calcitonin measurement to detect medullary thyroid carcinoma in nodular goiter: German evidence-based consensusn recommendation. Exp Clin Endocrinol Diabetes 112:52--58
22. Kebebew E, Ituarte PHG, Siperstein AE, Duh QY, Clark OH (2000) Medullary thyroid carcinoma: Clinical characteristics, treatment, prognostic factores, and a comparison of staging systems. Cancer 88:1139--1148
23. Machens A, Nicolli-Sire P, Hoegel J, Frank-Raue K, van Vroonhoven TJ, Roeher HD, Wahl RA, LameschP, Raue F, Conte-Delvox B, Dralle H (2003) Early malignant progression of hereditary medullary thyroid cancer. New Engl J Med:349:1617--1525
24. Moers AM, Lansvater RM, Schaap C, Jansen-Schillhorn von Veen JM, Valk IAJ de, Blijham GH, Höppner JWM, Vroom TM, Amstel HKP van, Lips CJM (1996) Familial medullary thyroid carcinoma: not a distinct entity? Genotype-phenotype correlation in a large family. Am J Med 101:635–641
25. Mulligan LM, Marsh DJ, Robinson BG, Schuffenecker I, Zedenius J, Lips CJ, Gager RF, Takai SI, Noll WW, Fink M (1995) Genotype-phenotype correlation in multiple endocrine neoplasia type 2: report of the International RET Mutation Consortium. J Intern Med 238:343–346
26. O'Riordian D, O'Brien T, Crotty TB, Garib H, Grant CS, Heerden JA van (1995) Multiple endocrine neoplasia type 2b: more than an endocrine disorder. Surgery 118:936–942
27. Pacini F, Fontanelli M, Fugazzola L, Elisei R, Romei C, Di Coscio G, Miccoli P, Pinchera A (1994) Routine measurement of serum calcitonin in nodular thyroid diseases allows the preoperative diagnosis of unsuspected sporadic medullary thyroid carcinoma. J Clin Endocrinol Metab 78:826–829
28. Raue F (1998) German medullary thyroid carcinoma/multiple endocrine neoplasia registry. Langenbecks Arch Surg 383:334–336
29. Raue F, Grauer A (1994) Determination of tumor markers in diagnosis and follow-up of patients with medullary thyroid carcinoma. Exp Clin Endocrinol 102 [Suppl 2]:67–73
30. Raue F, Kotzerke J, Reinwein D, Schröder S, Röher HD, Deckart H, Höfer R, Ritter M, Seif F, Buhr HJ, Beyer J, Schober O, Becker W, Neumann H, Calvi J, Winter J, Vogt H, and the German Medullary Thyroid Carcinoma Study Group (1993) Prognostic factors in medullary thyroid carcinoma: evaluation of 741 patients from the German medullary thyroid carcinoma register. Clin Invest 71:7–12
31. Raue F, Frank-Raue K, Grauer A (1994) Multiple endocrine neoplasia type 2, clinical features and screening. Endocrinol Metab Clin North Am 23:137–156
32. Raue F, Kraimps JL, Dralle H, Cougard P, Proye C, Frilling A, Limbert E, LLenas LF, Niederle B (1995) Primary hyperparathyroidism in multiple endocrine neoplasia type 2A. J Intern Med 238:369–373
33. Rieu M, Lame M-C, Richard A, Lissak B, Sambort B, Vuong-Ngoc P, Berrod J-L, Fombeur J-P (1995) Prevalence of sporadic medullary thyroid carcinoma: the importance of routine measurement of serum calcitonin in the diagnostic evaluation of thyroid nodules. Clin Endocrinol 42:453–460
34. Russo D, Chiefari E, Meringolo D, Bianchi D, Bellanova B, Filetti S (1997) A case of metastatic medullary thyroid carcinoma: early identification before surgery of an RET proto-

oncogene somatic mutation in fine needle aspirate specimens. J Clin Endocrinol Metab 82:3378–3382
35. Santoro M, Carlomagno F, Romano A, et al. (1995) Activation of RET as a dominant transforming gene by germline mutations of MEN 2A and MEN 2B. Science 267:381–383
36. Schilling T, Bürck J, Sinn H, Clemens A, Otto H, Höppner W, Herfarth C, Ziegler R, Schwab M, Raue F (2001) Prognostic value of codon 918 (ATG-ACG) RET protooncogene mutations in sporadic medullary thyroid carcinoma. Int J Cancer 95:62--66
37. Schröder S, Holl K, Padberg BC (1992) Pathology of sporadic and hereditary medullary thyroid carcinoma. Rec Res Cancer Res 125:19–45
38. Scopsi L, Sampietro G, Boracchi P, Del Bo R, Gullo M, Placucci M, Pilotti S (1996) Multivariate analysis of prognostic factors in sporadic medullary carcinoma of the thyroid. Cancer 78:2173–2183
39. Smith DP, Houghton C, Ponder BA (1997) Germline mutation of RET codon 883 in two cases of de novo MEN 2B. Oncogene 15:1213–1217
40. Vasen, HF, van der Feltz M, Raue F, Nieuwenhuyzen Kruseman A, Koppeschaar HPF, Pieters G, Seif f J, Blum WF, Lips CJM (1992) The natural course of multiple endocrine neoplasia type 2 b. Arch Intern Med 152:1250–1252
41. Vierhapper H, Raber W, Bieglmayer C, Kaserer K, Weinhäusl A, Niederle B (1997) Routine measurement of plasma calcitonin in nodular thyroid diseases. J Clin Endocrinol Metab 82:1589–1593
42. Wohllk N, Cote GJ, Bugalho MMJ, Ordonez N, Evans DB, Goepfert H, Khorana S, Schultz P, Richards S, Gagel RS (1996) Relevance of RET proto-oncogene mutations in sporadic medullary thyroid carcinoma. J Clin Endorinol Metab 81:3740–3745
43. Zedenius J, Wallin G, Hamberger B, Nordenskjöld M, Weber G, Larsson C (1994) Somatic and MEN 2A de novo mutations identified in the RET proto-oncogene by screening of sporadic MTC's. Hum Mol Genet 3:1259–1262
44. Zedenius J, Larsson C, Bergholm U, Bovée J, Svensson A, Hallergren B, Grimelius L, Bäckdahl M, Weber G, Wallin G (1995) Mutations of codon 918 in the RET proto-oncogene correlate to poor prognosis in sporadic medullary thyroid carcinoma. J Clin Endocrind Metab 80:3088–3090

Chapter 18

Imaging in Medullary Thyroid Cancer 18

T.M. Behr and W. Becker

18.1 Introduction

Medullary thyroid cancer (MTC) results from malignant de-differentiation of the parafollicular cells ("C cells") in the thyroid [2]. It was recognized in 1959 by Hazard as a clinicopathological entity that is different from other forms of differentiated thyroid cancer [17], originating from the iodine-processing thyrocytes. Over the subsequent decade, investigators identified and described the parafollicular C cell, which produces calcitonin, which is involved in the regulation of calcium homeostasis and bone metabolism [13]. In 1966 and 1967, Williams suggested that MTC arises from this C cell population [38]. This hypothesis could be confirmed by several subsequent investigators who documented elevated serum calcitonin levels in MTC patients. In the 1970s, Wells and co-workers established a provocative test, the pentagastrin stimulation test, which rendered calcitonin one of the most sensitive and specific tumor markers in oncology [37].

MTC accounts for between 3% and 12% of all thyroid cancers [2]. Genetic studies in the 1980s and 1990s demonstrated that it does occur in distinct familial syndromes. Whereas 60%–80% of all MTC cases are sporadic, 20%–40% were demonstrated to be associated with mutations in the *RET* proto-oncogene (either as isolated MTC or in the context of a hereditary multiple endocrine neoplasia [MEN] syndrome) [1, 2, 27].

Embryologically, the parafollicular C cells arise from the neural crest and, thus, are identified as APUD cells with a high content of chromogranin and neuron-specific enolase. C cells secrete a variety of proteins and peptides, including the characteristic calcitonin, but also ACTH, serotonin, prostaglandins, vasoactive intestinal peptide (VIP), somatostatin, and a variety of other endocrine substances [2, 38]. Malignant C cells additionally secrete procalcitonin, which precipitates as stromal amyloid around the tumor cells. An extraordinarily high percentage of MTCs express and secrete high amounts of carcinoembryonic antigen, and occasionally also CA 19-9 [2, 28, 36].

Since the C cells are located primarily in the upper and middle thirds of the thyroid gland, with a particular concentration laterally and posteriorly, MTC primary tumors are usually found in this location (cf. Fig. 18.1). This has also important implications for the lymphatic drainage and for the location of lymph node metastases (see below; cf. Fig. 18.7c).

The 5-year survival of MTC patients is, at approximately 70% (10-year survival rates are approximately 30%), clearly worse than the survival rates of patients with other forms of differentiated thyroid tumors [2, 12, 34]. One of the major reasons is probably the fact that, with the exception of anecdotically reported mixed medullary/follicular thyroid cancers [23, 26], MTCs do not take up and do not concentrate radioiodine. This is the reason why, in contrast to the outstanding role of radioiodine in the staging, follow-up, and therapy of other forms of differentiated thyroid cancer, it is more or less useless in MTC patients [2].

Frequently, MTC remains occult or only slowly progressive for many years. It is diagnosed incidentally in a multinodular goiter or, occasionally, after a long diagnostic odyssey in patients with persistent and therapy-refractory diarrhea [19]. Frequently, postsurgically persisting tumor marker levels indicate the presence of metastatic disease, although imaging is unable to identify the responsible lesions ("occult disease"). Usually, even metastatic MTC remains clinically inapparent for many years, before eventually changing into an accelerated, more rapidly metastasizing form with endocrine symptomatology which may be hard to influence therapeutically. Therefore, the management of patients with MTC encounters three distinct clinical scenarios: (a) diagnosing and identifying the primary tumor, (b) identifying responsible lesions in patients with persistently elevated tumor marker levels following surgery (occult disease), and (c) staging of the manifest metastatic situation. This chapter intends to critically review the currently available radiological imaging modalities which can be used for primary staging or restaging of MTC patients in these different clinical settings.

18.2 Diagnosis and Localization of the Medullary Thyroid Primary Tumor; Presurgical Staging

Since MTCs cause symptoms only in very advanced tumor stages, most of them are diagnosed incidentally. Usually, MTC primaries appear as scintigraphically cold, sonographically hypodense nodules (Fig. 18.1). With respect to these sonographic and scintigraphic features, there is no difference between medullary and other forms of thyroid malignancies. For differentiation, fine-needle aspiration cytology may help to establish the diagnosis preoperatively (Fig. 18.1c, d). Also serum calcitonin determination may be helpful in differential diagnosis.

Fig. 18.1 a–d MTC in a 59-year-old woman with a history of colorectal cancer and rising serum CEA levels (7.5 ng/ml at the time of presentation). **a** Ultrasonography of the neck shows a solid, hypoechoic nodule in the right lobe of the thyroid (*lower panel*), corresponding to a scintigraphically cold area in the pertechnetate scan (*upper panel*)

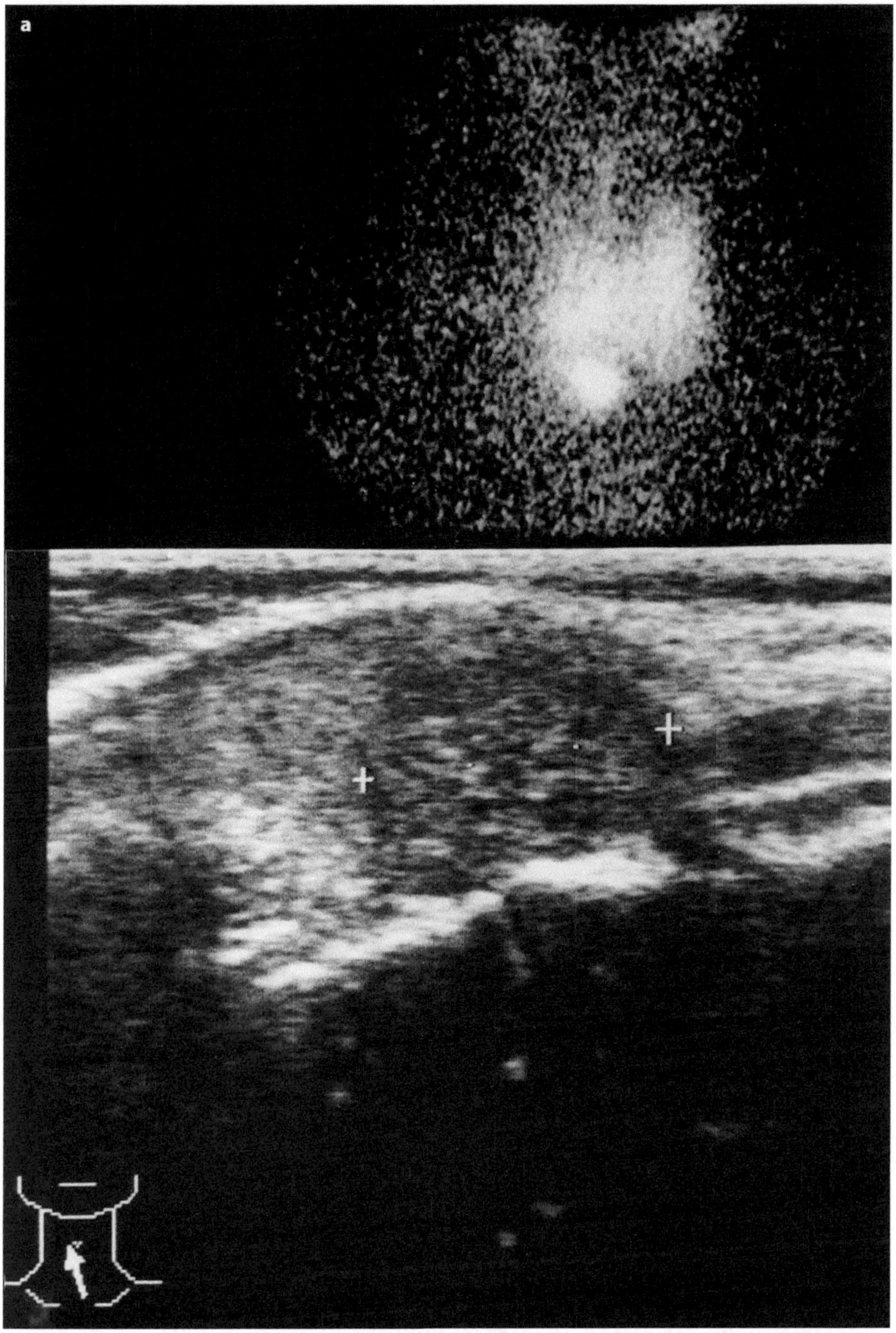
a

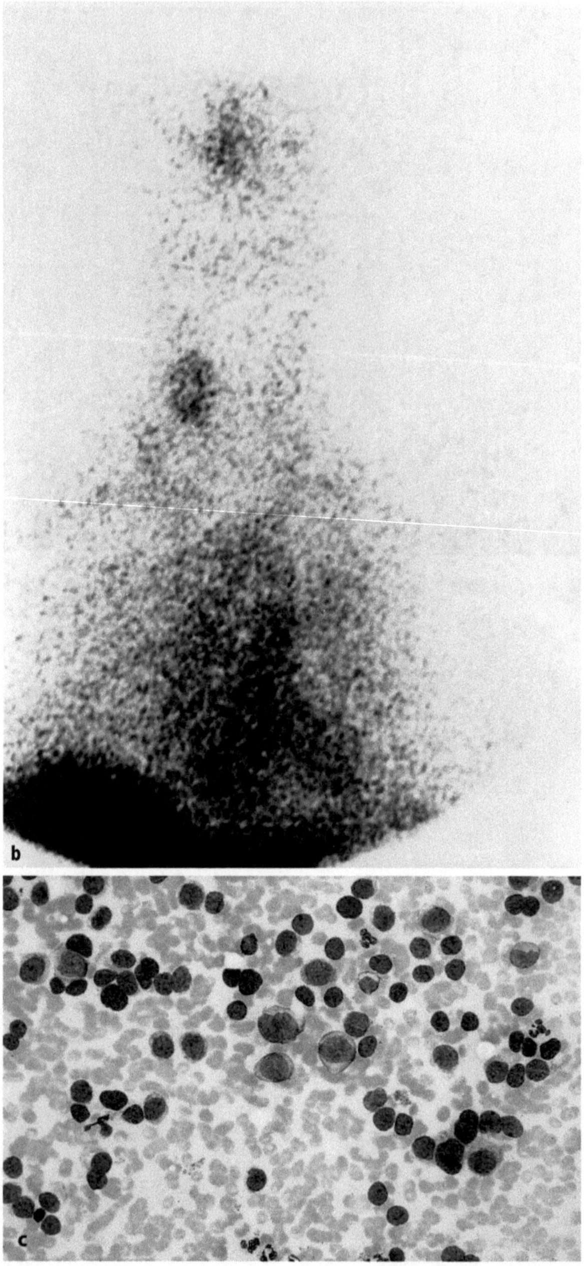

Fig. 18.1 b–c **b** Immunoscintigraphy with a ^{99m}Tc-labeled anti-CEA antibody, clone BW431/26, shows intense antibody accumulation in this nodule in the right lobe of the thyroid. **c** Fine-needle aspiration cytology

Interestingly, Pacini and co-workers published a study in 1994, investigating whether routine measurement of serum calcitonin could improve the preoperative diagnosis of sporadic MTC [29]. Almost 1,500 consecutive patients,

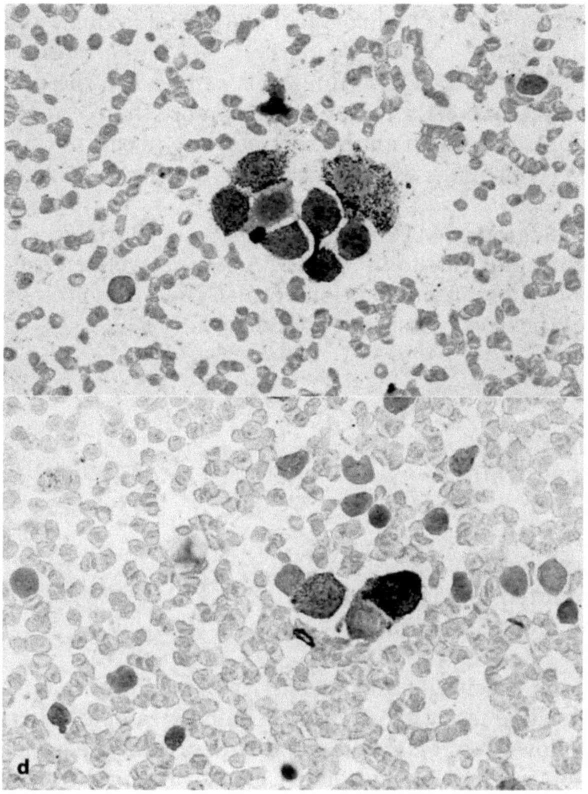

Fig. 18.1 d Immunohistochemical staining show calcitonin (*upper panel*) and chromo-granin-A (*lower panel*) expressing cells, proving their neuroendocrine origin, which is in accordance with a primary MTC

presenting for nodular thyroid disease during 1 year, were submitted to serum calcitonin determination and fine-needle aspiration cytology. The clinical diagnosis was nontoxic nodular goiter in 86% of these patients, toxic multinodular goiter in 5%, autonomously functioning thyroid nodule in another 5%, and autoimmune thyroid disease with nodules in the remaining 4%. As controls, almost 200 patients with nonnodular thyroid disease and more than 30 normal subjects were included. Patients with fine-needle biopsy suspicious of any kind of thyroid carcinoma and patients with elevated basal and pentagastrin-stimulated serum calcitonin, regardless of the results of biopsy, were submitted to surgery. Eight (0.6%) patients (seven with nontoxic nodular goiter and one with thyroid autonomy) had elevated basal serum calcitonin levels. The pentagastrin test was abnormal in all of them. Fine-needle biopsy was suggestive of MTC in two, thyroid carcinoma in one, and benign nodule in three, and was inadequate in two. By histology, immunohistochemistry, and Northern blot analysis of total tumor RNAs, MTC was confirmed in all patients, including the one with thyroid autonomy, who had the association of microfollicular adenoma and a small MTC in the same lobe. The authors concluded that these results indicate that serum calcitonin measurement is useful for the screening of sporadic MTC in patients with thyroid nodules. The prevalence of MTC, diagnosed by serum calcitonin measurement, was surprisingly high: 0.6% of all thyroid nodules and 16% of all thyroid carcinomas [29].

Occasionally, pathologically elevated CEA serum levels can lead to the diagnosis of MTC as well. In no less than eight out of 235 (i.e., more than 3%) colorectal cancer patients who presented with an unexplained rise in serum CEA levels, we found an occult MTC primary as the reason for the tumor marker elevations (Fig. 18.1) [5].

Summarizing, presurgical staging of MTC includes, besides a thorough clinical examination, thyroid hormone, calcitonin, and CEA serum level determinations and ultrasonography of the neck, and optionally also chest radiography and computed tomography of the neck, chest, and abdomen.

18.3 Imaging and Disease Localization in the Follow-up of Patients with MTC

18.3.1 Conventional Radiological Techniques (Ultrasonography, X-ray, Computed Tomography, Magnetic Resonance Imaging, Bone Scanning)

Due to the extraordinarily high sensitivity and specificity of calcitonin, especially in the context of provocative tests, regular serum calcitonin determinations play a key role in the follow-up of MTC patients. Other peptides (e.g., somatostatin) and tumor markers, with the exception of CEA, have been shown to be much less sensitive, and thus do not play a relevant clinical role. Frequently, elevated calcitonin levels indicate the persistence or presence of malignant C cells even though all conventional imaging procedures [ultrasonography, X-ray, computed tomography (CT), magnetic resonance imaging (MRI)] fail to localize responsible lesions ("occult disease," cf. Fig. 18.2). This is mainly due to the fact that the total tumor mass is very small, with diffuse (micro-)metastatic spread to the lung, liver, or bone marrow, and with individual lesions being too small to be detectable by conventional radiological methods [2, 6].

Local recurrences and cervical lymph node metastases are usually detectable by ultrasonography, whereas in many cases, mediastinal and hilar lymph node metastases correspond to normally sized lymph nodes, escaping radiological diagnosis (the sometimes encountered calcifications are ambiguous, allowing for several differential diagnoses) (Fig. 18.2). Pulmonary lymphangiosis frequently escapes radiological diagnosis, as is the case in other forms of differentiated thyroid cancer, so that only biopsy is able to clearly prove its presence. In bone scanning, due to their low metabolic activity, bone metastases are difficult to distinguish from other, nonneoplastic processes, such as degenerative changes [2, 6]. Often, liver metastases are hypervascular so that they are solely visualized by CT without intravenous contrast agent, becoming isointense to the normal liver parenchyma after i.v. injection of contrast dye (Fig. 18.3a) [20].

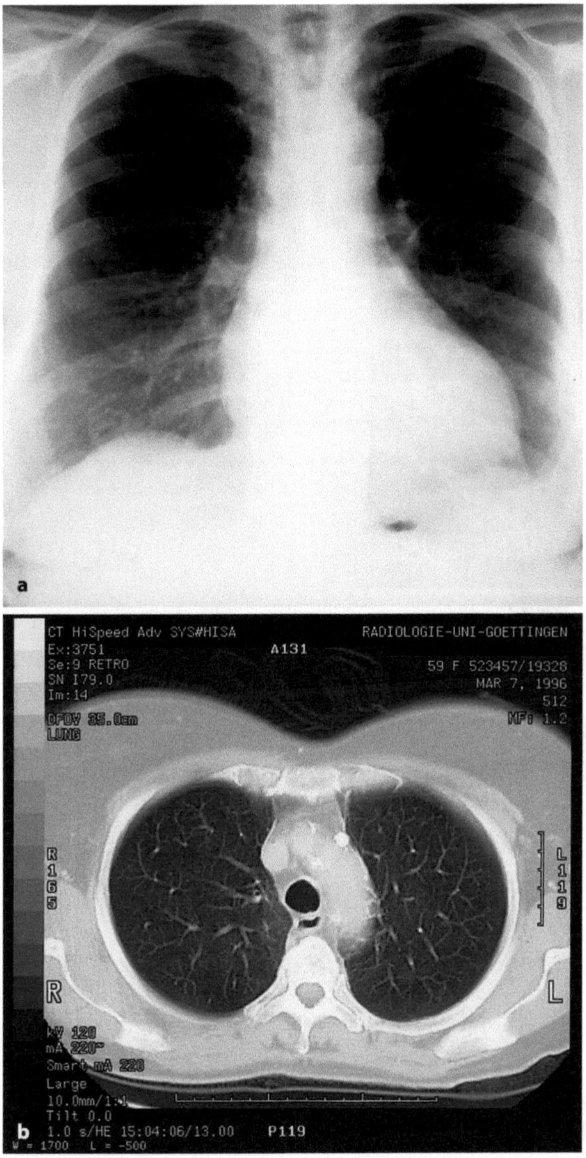

Fig. 18.2 a–d Metastatic involvement of mediastinal lymph nodes in a woman with occult metastatic MTC. Whereas the chest radiograph (**a**) is without pathological findings and a CT scan of the chest (**b**) merely shows some nonspecific calcified lymph nodes, somatostatin receptor scintigraphy (**c**) shows typical bilateral lymph node involvement ("chimney sign"). By contrast, FDG-PET (**d**) is false-negative

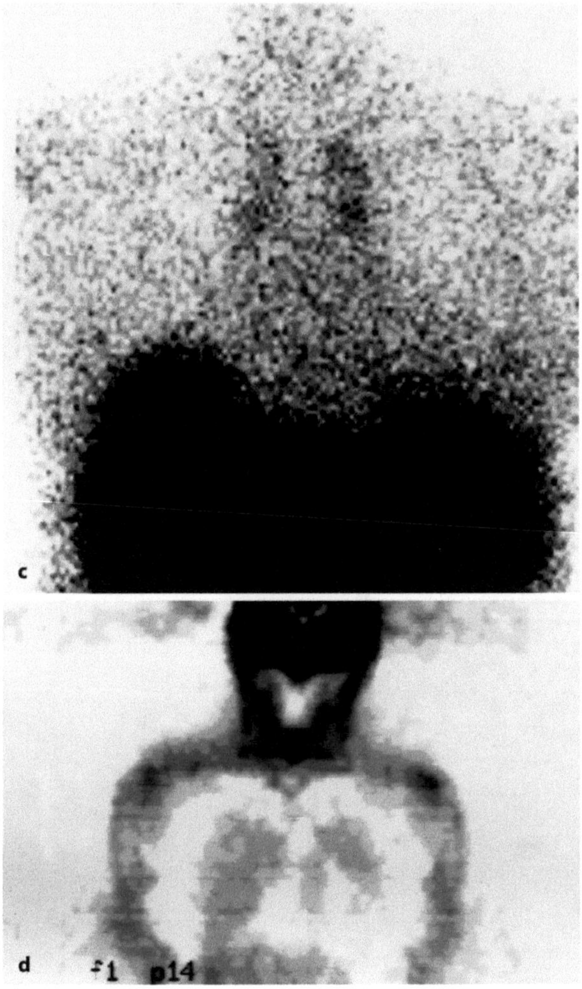

Fig. 18.2 c–d.

18.3.2 Traditional Scintigraphic Techniques [^{201}Tl Chloride, ^{99m}Tc-(V)-DMSA, $^{123/131}$I-MIBG, etc.]

In contrast to other forms of differentiated thyroid cancer, MTC usually does not concentrate radioiodine, with the very rare exception of mixed medullary follicular carcinomas [23, 26]. There is a multitude of studies on the diagnostic sensitivities and accuracies of a range of more or less non-MTC-specific tumor-seeking radiopharmaceuticals, such as ^{201}Tl chloride (uptake as K^+ analog via Na^+/K^+-ATPase) [2], ^{99m}Tc-labeled phosphonates (specific uptake in osteoblastic bone lesions or in calcifications of soft tissue metastases) [2], ^{67}Ga citrate [transchelation of gallium as iron analog into transferrin, uptake via CD71 (transferrin receptors)] or

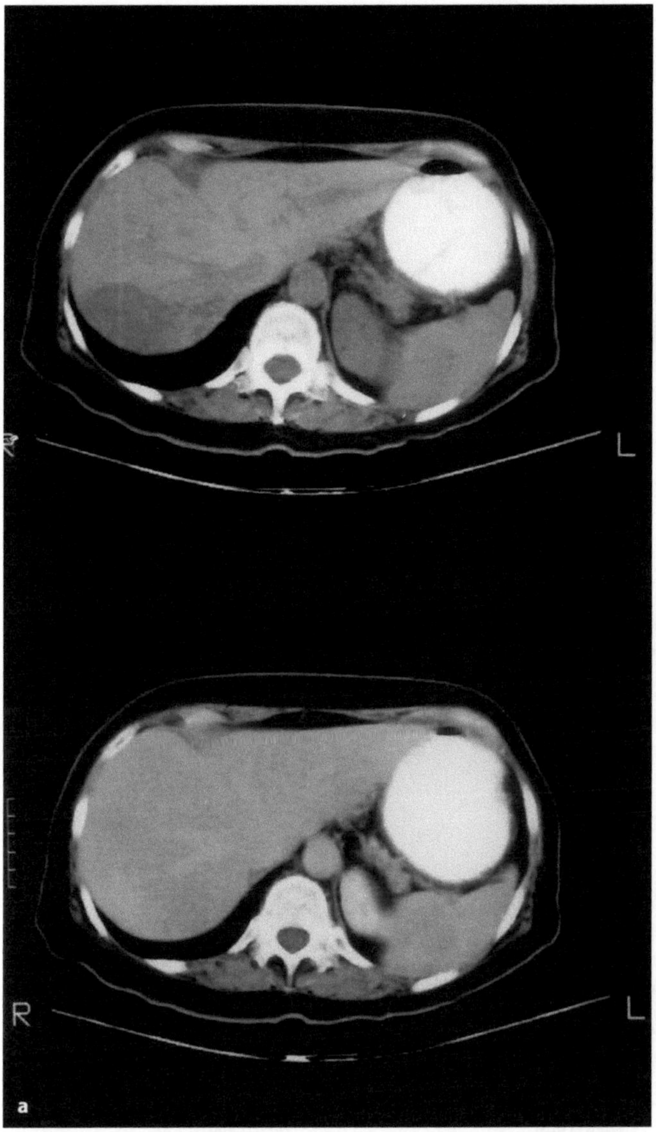

Fig. 18.3 a–c Imaging and therapeutic response with ^{131}I-labeled anti-CEA antibodies in a 72-year-old woman with advanced metastatic MTC (local recurrence and lung, pleural, and liver metastases). **a** Hypervascular liver metastasis is visible as hypodense lesions in the plain CT scan (*upper panel*) but becomes isointense to the normal liver parenchyma, and thus invisible, in the contrast-enhanced CT scan (*lower panel*)

^{99m}Tc-(V)-dimercaptosuccinic acid (DMSA) [18]. ^{123}I- or ^{131}I-metaiodobenzylguanidine ($^{123/131}$I-MIBG) is chemically related to the anti-sympathomimetic drug guanethidine, which is taken up by neuroendocrine cells via the norepinephrine

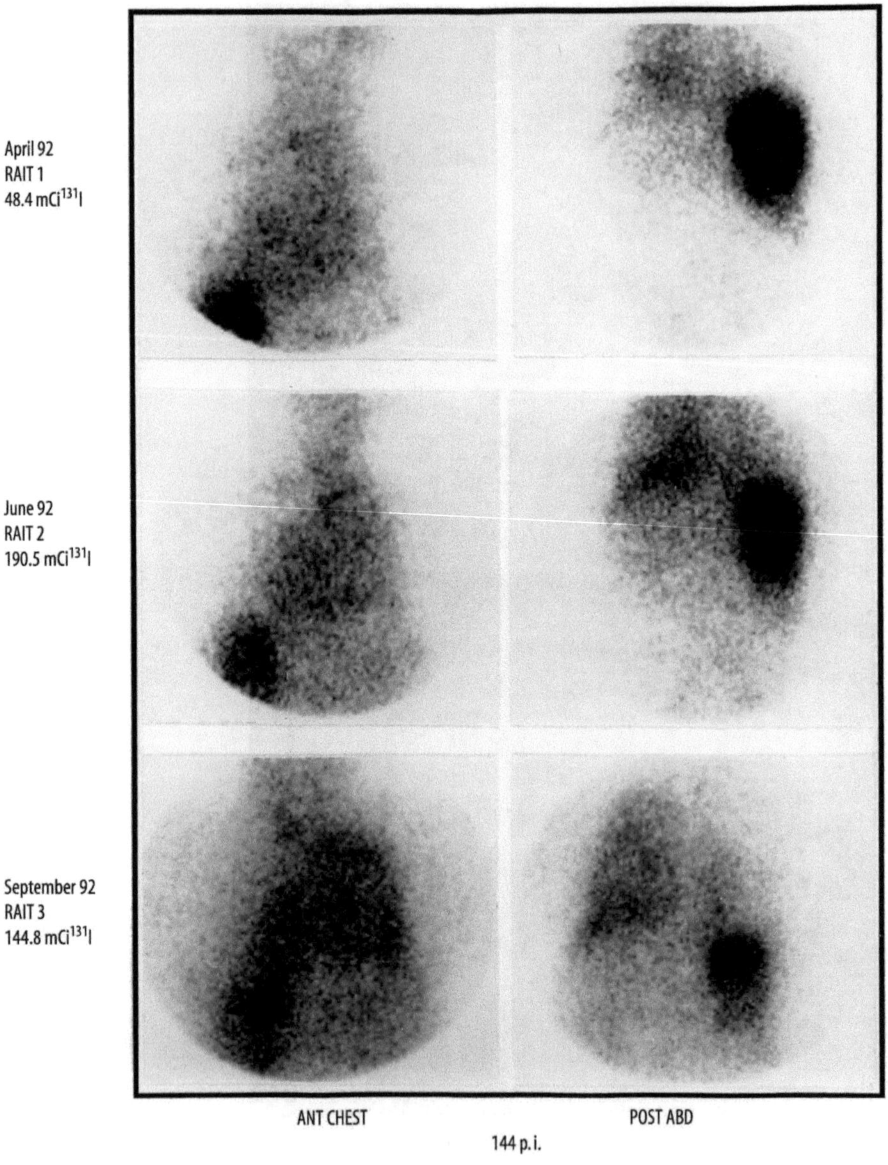

Fig. 18.3 b Tumor targeting in the same patient on the occasion of three therapy injections (144 h p.i. each)

reuptake mechanism. MIBG is stored intracellularly in chromaffin granules [3]. However, in contrast to pheochromocytoma and neuroblastoma, its uptake is rather low in MTC. Summarizing, all these scintigraphic techniques are more or less nonspecific and have yielded variable results clinically.

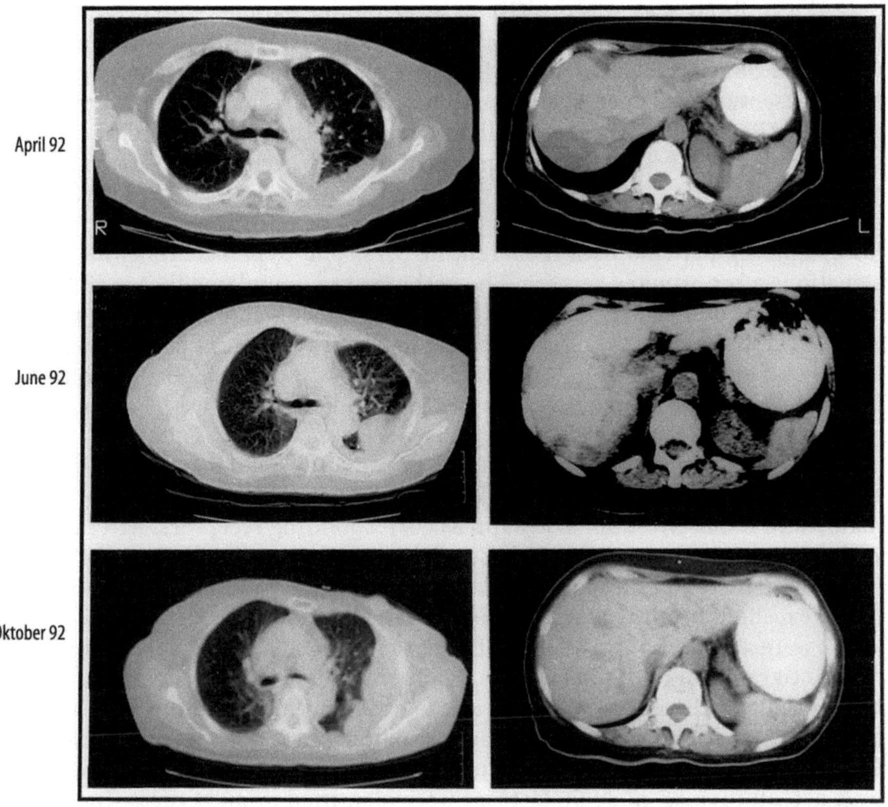

Fig. 18.3 c The large hyperperfused liver metastasis disappeared completely 1 month after the third therapy injection, having received a total dose of approximately 65 Gy, whereas the pleural effusion is progressing (thus representing a mixed response)

18.3.3 Modern Nuclear Medical Techniques (Anti-CEA Immunoscintigraphy, Somatostatin Receptor Scintigraphy, Positron Emission Tomography)

After some disappointing results of immunoscintigraphy [30], more modern approaches with high-affinity antibodies were able to show excellent results in manifest as well as occult metastatic disease. Juweid et al. reported on 26 patients with known or occult MTC who were studied with radiolabeled anti-CEA antibodies [20, 22]. The targeting results of ^{99m}Tc-, ^{123}I-, and ^{131}I-labeled anti-CEA antibodies indicated that all these reagents were capable of detecting established and occult MTC. The sensitivity for detection of known sites of disease ranged from 76% to 100% for the various anti-CEA antibodies used, when compared with CT, MRI, bone scan, or other imaging modalities [20–22]. Moreover, the antibody scan was positive in seven of nine patients with occult disease (patients with negative conventional imaging studies, but who had elevated calcitonin and/or CEA levels). Three of these seven patients underwent surgery and the disease was confirmed by histopathology in all three. The authors concluded that anti-CEA antibodies are excellent agents for imaging recurrent, residual, or metastatic MTC. The high lesion sensitivity in patients with known lesions, combined with the ability to detect disease, may make these agents ideal for staging patients, for monitoring disease pretherapy or posttherapy, and especially for evaluating patients with recurrent or persistent hypercalcitonemia or CEA elevations after primary surgery. The authors even postulated that radiolabeled anti-CEA antibodies may achieve a role in diagnosing and monitoring patients with MTC similar to that of radioiodine in the evaluation of patients with differentiated thyroid cancer. Initially promising results were also reported by the same authors with the therapeutic use of radiolabeled anti-CEA antibodies (Fig. 18.3) [21].

Enthusiastic hopes accompanied the introduction of somatostatin receptor scintigraphy [15, 16]. In vitro data had shown that MTCs not only produce somatostatin themselves, but also express corresponding receptors. After initially very optimistic reports indicating sensitivities of more than 90% in known as well as occult MTC, subsequent studies were unable to reproduce these apparently excellent results in larger series of patients.

We were able to show in a series of almost 30 patients that somatostatin receptor scintigraphy of occult MTC has a good sensitivity which is superior to that of conventional radiological methods in the neck and mediastinum (cf. Figs. 18.2 and 18.4). We found a typical metastatic pattern: in patients with persistently elevated calcitonin levels in the immediate postsurgical period, cervical or supraclavicular lymph node metastases were identified in most cases. In patients with postsurgically normalized, but slowly increasing calcitonin levels, bilateral "chimney-shaped" mediastinal lymph node involvement was found, for which we coined the term "chimney-sign" (Figs. 18.2, 18.5 and 18.6) [6, 7].

In this context, we recently compared the sensitivity and diagnostic accuracy of immunoscintigraphy with anti-CEA antibodies and somatostatin analogs for the detection of recurrent or metastatic MTC [4, 6]. Additionally, we tried to assess whether there may be correlations between the scintigraphic behavior in both imaging modalities and the prognosis [4, 6]. A total of 26 patients with MTC were examined. Ten suffered from known disease, 14 from occult metastatic MTC, and two patients were free of disease at the time of presentation (as indicated by normal serum calcitonin after pentagastrin stimulation). All patients underwent conventional radiological evaluation (ultrasonography, CT, MRI) and/or biopsy within 4 weeks. Additional imaging was performed with ^{99m}Tc-(V)-DMSA, ^{123}I-MIBG, ^{201}Tl chloride, ^{99m}Tc-methylene diphosphonate (MDP), and/or ^{18}F-fluorodeoxyglucose positron emission tomography (FDG-PET). Clinical follow-up for up to 10 years was obtained in all cases.

All patients with established disease had elevated plasma CEA (range 6.8–345 ng/ml) and calcitonin levels (92–11,497 pg/ml), whereas in 9/14 occult cases, CEA levels were, at ≤5 ng/ml, normal (overall range in occult disease patients: CEA 0.6–829 ng/ml; calcitonin 72–2,920 pg/ml). In patients with known

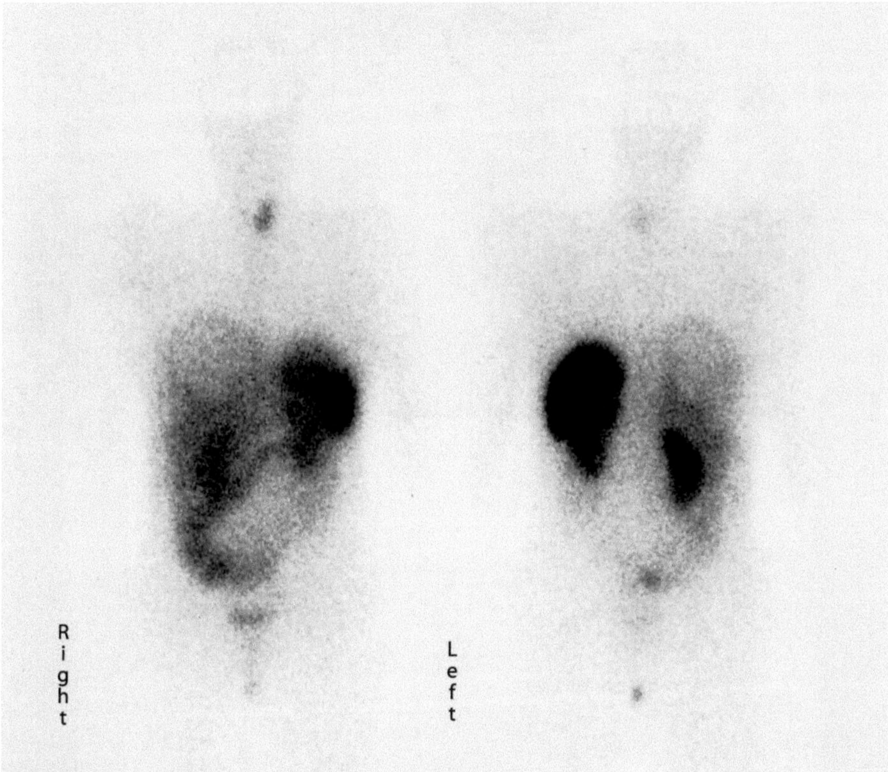

Fig. 18.4 Thirty-year-old woman with primary and metastatic MTC. Somatostatin receptor scintigraphy shows good ^{111}In-DTPA-octreotide uptake in the primary tumor in the left lobe of the thyroid, but no somatostatin receptor expression in a large liver metastasis (scan at 24 h p.i.). This is in accordance with the known loss of somatostatin receptor expression in dedifferentiating MTC

disease, the overall lesion-based sensitivity was 86% for anti-CEA immunoscintigraphy. In contrast, octreotide was unable to target any tumor in patients with rapidly progressing disease, or to detect distant metastases (resulting in an overall sensitivity of only 47%) (Figs. 18.4 and 18.6). However, in all patients with occult MTC, anti-CEA monoclonal antibodies as well as octreotide were able to localize at least one lesion (patient-based sensitivity virtually 100%). In patients with persistent hypercalcitoninemia following surgery, cervical lymph node metastases were identified as the most frequent site of disease, whereas in patients with occult and slowly progressing disease several years after primary surgery, immunoscintigraphy and octreotide showed bilateral involvement of mediastinal lymph nodes ("chimney sign") [7] (Figs. 18.2, 18.5 and 18.6); however, tumor/nontumor ratios were usually higher with octreotide in these cases. With anti-CEA antibodies, highest tumor/nontumor ratios were observed in clinically aggressive, rapidly progressing disease.

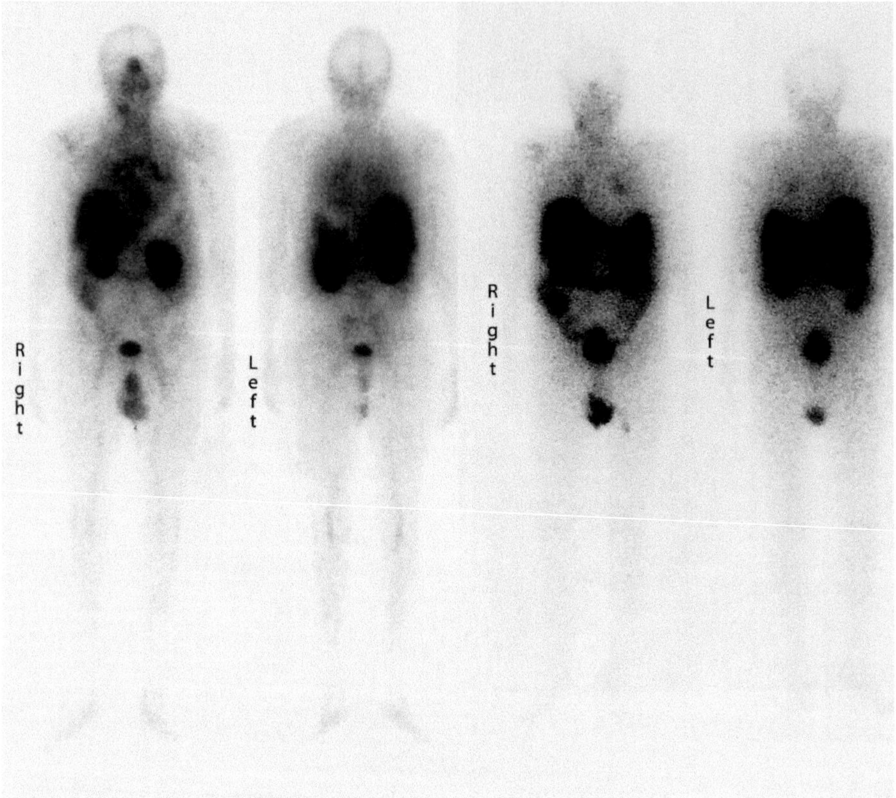

Fig. 18.5 Bilateral mediastinal lymph node involvement ("chimney sign") in a patient with the primary tumor in situ in the upper parts of the right lobe of the thyroid [*left panel*: anti-CEA immunoscintigraphy with ^{99m}Tc-labeled Fab' fragments, clone NP-4 (CEAScan); *right panel*: ^{111}In-DTPA-octreotide somatostatin receptor scintigraphy; both scans at 24 h p.i.]

We concluded from these data that for the detection of occult MTC, anti-CEA immunoscintigraphy and octreotide seem to have a sensitivity which is superior to conventional diagnostic modalities, especially when used in combination. However, better detectability with anti-CEA antibodies (probably corresponding to a higher tissue CEA expression) seems to be associated with more aggressive forms of MTC, whereas somatostatin receptor expression at normal plasma CEA levels and weaker antibody targeting is associated with a more benign clinical course [4, 6]. These data are in good accordance with the study of Busnardo et al. [14], who showed rising CEA and, at the same time, constant or decreasing serum calcitonin levels to be associated with a bad prognosis. These data also confirm the data of Mendelsohn et al. [25], who analyzed the relationship of tissue CEA and calcitonin expression to tumor virulence immunohistochemically; these authors found a clear increase in CEA and decrease in calcitonin expression with progressing dedifferentiation. Finally, our

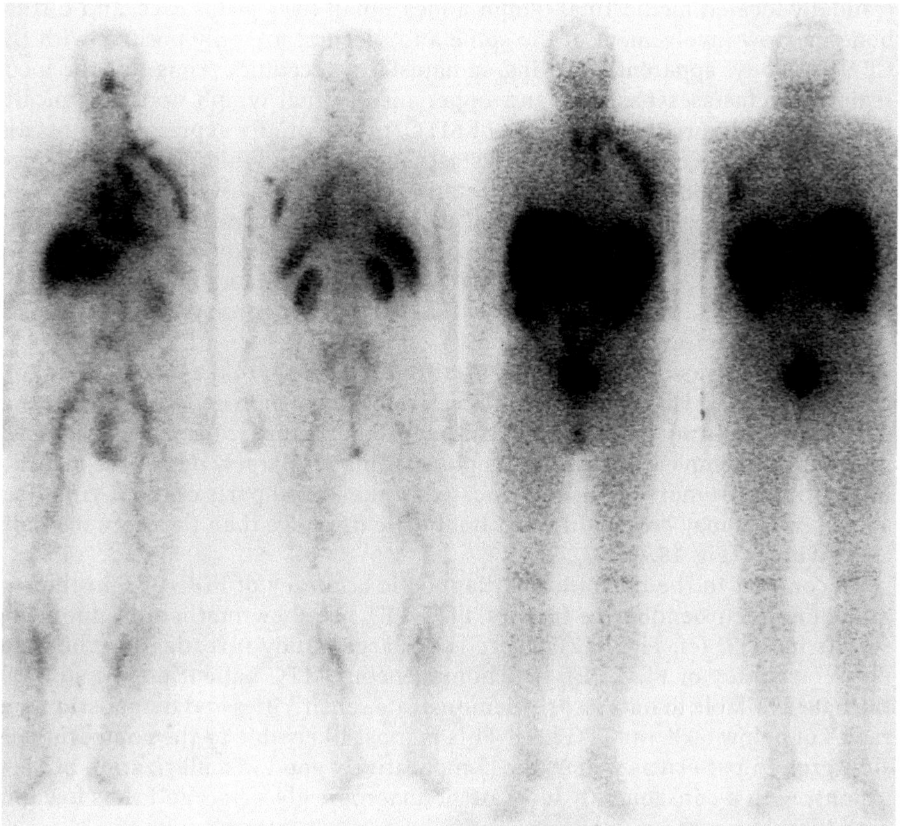

Fig. 18.6 Whole-body scans of a 67-year-old male with primary and metastatic MTC (*left panel*: ^{99m}Tc-anti-CEA IgG$_1$, clone BW431/26; *right panel*: ^{111}In-DTPA-octreotide; both scans at 24 h p.i.). Again, the primary tumor (in the cranial parts of the left lobe of the thyroid) seems to express both CEA and somatostatin receptors, as is the case for left supraclavicular and axillary lymph nodes, whereas more distant metastases (caudally located mediastinal lymph nodes, small liver metastases, and diffuse bone marrow involvement of the spine and sacrum) are merely positive with the CEA antibody, apparently lacking somatostatin receptors as a sign of their dedifferentiation

scintigraphic in vivo findings confirm in vivo the receptor autoradiographic in vitro data of Reubi et al. [32], who demonstrated the loss of somatostatin receptor expression in dedifferentiated MTC.

These scintigraphic findings even hold true within the same patient. As an illustration, Fig. 18.6 shows whole-body scans of a 67-year-old male with primary and metastatic MTC. The primary tumor (in the cranial parts of the left lobe of the thyroid) seems to express both CEA and somatostatin receptors, as is the case for left supraclavicular and axillary lymph nodes. In contrast, the chimney-shaped [7] cranial mediastinal lymph node involvement exhibits much stronger somatostatin receptor than CEA expression, whereas more distant metastases (caudally located mediastinal lymph nodes, small liver metastases, and diffuse bone marrow involvement of the spine and sacrum) are only positive with the CEA antibody, apparently lacking somatostatin receptors. Thus: (a) the locoregional metastases (cervical and upper mediastinal lymph nodes), typically found in slowly progressing forms of MTC, preferentially express somatostatin receptors; (b) the more distant metastases (axillary and midmediastinal lymph nodes) express both CEA and somatostatin receptors; (c) lesions which originate from hematogenous spread and which are typical for aggressive metastatic MTC (liver and bone marrow) exclusively express CEA as a marker of their dedifferentiation [25]. Thus, scintigraphic visualization of MTC allows not only for lesion localization, but also for prediction of the patient's prognosis by means of tissue characterization in vivo [4].

Why, in contrast to other forms of differentiated thyroid cancer, MTC more frequently metastasizes in the more laterally located lymph node areas in the mediastinum, resulting in the typical chimney-shaped appearance in scintigraphic scans, is not completely clear at this point. It may be largely due to the fact that MTC primary tumors are usually located in the lateral parts of the thyroid (see above), which may have a different lymphatic drainage than the more medially located areas (Fig. 18.7).

In contrast to the outstanding diagnostic accuracy of FDG-PET in the staging of nonneuroendocrine tumors, FDG-PET has shown rather disappointing results in MTC (cf. Fig. 18.2). There is no larger study investigating the diagnostic accuracy of FDG-PET in a homogeneous MTC patient population, but the data available to date clearly demonstrate sensitivities and diagnostic accuracies of below 60% in MTC [24]. This is most likely due to the comparatively slow growth pattern as well as the comparatively good vascularization of MTC lesions, with a consequently low rate of anaerobic glycolysis and thus low glucose turnover.

18.4 Future Developments: Will Cholecystokinin-B/ Gastrin Receptor Scintigraphy Allow for More Sensitive Staging of MTC?

The high sensitivity of pentagastrin stimulation in detecting primary or metastatic MTC suggests widespread expression of the corresponding receptor type on human MTC cells [8, 37]. Indeed, autoradiographic studies have demonstrated cholecystokinin (CCK)-B/gastrin receptors not only in over 90% of MTCs, but also in a high percentage of small cell lung cancers [31, 33] and potentially a variety of gastrointestinal adenocarcinomas [35]. In a pilot study, we demonstrated the feasibility of using radiolabeled gastrin-I to target CCK-B receptor expressing tissues in vivo in animals and patients [8]. The aim of our subsequent work was to systematically optimize, in a preclinical model, suitable radioligands for targeting CCK-B receptors in vivo. For this purpose, a variety of CCK/gastrin-related peptides, all having in common the C-terminal CCK-receptor binding tetrapeptide sequence Trp-Met-Asp-PheNH_2 or derivatives thereof, were studied

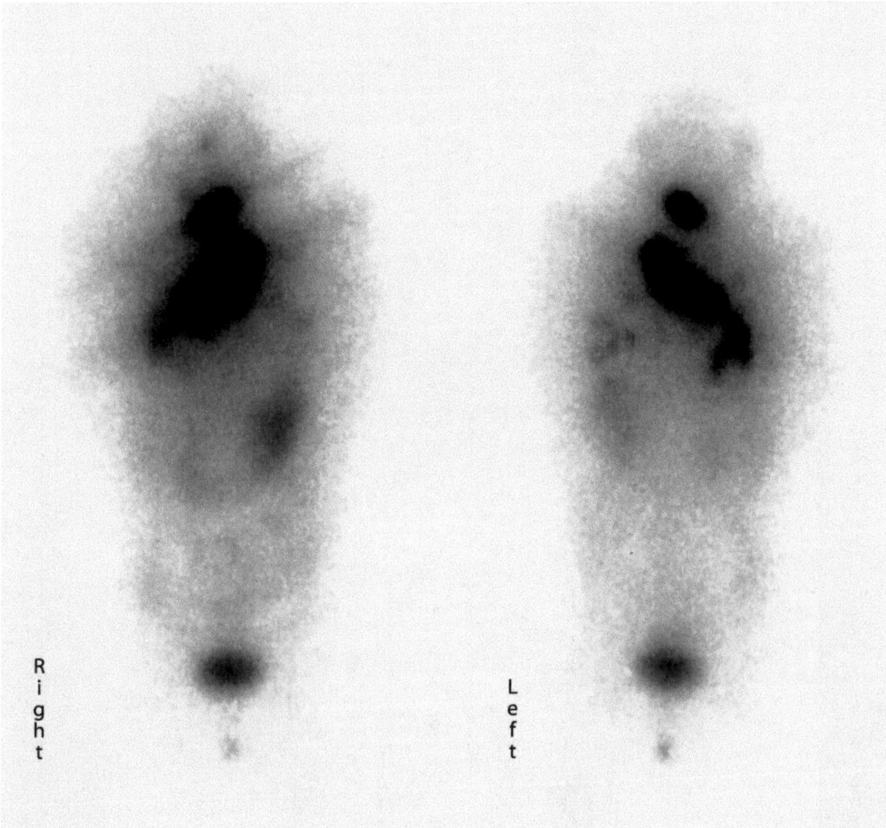

Fig. 18.7 a–c Differences in the lymphatic drainage between medullary and other forms of differentiated thyroid cancer. In papillary (a) as well as follicular (**b**) thyroid cancer (both $Na^{131}I$ posttherapy scans), mediastinal lymph node metastases are more randomly distributed, whereas in MTC (**c**), a typical bilateral lymph node involvement ("chimney sign") is commonly found (cf. Figs. 16.2, 16.5 and 16.6). This most likely reflects the different localization of the primary tumors (MTC is located more laterally than the other histological types; cf. the *hatched area*) and their respective draining lymph nodes, which, in the case of MTC, are localized more laterally in relation to the large vessels in the mediastinum

[9, 10]. They were radioiodinated by the Iodogen or Bolton-Hunter procedures. The peptides tested were members of the gastrin or CCK families, or possessed characteristics of both, which differ by the intramolecular position of a tyrosyl moiety (occurring in native or sulfated form). Their stability and affinity were studied in vitro and in vivo; their biodistribution and therapeutic efficacy were tested in nude mice bearing subcutaneous human MTC xenografts. DTPA derivatives of suitable peptides were synthesized and evaluated, labeled with ^{111}In.

All members of the CCK or gastrin family were stable in serum (with $t_{1/2}$'s of several hours at 37°C); nevertheless, the highest stability was found for those

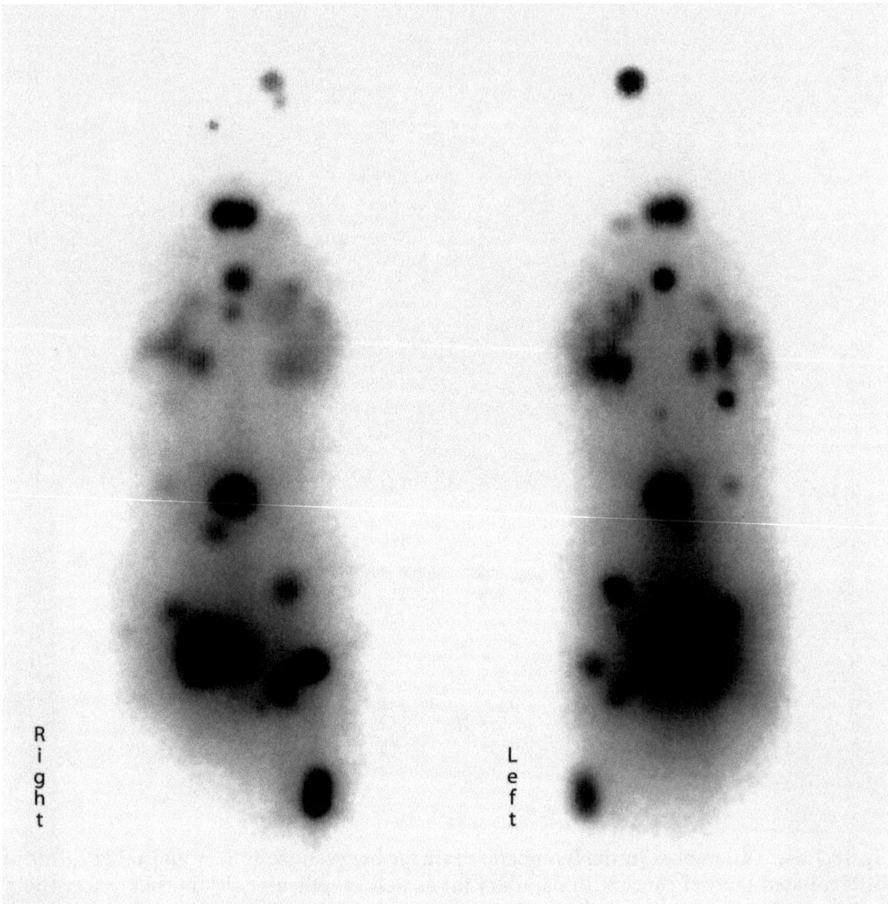

Fig. 18.7 b

peptides which bear N-terminal pGlu residues (e.g., big gastrin, gastrin-I, cerulein, etc.) or D-amino acids [9, 10]. In accordance with their comparatively low affinity, nonsulfated members of the CCK family showed fairly low uptake in the tumor and other CCK-B receptor-expressing tissues (e.g., the stomach). Sulfated CCK derivatives performed significantly better, but additionally displayed a high uptake in normal, CCK-A receptor-expressing tissues (such as the liver/gallbladder, pancreas, and bowel). Best tumor uptake and tumor-to-nontumor ratios were obtained with members of the gastrin family, probably due to their selectivity and affinity for the CCK-B receptor subtype. Pilot therapy experiments in MTC-bearing animals showed significant antitumor efficacy as compared to untreated controls. ^{111}In-labeled DTPA derivatives of minigastrin showed excellent targeting of CCK-B receptor-expressing tissues in animals and a normal human volunteer [9, 10].

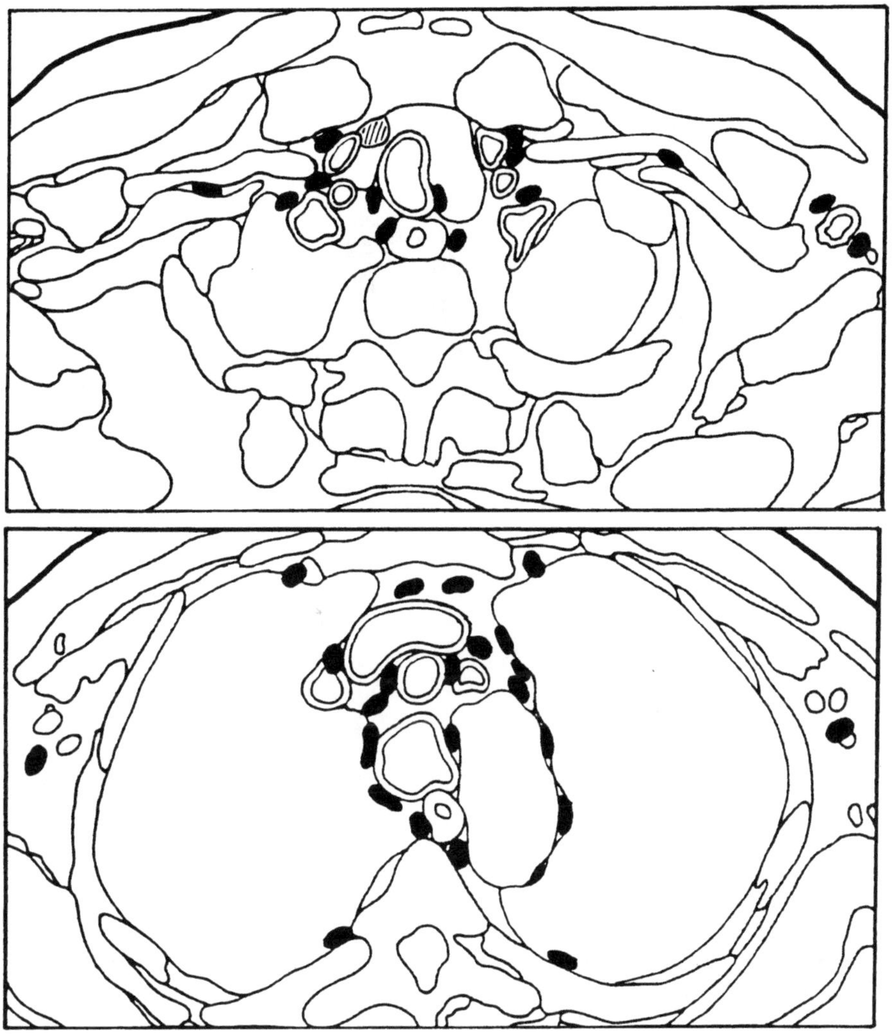

Fig. 18.7 c

These data suggested that CCK/gastrin analogs may be a useful new class of receptor binding peptides for the diagnosis and therapy of CCK-B receptor-expressing tumors, such as MTC or small cell lung cancer. Nonsulfated gastrin derivatives may be preferable due to their CCK-B receptor selectivity, and hence lower accumulation in normal CCK-A receptor-expressing organs.

Subsequently, 35 patients with metastatic MTC were studied [11]. All had undergone ultrasonography, whole-body CT, and MRI, as well as bone scanning and somatostatin receptor scintigraphy. As a result, 19 had known disease, and 16 occult disease. CCK-B receptor scintigraphy was performed with 3–5 mCi of

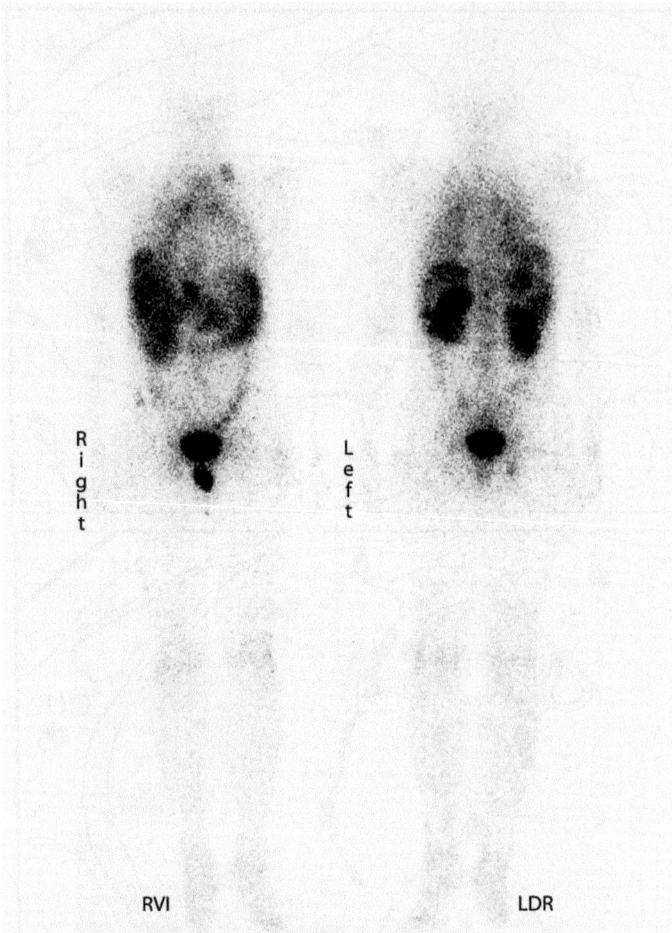

Fig. 18.8 Cholecystokinin-B/gastrin receptor scintigraphy with ^{111}In-labeled DTPA-D-Glu^{1}-minigastrin in a 34-year-old patient with advanced metastatic MTC, showing intense uptake in lymph node, diffuse lung, bone (marrow), and liver metastases. Physiological uptake is confined to the stomach, as the organ with the highest normal CCK-B receptor expression, and the kidneys, as excretory organs

a ^{111}In-labeled DTPA derivative of minigastrin (13 amino acids long; affinity in the n*M* range). Whole-body scans were performed at 10 min and 1, 4, and 24 h, and SPECT at 4 and 24 h p.i. The normal organ uptake of the radiopeptide was confined to the stomach (and to a much lesser extent, the gallbladder) as a result of CCK-B receptor-specific binding, and to the kidneys as excretory organs. No physiological uptake was observed in any other organ, such as the liver or spleen. All tumor manifestations known from conventional imaging were visualized as early as 1 h p.i., with increasing tumor-to-background ratios over time; at least one lesion was detected in 15/16 patients with occult disease (patient-based sensitivity 94%; eight cases surgically confirmed, seven remaining unconfirmed positive). Among them were local recurrences and lymph node, pulmonary, hepatic, splenic, and bone metastases (Fig. 18.8). We concluded that these data suggest that CCK-B receptor ligands are a promising new class of receptor binding peptides for the staging of MTC.

18.5 Conclusion

Imaging of MTC and especially of its (occult) metastatic forms remains a challenge which has not been satisfactorily solved. The new molecular targeting approaches, such as cholecystokinin-B/gastrin receptor binding peptides, offer a novel and promising tool. However, larger clinical studies are warranted before their potential future role can be appreciated more adequately. On the other hand, these molecular targeting approaches may also offer new therapeutic options in this otherwise therapy-resistant cancer type.

References

1. Ambrosch A, Pfützner A, Ponder BAJ, Beyer J, Luley C, Lehnert H (1995) Multiple endokrine Neoplasie Typ 2A – Genetisches Screening bei familiärem Tumorsyndrom. Dtsch Med Wochenschr 120:615–619
2. Becker W, Spiegel W, Reiners C, Börner W (1986) Besonderheiten bei der Nachsorge des C-Zell-Karzinoms. Nuklearmediziner 9:167–181
3. Becker W, Börner W, Reiners C (1989) Tc-99m-(V)-DMSA: the new sensitive and specific radiopharmaceutical for imaging metastases of medullary thyroid carcinomas? Horm Metab Res Suppl 21:38–42
4. Behr TM, Becker W (1999) Metabolic and receptor imaging of metastatic medullary thyroid cancer: does anti-CEA and somatostatin-receptor scintigraphy allow for diagnostic predictions? Eur J Nucl Med 26:70–71
5. Behr TM, Becker W (1999) Erhöhte Serum-CEA-Spiegel als Erstmanifestation eines medullären Schilddrüsenkarzinoms. Dtsch Med Wochenschr 124:303–394
6. Behr TM, Gratz S, Markus PM, Dunn RM, Hüfner M, Schauer A, Fischer M, Munz DL, Becker H, Becker W (1997) Anti-carcinoembryonic antigen antibodies versus somatostatin analogs in the detection of metastatic medullary thyroid carcinoma: are carcinoembryonic antigen and somatostatin receptor expression prognostic factors? Cancer 80:2436–2457
7. Behr TM, Gratz S, Markus PM, Hüfner M, Schauer A, Becker H, Becker W (1997) Enhanced bilateral somatostatin receptor expression in mediastinal lymph nodes ("chimney sign") in occult metastatic medullary thyroid cancer: a typical sign of tumor manifestation? Eur J Nucl Med 24:184–191
8. Behr TM, Jenner N, Radetzky S, Béhé M, Gratz S, Yücekent S, Raue F, Becker W (1998) Targeting of cholecystokinin-B/gastrin receptors in vivo: preclinical and initial clinical evaluation of the diagnostic and therapeutic potential of radiolabeled gastrin. Eur J Nucl Med 25:424–430
9. Behr TM, Béhé M, Angerstein C, Gratz S, Mach R, Hagemann L, Jenner N, Stiehler M, Frank-Raue K, Raue F, Becker W (1999) Cholecystokinin-B/gastrin receptor binding peptides: preclinical development and evaluation of their diagnostic and therapeutic potential. Clin Cancer Res 5:3124–3138

10. Behr TM, Jenner N, Béhé M, Angerstein C, Gratz S, Raue F, Becker W (1999) Radiolabeled peptides for targeting of cholecystokinin-B/gastrin receptor expressing tumors: from preclinical development to initial clinical results. J Nucl Med 40:1029–1044
11. Behr TM, Béhé M, Angerstein C, Hüfner M, Becker W (2000) Cholecystokinin-B/gastrin-receptor binding peptides for the staging of known and occult metastatic medullary thyroid cancer. Eur J Nucl Med 27:in press
12. Bergholm U, Bergström R, Ekbom A (1997) Long-term follow-up of patients with medullary carcinoma of the thyroid. Cancer 79:132–138
13. Brunt LM, Wells SA Jr (1987) Advances in the diagnosis and treatment of medullary thyroid carcinoma. Endocr Surg 67:263
14. Busnardo B, Girelli ME, Simioni N, Nacamulli D, Bosetto E (1984) Nonparallel patterns of calcitonin and carcinoembryonic antigen levels in the follow-up of medullary thyroid carcinoma. Cancer 53:278–285
15. Dörr U, Frank-Raue K, Raue F, Buhr HJ, Hehrmann R, Iser G, Bihl H (1993) Localization of recurrences from medullary thyroid carcinoma by somatostatin-receptor-scintigraphy (abstract). Eur J Nucl Med 20:843
16. Dörr U, Würstlin S, Frank-Raue K, Raue F, Hehrmann R, Iser G, Scholz M, Guhl L, Buhr HJ, Bihl H (1993) Somatostatin receptor scintigraphy and magnetic resonance imaging in recurrent medullary thyroid carcinoma: a comparative study. In: Bihl H, Dörr U (eds) Somatostatin receptor imaging. (Hormone and Metabolic Research Suppl. vol 27). Thieme, Stuttgart New York, pp 48–55
17. Hazard JB, Hawk WA, Crile G (1959) Medullary (solid) carcinoma of the thyroid: a clinicopathological entity. J Clin Endocrinol Metab 19:152
18. Hilditch TE, Connell JMC, Elliott AT, Murray T, Reed NS (1986) Poor results with technetium-99m (V) DMSA and iodine-131 MIBG in the imaging of medullary thyroid carcinoma. J Nucl Med 27:1150–1153
19. Jensen RT (1999) Overview of chronic diarrhea caused by functional neuroendocrine neoplasms. Semin Gastrointest Dis 10:156–172
20. Juweid ME, Sharkey RM, Behr T, Swayne LC, Rubin AD, Hanley D, Markowitz A, Siegel J, Goldenberg DM (1995) Targeting and initial radioimmunotherapy of medullary thyroid cancer with ^{131}I-labeled monoclonal antibodies to carcinoembryonic antigen. Cancer Res. 55:5946–5951
21. Juweid ME, Sharkey RM, Behr T, Swayne LC, Herskovic T, Pereira M, Rubin AD, Hanley D, Dunn RM, Siegel J, Goldenberg DM (1996) Radioimmunotherapy of medullary thyroid carcinoma with ^{131}I-labeled anti-CEA antibodies. J Nucl Med 37:875–881
22. Juweid ME, Sharkey RM, Behr T, Swayne LC, Rubin AD, Herskovic T, Hanley D, Markowitz A, Dunn RM, Siegel J, Kamal T, Goldenberg DM (1996) Improved detection of medullary thyroid cancer with radiolabeled antibodies to carcinoembryonic antigen. J Clin Oncol 14:1209–1217
23. Kameda Y, Ikeda K, Ikeda A (1981) Uptake of radioiodine in follicles of dog C-cell complexes studied by autoradiograph and immunoperoxidase staining. Anat Rec 200:461–470
24. Köster C, Ehrenheim C, Burchert W, Oetting G, Hundeshagen H (1996) ^{18}F-FDG-PET, MRT und CT in der Nachsorge des medullären Schilddrüsenkarzinoms. Nucl Med 35: A60
25. Mendelsohn G, Wells Jr SA, Baylin SB (1984) Relationship of tissue carcinoembryonic antigen and calcitonin to tumor virulence in medullary thyroid carcinoma. Cancer 54:657–662
26. Nusynowitz ML, Pollard E, Benedetto AR, Lecklitner ML, Ware RW (1982) Treatment of medullary carcinoma of the thyroid with I-131. J Nucl Med 23:143–146
27. O'Riordain DS, O'Brien T, Weaver AL, Gharib H, Hay ID, Grant CS, van Heerden JA (1994) Medullary thyroid carcinoma in multiple endocrine neoplasia types 2A and 2B. Surgery 116:1017

28. Pacini F, Basolo F, Elisei R, Fugazzola L, Cola A, Pinchera A (1991) Medullary thyroid cancer. An immunohistochemical and humoral study using six separate antigens. Am J Clin Pathol 95:300–308
29. Pacini F, Fontanelli M, Fugazzola L, Elisei R, Romei C, Di Coscio G, Miccoli P, Pinchera A (1994) Routine measurement of serum calcitonin in nodular thyroid diseases allows the preoperative diagnosis of unsuspected sporadic medullary thyroid carcinoma. J Clin Endocrinol Metab 78:826–829
30. Reiners C, Eilles C, Spiegel W, Becker W, Börner W (1986) Immunoscintigraphy in medullary thyroid cancer using an ^{123}I- or ^{111}In-labelled monoclonal anti-CEA antibody fragment. Nucl Med 25:227–231
31. Reubi JC, Waser B (1996) Unexpected high incidence of cholecystokinin/gastrin receptors in human medullary thyroid carcinomas. Int J Cancer 67:644–647
32. Reubi JC, Chayvialle JA, Franc B, Cohen R, Calmettes C, Modigliani E (1991) Somatostatin receptors and somatostatin content in medullary thyroid carcinomas. Lab Invest 64:567–573
33. Reubi JC, Schaer JC, Waser B (1997) Cholecystokinin(CCK)-A and CCK-B/gastrin receptors in human tumors. Cancer Res. 57:1377–1386
34. Samaan NA, Schultz PN, Hickey RC (1988) Medullary thyroid carcinoma: prognosis of familial versus sporadic disease and the role of radiotherapy. J Clin Endocrinol Metab 67:801–808
35. Smith JP, Stock EA, Wotring MG, McLaughlin PJ, Zagon IS (1996) Characterization of the CCK-B/gastrin-like receptor in human colon cancer. Am J Physiol 271:R797–R805
36. Vierbuchen M, Schröder S, Larena A, Uhlenbruck G, Fischer R (1994) Native and sialic acid masked Lewis(a) antigen reactivity in medullary thyroid carcinoma. Distinct tumour-associated and prognostic relevant antigens. Virchows Arch 424:205–211
37. Wells SA Jr, Baylin SB, Linehan WM, et al. (1978) Provocative agents and the diagnosis of medullary carcinoma of the thyroid gland. Ann Surg 188:139.
38. Williams ED (1966) Histogenesis of medullary carcinoma of the thyroid. J Clin Pathol 19:114

Chapter 19

Therapy for Medullary Thyroid Cancer

O. Gimm and H. Dralle

19.1 Introduction

In 1959, Hazard described a thyroid carcinoma characterized by a nonfollicular histological pattern, the presence of amyloid in the stroma, and a high incidence of lymph node metastases as a clinicopathological entity [20]. This histological subtype of thyroid carcinoma has already been described by Horn in 1951 [22], and the description of thyroid tumors with amyloid deposition was made at the beginning of the twentieth century [23]. But it was Hazard who clearly identified it as an individual entity to be distinguished from other types of thyroid carcinoma. Hazard also proposed the term "medullary thyroid carcinoma" (MTC).

The incidence of MTC is not well known. The only population-based studies were made shortly after MTC had been identified as an entity [4, 21]. The low incidence of 3.6–3.8% of MTC in those studies is, hence, at least in part most likely due to misdiagnosis of MTC as anaplastic carcinoma. In contrast, recent studies which emphasized the necessity of measuring calcitonin levels in patients with thyroid nodules reported the incidence of MTC as high as 16–40% [36, 39, 42]. In general, MTC is believed to comprise about 5–10% of all thyroid malignancies.

In contrast to differentiated thyroid carcinoma, MTC derives from the parafollicular C-cells (see Chap. 2). Hence, it does not take up radioiodine and is, therefore, not susceptible to radioiodine treatment. Surgery is still the treatment of choice for the primary tumor and local metastases.

19.2 Sporadic Versus Familial Medullary Thyroid Carcinoma

The majority (75%) of MTCs are sporadic [38]. These tumors are often unifocal but almost always larger than 1 cm in diameter at the time of diagnosis. At this time, about 50–80% of patients have lymph node metastases [19].

About a quarter of patients with MTCs do have a familial form. More than 95% of these patients harbor a germline mutation in the proto-oncogene *RET*, which is almost always a missense mutation (see Chap. 17) [13]. The remaining patients, less than 5%, have a family history or accompanying diseases suggestive of MEN 2 but no germline *RET* mutation. Clinically, three familial forms of MTC are distinguished: familial MTC only (FMTC), MTC as part of multiple endocrine neoplasia type 2A (MEN 2A–MTC, pheochromocytoma, hyperparathyroidism), and MTC as part of MEN 2B (MTC, pheochromocytoma, marfanoid habitus, intestinal ganglioneuromatosis, mucosal neuromas, corneal nerve fibers). In a given family, the "index patient" is that person who was first identified as having MTC or, less likely, one of the accompanying diseases as part of MEN 2, i.e., the diagnosis MTC is made and subsequent analysis revealed a mutation in the proto-oncogene *RET*. These individuals often present with multifocal tumors of which the largest one is almost always larger than 1 cm in diameter. Like patients with sporadic MTC, they often present with lymph node metastases. "Screening patients" are those members of a given family who are identified as harboring the same germline mutation as the index patient. It is estimated that *RET* mutation carriers have a risk of 70% of developing clinically significant MTC by the age of 70 years [37]. Every single thyroid C-cell harbors the potency to become malignant. This is the rationale for advocating removal of the total thyroid gland in every patient with FMTC/MEN 2-specific *RET* mutation. Patients can be screened at a very young age. The genetically determined development of C-cell neoplasia might therefore still be at the beginning, when solely C-cell hyperplasia (increased number of C cells) or even a normal thyroid gland is found histologically. The risk of lymph node metastases is only given once C-cell carcinoma (i.e., MTC) has developed.

Family members of FMTC/MEN 2 families are often referred to as "gene carriers." This term is incorrect, since we all "carry" the gene and therefore pose a threat. The correct term would be "FMTC/MEN 2-specific *RET* mutation carriers." Since this term is very long and awkward, the term "*RET* mutation carriers" or just "mutation carriers" might be used instead.

19.3 Therapy

Among solid tumors, MTC is almost unique regarding its production of a quite specific tumor marker. This tumor marker, calcitonin, is not only helpful in making the diagnosis (see Chap. 17), but also in assessing the therapeutic success. It has been shown that pre- and early postoperative calcitonin levels in a given individual correlate very well with the remaining tumor burden [43]. In some instances [e.g., extrathyroidal tumor extension (pT4 tumor), lymph node metastases in all four locoregional lymph compartments, presence of distant metastases], "biochemical cure" (i.e., calcitonin levels within normal basal limits and after stimulation with either pentagastrin or calcium or both) cannot be expected despite extensive surgery [17]. The indication to operate on these patients is, however, still almost always given, since MTC is generally a slowly progressing tumor and tumor-related complications (e.g., airway obstruction) must be avoided.

19.3.1
Surgical Treatment

Surgery is the treatment of choice for MTC, no matter whether MTC is sporadic or familiar, primary or recurrent, restricted to the thyroid gland or extending beyond it. To facilitate the identification, preparation, and preservation of important structures (e.g., parathyroid glands, recurrent laryngeal nerve), the use of magnifying glasses, bipolar coagulation forceps, and neuromonitoring is recommended [9, 34].

19.3.1.1
Thyroid gland

MTC is often multifocal (sporadic MTC 10–20%, familial MTC 80–90%) [41] and not susceptible to radioiodine ablation. Hence, most investigators recommend total thyroidectomy in any patient with MTC. However, a unifocal approach in sporadic cases has been proposed by some authors [30].

19.3.1.2
Lymph node metastases

Multivariate analysis of long-term follow-up data showed that lymph node metastases are of prognostic value in MTC [2, 7]. Based on anatomical structures, four locoregional lymph node compartments have been defined [11]:

- Cervicocentral compartment (C1). This compartment is limited laterally by the carotid sheaths, cranially by the hyoid bone, and caudally by the brachiocephalic vein, and includes the cervical paratracheoesophageal lymph nodes.
- Cervicolateral compartments (C2, right; C3, left). These compartments extend laterally from the carotid sheath to the trapezoid muscle, and caudally from the subclavian vein up to the hypoglossal nerve.
- Mediastinal compartment (C4). The mediastinal compartment lies retrosternally and includes the lymph nodes between the brachiocephalic vein and the tracheal bifurcation in the upper anterior and posterior mediastinum.

This classification has been proved useful both for defining the extent of lymphadenectomy (compartment-oriented lymphadenectomy) [8, 14] and for comparing patterns of metastasis [17, 19]. Once, the decision to operate on a compartment is made, the whole compartment, i.e., lymph nodes and the surrounding adipose and connective tissue should be removed en-bloc. The technique has been termed "systematic compartment-oriented lymphadenectomy" or "compartment-oriented microdissection" [9]. The reason for advocating this technique is that pre- and/or intraoperative detection of lymph nodes can be impossible, since they tend to be small.

Routine lymphadenectomy of the cervicocentral compartment (C1) as part of total thyroidectomy is recommended and widely accepted for the following reasons:

1. Lymph node metastases derived from MTC have a prognostic influence [2, 7].
2. About 50–80% of patients with sporadic MTC have lymph node metastases at the time of diagnosis, most often in the cervicocentral compartment [19]. Lymph node metastases are also found in almost 9% of patients with familial MTC who underwent screening procedures [25]. Among children and adolescents with FMTC/MEN 2A (younger than 20 years), lymph node metastases are still found in 4–6% [10, 35].
3. No adequate nonsurgical treatment modalities exist yet.

It is also widely accepted to dissect compartments which obviously contain lymph node metastases. No strategy has gained common acceptance in the absence of obvious lymph node involvement. The following algorithms have been proposed.

19.3.1.2.1 Inclusion of the cervicolateral compartments (C2 and/or C3)

1. Bilateral cervicolateral (C2 and C3) lymphadenectomy in any patient with clinical evidence of disease [29]
2. General inclusion of the ipsilateral cervicolateral (with regard to the site of the primary tumor) compartment (C2 or C3)
3. Inclusion of the cervicolateral compartments (C2 and/or C3) only in the presence of cervicocentral lymph node metastases
4. Inclusion of the ipsilateral cervicolateral compartment (C2 or C3) if the primary tumor is >2 cm in diameter [31]

19.3.1.2.2 Inclusion of the mediastinal compartment (C4)

1. More than three lymph node metastases in the cervicocentral compartment (C1) [18]
2. Lymph node metastases in one of the cervicolateral compartments (C2 and/or C3) [18]
3. Lymph node metastases in the cervicomediastinal transition.

Based on the results reported [3, 8, 12, 17, 19, 31, 32], the following approach is currently recommended:

1. Total thyroidectomy and lymphadenectomy of the three cervical (cervicocentral, cervicolateral right and left) compartments is performed in any patient with primary MTC. The only exception to perform a less extended operation is given in a young *RET* mutation carrier; see below)
2. Since involvement of the mediastinal compartment rarely (<10%) enables "biochemical cure" and since dissection of this compartment via a transsternal approach inherits a higher morbidity rate, dissection is nowadays recommended if mediastinal metastases are proven by imaging techniques.

19.3.1.3
Distant metastases

Surgical treatment of distant metastases derived from MTC is rarely, if ever, curative. Hence, the indications to operate are prevention of local complications and alleviation of symptoms. For example, removal of asymptomatic retrosternal lymph node metastases via a transsternal approach is most likely unjustified if multiple, progressing distant metastases are present also.

19.3.1.4
Reoperation

Persistent or recurrent disease is quite frequent in MTC [17, 33, 41]. The first sign of persistent or recurrent disease is an elevated calcitonin level. Calcitonin is a sensitive tumor marker of MTC. It serves as a useful tool both at primary diagnosis and during follow-up (see Chap. 17). Indeed, calcitonin levels may already be elevated when imaging techniques fail to show evidence of tumor. The surgeon might therefore be confronted with the following situations:

1. Calcitonin levels are within normal range (basal and after injection of provocative reagents), but the primary operation was "incomplete" (less than total thyroidectomy and cervicocentral lymphadenectomy): If the patient turns out to have MTC as part of FMTC/MEN 2, the indication to reoperate is clearly given, since every single C cell carries the potency to become malignant. In sporadic cases, the indication to perform reoperation is less clear. In the case of a small primary tumor (<2 cm), no reoperation but thorough follow-up is recommended. If compliance cannot be reassured or if primary tumors are large (>2 cm), reoperation should be performed.
2. Elevated calcitonin levels without proved tumor persistence or recurrence: This is another challenging situation. Elevated calcitonin levels and in particular rising calcitonin levels after injection of provocative reagents almost always indicate persistent or recurrent tumor. If previous operation consisted of less than total thyroidectomy and/or cervicocentral (C1) lymphadenectomy, it is almost certain that tumor remnants can be found in compartment C1. Further effort should be undertaken to exclude or confirm the presence of distant metastases, since their presence may alter the extent of reoperation.
3. Elevated calcitonin levels and proved local tumor persistence or recurrence: The indication to reoperate in these patients is almost always given.
4. Caution must be exercised if imaging techniques are suggestive of tumor but calcitonin levels are within normal levels. Two explanations are possible. Scarring tissue might be mistaken as tumor or the tumor is dedifferentiated and has lost its ability to synthesize and/or secrete calcitonin. Fine-needle aspiration cytology with immunohistochemistry staining (e.g., calcitonin, CEA, chromogranin) should be performed.

In any case, if reoperation is indicated it should at least consist of completion thyroidectomy and cervicocentral lymphadenectomy if not performed previously. We recommend performing a bilateral cervicolateral lymphadenectomy in addition. Otherwise, the same considerations to limit or extend the extent of lymph node dissection beyond the cervicocentral compartment that apply at primary therapy also apply at reoperation.

19.3.2 Special Therapeutic Considerations in Familial MTC

The identification of *RET* as the disease causing gene of familial MTC in 1993 has changed the diagnostic strategy. Since then, patients at risk for MTC can be identified at an asymptomatic stage (see Chap. 17). However, due to the nature of this subject, our knowledge is limited and recommendations regarding therapeutic strategies are so far based on relatively small numbers of patients and short follow-up periods.

19.3.2.1 Thyroid gland

The identification of *RET* mutation carriers is nowadays often made before clinical disease is present. In these cases, the removal of the thyroid gland is often referred to as “prophylactic thyroidectomy.” In many instances, however, histopathological analysis of these thyroid glands already revealed the presence of MTC [10]. Some investigators find that the term “prophylactic thyroidectomy” is misleading in these cases. Instead, they propose to use the term “early thyroidectomy.” No matter what one considers to be the correct term, most surgeons recommend performance of a prophylactic/early thyroidectomy at the age of 4–6 years [5, 10, 44], when the risk of MTC and, in particular, of metastases is low. Others recommend performing thyroidectomy when calcitonin levels turn pathological. This strategy, however, inherits some pitfalls. On the one hand, calcitonin can be pathological when only C cell hyperplasia is present [10] and surgery at a young age inherits an increased risk of complications. On the other hand, calcitonin levels can still be normal despite the presence of MTC [10, 44] (false-negative). Therefore, calcitonin level does not seem to be a good indicator of when to operate. Recently, several studies have shown that a genotype-phenotype correlation exists [27, 45], i.e., some mutations (e.g., E768D, Y791F) inherit a lower risk of transformation from C cell hyperplasia to MTC than other mutations (e.g., C634R). In these instances, surgery may be postponed unless calcitonin level turns pathological.

19.3.2.2 Lymph node metastases

Similar to patients with sporadic MTC, a cervicocentral lymphadenectomy is generally recommended in addition to total thyroidectomy. Since familial MTC is often multifocal and bilateral, a bilateral cervicolateral (compartment C2 and C3) is highly recommended to avoid unnecessary reoperations.

Despite apparent differences between sporadic and hereditary MTC, therapeutic recommendations do obviously not differ a lot. It remains to be shown whether cervicocentral lymphadenectomy, which carries an increased morbidity, can be avoided in some cases. For instance, lymph node involvement seems to be extremely rare if stimulated calcitonin is within normal limits or if patients are younger than 10 years. Also, patients harboring some *RET* mutations (e.g., E768D, Y791F) seem to develop lymph node metastases at a later age. Therefore, in these patients, routine inclusion of the cervicocentral compartment might not be necessary. However, further analysis of larger series will be necessary to provide general recommendations.

19.3.3 Nonsurgical Treatment Modalities

Nonsurgical treatment modalities should only be used if surgery is not feasible.

19.3.3.1 Octreotide

Octreotide is a synthetic somatostatin analog. It has been shown to be useful in the diagnosis of MTC, since 40–60% of primary MTCs are found to be somatostatin receptor-positive by immunohistochemical means (see Chap. 17). Octreotide, however, has not fulfilled the expectations regarding treatment of MTC beyond the thyroid gland [15]. At least, in patients with symptoms related to excessive calcitonin secretion (e.g., diarrhea), octreotide may be of help [28].

19.3.3.2 Radioactive iodine

Radioiodine is a tremendously helpful tool in the diagnosis and treatment of follicular thyroid cancer (see Chap. 6). Since MTC does not derive from the follicular thyroid cells, it does not accumulate radioiodine. Some progress has been made using radioiodine labeled anti-CEA monoclonal antibodies (anti-CEA MAbs). They have not only been proved to be useful in detecting but also showed to be suitable to treat metastatic disease [24]. In combination with chemotherapeutic agents, anti-CEA MAbs showed synergistic therapeutic efficacy [1] which has been confirmed more recently [40]. Clinical studies have still not been reported.

19.3.3.3
External radiation

External radiation should be avoided for as long as possible. There is no need for prophylactic radiation, and the distressing long-term side effects of cough and dryness should not be underestimated. Also, assessment of local tumor recurrence both clinically and by imaging techniques as well as reoperation can be difficult due to scarring of the neck. If surgery cannot be performed, however, radiation may be helpful in treating symptomatic and/or rapidly progressing local and distant disease.

19.3.3.4
Chemotherapy

MTC has been shown to be almost unresponsive to chemotherapy. Partial responses and long-term disease control could only be achieved in rare instances. In general, combination chemotherapy seems to be superior to monotherapy. Various combinations (e.g., doxorubicin and cisplatin; 5-fluorouracil and streptozocin; cyclophosphamide and vincristine; and dacarbazine) have been investigated. Combined radiochemotherapy has been shown to improve treatment outcome in a nude mouse model but clinical experience is lacking [1]. In patients with multiple symptomatic liver metastases, chemoembolization has been shown to be of help [26].

In summary, the available nonsurgical treatment modalities for MTC are limited and of low efficacy. Chemotherapy per se will most likely not be the answer. Curative agents will have to target the molecular. Recently, it has been shown that MDM 2, an oncoprotein that physically interacts with the *p53* tumor suppressor gene product, promotes apoptosis in p53-deficient human MTC cells [6]. It remains to be shown whether this knowledge will be of help in developing new therapeutic tools.

19.3.3.5
Psychological support

From the clinical point of view, it seems to be justified to screen patients with MTC and relatives of mutations carriers for germline *RET* mutations. The psychological impact, however, is often neglected. It is therefore not surprising that a study from France about the psychological impact of genetic testing in familial MTC revealed a high level of frustration and latent discontent [16]. The discontent was related either to the management of genetic information given by the clinicians and its psychological consequences or simply to the knowledge of the genetic risk of cancer. Surgeons, endocrinologists, oncologists, radiologists, geneticists, and genetic counselors have to keep in mind that we are not just treating a disease but also an individual. Much more effort should, hence, be put into the interaction between clinicians and the potentially affected individual.

References

1. Behr TM, Wulst E, Radetzky S, Blumenthal RD, Dunn RM, Gratz S, Rave-Frank M, Schmidberger H, Raue F, Becker W (1997) Improved treatment of medullary thyroid cancer in a nude mouse model by combined radioimmunochemotherapy: doxorubicin potentiates the therapeutic efficacy of radiolabeled antibodies in a radioresistant tumor type. Cancer Res 57:5309–5319
2. Bergholm U, Bergstrom R, Ekbom A (1997) Long-term follow-up of patients with medullary carcinoma of the thyroid. Cancer 79:132–138
3. Chi DD, Moley JF (1998) Medullary thyroid carcinoma: genetic advances, treatment recommendations, and the approach to the patient with persistent hypercalcitoninemia. Surg Oncol Clin North Am 7:681–706
4. Christensen SB, Ljungberg O, Tibblin S (1984) A clinical epidemiologic study of thyroid carcinoma in Malmo, Sweden. Curr Probl Cancer 8:1–49
5. Decker RA, Geiger JD, Cox CE, Mackovjak M, Sarkar M, Peacock ML (1996) Prophylactic surgery for multiple endocrine neoplasia type IIa after genetic diagnosis: is parathyroid transplantation indicated? World J Surg 20:814–820; discussion 820–811
6. Dilla T, Velasco JA, Medina DL, Gonzalez-Palacios JF, Santisteban P (2000) The MDM 2 oncoprotein promotes apoptosis in p53-deficient human medullary thyroid carcinoma cells. Endocrinology 141:420–429
7. Dottorini ME, Assi A, Sironi M, Sangalli G, Spreafico G, Colombo L (1996) Multivariate analysis of patients with medullary thyroid carcinoma. Prognostic significance and impact on treatment of clinical and pathological variables. Cancer 77:1556–1565
8. Dralle H, Damm I, Scheumann GF, Kotzerke J, Kupsch E, Geerlings H, Pichlmayr R (1994) Compartment-oriented microdissection of regional lymph nodes in medullary thyroid carcinoma. Surg Today 24:112–121
9. Dralle H, Gimm O (1996) Lymph node excision in thyroid carcinoma. Chirurg 67:788–806
10. Dralle H, Gimm O, Simon D, Frank-Raue K, Gortz G, Niederle B, Wahl RA, Koch B, Walgenbach S, Hampel R, Ritter MM, Spelsberg F, Heiss A, Hinze R, Hoppner W (1998) Prophylactic thyroidectomy in 75 children and adolescents with hereditary medullary thyroid carcinoma: German and Austrian experience. World J Surg 22:744–750; discussion 750–741
11. Dralle H, Scheumann GF, Kotzerke J, Brabant EG (1992) Surgical management of MEN 2. Rec Res Cancer Res 125:167–195
12. Dralle H, Scheumann GF, Proye C, Bacourt F, Frilling A, Limbert F, Gheri G, Henry JF, Berner M, Niederle B et al (1995) The value of lymph node dissection in hereditary medullary thyroid carcinoma: a retrospective, European, multicentre study. J Intern Med 238:357–361
13. Eng C, Clayton D, Schuffenecker I, Lenoir G, Cote G, Gagel RF, van Amstel HK, Lips CJ, Nishisho I, Takai SI, Marsh DJ, Robinson BG, Frank-Raue K, Raue F, Xue F, Noll WW, Romei C, Pacini F, Fink M, Niederle B, Zedenius J, Nordenskjold M, Komminoth P, Hendy GN, Gharib H, Thibodeau SN, Lacroix A, Frilling A, Ponder BA, Mulligan LM (1996) The relationship between specific *RET* proto-oncogene mutations and disease phenotype in multiple endocrine neoplasia type 2. International RET mutation consortium analysis. JAMA 276:1575–1579
14. Fleming JB, Lee JE, Bouvet M, Schultz PN, Sherman SI, Sellin RV, Friend KE, Burgess MA, Cote GJ, Gagel RF, Evans DB (1999) Surgical strategy for the treatment of medullary thyroid carcinoma. Ann Surg 230:697–707
15. Frank-Raue K, Ziegler R, Raue F (1993) The use of octreotide in the treatment of medullary thyroid carcinoma. Horm Metab Res [Suppl] 27:44–47
16. Freyer G, Dazord A, Schlumberger M, Conte-Devolx B, Ligneau B, Trillet-Lenoir V, Lenoir GM (1999) Psychosocial impact of genetic testing in familial medullary-thyroid carcinoma: a multicentric pilot-evaluation. Ann Oncol 10:87–95

17. Gimm O, Dralle H (1997) Reoperation in metastasizing medullary thyroid carcinoma: is a tumor stage-oriented approach justified? Surgery 122:1124–1130; discussion 1130–1121
18. Gimm O, Dralle H (1999) C-cell cancer – prevention and treatment. Langenbecks Arch Surg 384:16–23
19. Gimm O, Ukkat J, Dralle H (1998) Determinative factors of biochemical cure after primary and reoperative surgery for sporadic medullary thyroid carcinoma. World J Surg 22:562–567; discussion 567–568
20. Hazard JB, Hawk WA, Crile G (1959) Medullary (solid) carcinoma of the thyroid – a clinicopathological entity. J Clin Endocrinol Metab 19:152–161
21. Hoie J, Jorgensen OG, Stenwig AE, Langmark F (1988) Medullary thyroid cancer in Norway. A 30-year experience. Acta Chir Scand 154:339–343
22. Horn RC (1951) Carcinoma of the thyroid: description of a distinctive morphological variant and report of seven cases. Cancer 4:697–707
23. Jaquet AJ (1906) Ein Fall von metastasierenden Amyloidtumoren (Lymphosarcoma). Virchows Archiv (Pathol Anat) 185:251
24. Juweid M, Sharkey RM, Behr T, Swayne LC, Herskovic T, Pereira M, Rubin AD, Hanley D, Dunn R, Siegel J, Goldenberg DM (1996) Radioimmunotherapy of medullary thyroid cancer with iodine-131-labeled anti-CEA antibodies. J Nucl Med 37:905–911
25. Kebebew E, Tresler PA, Siperstein AE, Duh QY, Clark OH (1999) Normal thyroid pathology in patients undergoing thyroidectomy for finding a *RET* gene germline mutation: a report of three cases and review of the literature. Thyroid 9:127–131
26. Machens A, Behrmann C, Dralle H (2000) Chemoembolization of liver metastases from medullary thyroid carcinoma. Ann Intern Med 132:596–597
27. Machens A, Gimm O, Hinze R, Hoppner W, Boehm BO, Dralle H (2001) Genotype-phenotype correlations in hereditary medullary thyroid carcinoma: oncological features and biochemical properties. J Clin Endocrinol Metab 86:1104–1109
28. Mahler C, Verhelst J, de Longueville M, Harris A (1990) Long-term treatment of metastatic medullary thyroid carcinoma with the somatostatin analogue octreotide. Clin Endocrinol (Oxf) 33:261–269
29. Marzano LA, Porcelli A, Biondi B, Lupoli G, Delrio P, Lombardi G, Zarrilli L (1995) Surgical management and follow-up of medullary thyroid carcinoma. J Surg Oncol 59:162–168
30. Miyauchi A, Matsuzuka F, Hirai K, Yokozawa T, Kobayashi K, Ito Y, Nakano K, Kuma K, Futami H, Yamaguchi K (2002) Prospective trial of unilateral surgery for nonhereditary medullary thyroid carcinoma in patients without germline *RET* mutations. World J Surg 26:1023–1028
31. Moley JF (1995) Medullary thyroid cancer. Surg Clin North Am 75:405–420
32. Moley JF, DeBenedetti MK (1999) Patterns of nodal metastases in palpable medullary thyroid carcinoma: recommendations for extent of node dissection. Ann Surg 229:880–887; discussion 887–888
33. Moley JF, Dilley WG, DeBenedetti MK (1997) Improved results of cervical reoperation for medullary thyroid carcinoma. Ann Surg 225:734–740; discussion 740–733
34. Moley JF, Wells SA, Dilley WG, Tisell LE (1993) Reoperation for recurrent or persistent medullary thyroid cancer. Surgery 114:1090–1095; discussion 1095–1096
35. Niccoli-Sire P, Murat A, Baudin E, Henry JF, Proye C, Bigorgne JC, Bstandig B, Modigliani E, Morange S, Schlumberger M, Conte-Devolx B (1999) Early or prophylactic thyroidectomy in MEN 2/FMTC gene carriers: results in 71 thyroidectomized patients. Eur J Endocrinol 141:468–474
36. Pacini F, Fontanelli M, Fugazzola L, Elisei R, Romei C, Di Coscio G, Miccoli P, Pinchera A (1994) Routine measurement of serum calcitonin in nodular thyroid diseases allows the preoperative diagnosis of unsuspected sporadic medullary thyroid carcinoma (see Comments). J Clin Endocrinol Metab 78:826–829

37. Ponder BA, Ponder MA, Coffey R, Pembrey ME, Gagel RF, Telenius-Berg M, Semple P, Easton DF (1988) Risk estimation and screening in families of patients with medullary thyroid carcinoma. Lancet 1:397–401
38. Raue F, Kotzerke J, Reinwein D, Schroder S, Roher HD, Deckart H, Hofer R, Ritter M, Seif F, Buhr H et al (1993) Prognostic factors in medullary thyroid carcinoma: evaluation of 741 patients from the German Medullary Thyroid Carcinoma Register. Clin Invest 71:7–12
39. Rieu M, Lame MC, Richard A, Lissak B, Sambort B, Vuong-Ngoc P, Berrod JL, Fombeur JP (1995) Prevalence of sporadic medullary thyroid carcinoma: the importance of routine measurement of serum calcitonin in the diagnostic evaluation of thyroid nodules (see Comments). Clin Endocrinol (Oxf) 42:453–460
40. Stein R, Chen S, Reed L, Richel H, Goldenberg DM (2002) Combining radioimmunotherapy and chemotherapy for treatment of medullary thyroid carcinoma: effectiveness of dacarbazine. Cancer 94:51–61
41. Van Heerden JA, Grant CS, Gharib H, Hay ID, Ilstrup DM (1990) Long-term course of patients with persistent hypercalcitoninemia after apparent curative primary surgery for medullary thyroid carcinoma. Ann Surg 212:395–400; discussion 400–401
42. Vierhapper H, Raber W, Bieglmayer C, Kaserer K, Weinhausl A, Niederle B (1997) Routine measurement of plasma calcitonin in nodular thyroid diseases. J Clin Endocrinol Metab 82:1589–1593
43. Wells SA Jr, Baylin SB, Gann DS, Farrell RE, Dilley WG, Preissig SH, Linehan WM, Cooper CW (1978) Medullary thyroid carcinoma: relationship of method of diagnosis to pathological staging. Ann Surg 188:377–383
44. Wells SA Jr, Chi DD, Toshima K, Dehner LP, Coffin CM, Dowton SB, Ivanovich JL, DeBenedetti MK, Dilley WG, Moley JF et al (1994) Predictive DNA testing and prophylactic thyroidectomy in patients at risk for multiple endocrine neoplasia type 2A. Ann Surg 220:237–247; discussion 247–250
45. Yip L, Cote GJ, Shapiro SE, Ayers GD, Herzog CE, Sellin RV, Sherman SI, Gagel RF, Lee JE, Evans DB (2003) Multiple endocrine neoplasia type 2: evaluation of the genotype-phenotype relationship. Arch Surg 138:409–416; discussion 416

CHAPTER 20

Follow-up of Medullary Thyroid Cancer 20

T. SCHILLING and R. ZIEGLER

20.1 Distinction Between Sporadic and Familial Forms of Medullary Thyroid Cancer

A precondition for follow-up is to know whether the patients suffers from the sporadic or familial form of medullary thyroid cancer (MTC). Mutational analysis of the *RET* proto-oncogene helps to distinguish between both forms of MTC. In 11.6% of the apparent sporadic MTC patients, a mutation in the *RET* proto-oncogene is found. This means that these patients belong to the familial form of MTC, i.e., they suffer from multiple endocrine neoplasia (MEN) type 2 (Table 20.1) [2]. As the clinical presentation may be the same in both forms, every patient with medullary thyroid carcinoma should undergo a mutational analysis of *RET* proto-oncogene to distinguish between the sporadic and the familial form (Table 20.2). Patients suffering from MEN 2 have a 50–100% chance of developing pheochromocytoma and a 10–20% chance of developing hyperparathyroidism (Table 20.1).

20.2 Survival in Patients Suffering from MTC

The survival rate depends on the tumor stage on diagnosis. It decreases rapidly with increasing tumor stage (Table 20.3). The overall 5-year survival rate is approximately 80%, the 10-year survival rate is approximately 65%. If the tumor is restricted to the thyroid gland (stage I) the 5-year survival rate is nearly 100%. If local lymph node metastases are present (stage III), the 5-year survival rate decreases to 84%. The occurrence of distant metastases further lowers the 5-year survival to 46% [16]. Considering the same tumor stage, sporadic and familial forms of MTC do not differ in survival rates [17]. Due to the fact that familial MTC is diagnosed in an earlier tumor stage, the overall prognosis seems to be better compared with that of sporadic MTC patients.

Table 20.1 Multiple endocrine neoplasia (MEN) type 2 syndromes

Syndrome	Symptoms	Risk of development
Multiple endocrine neoplasia type 2A	Medullary thyroid carcinoma	100%
	Pheochromocytoma	50%
	Hyperparathyroidism	10–20%
Multiple endocrine neoplasia type 2B	Medullary thyroid carcinoma	100%
	Intestinal ganglioneuromatosis	100%
	Marfanoid habitus	100%
	Pheochromocytoma	50%
Familial medullary thyroid carcinoma	Familial occurrence of MTC without hyperparathyroidism and without pheochromocytoma	

MTC medullary thyroid carcinoma

Table 20.2 Difference in clinical diagnosis between sporadic and familiar medullary thyroid carcinoma (MTC)

	Sporadic MTC	Familial MTC
Leading symptom	Nodular goiter	Familial history
	Enlarged cervical lymph nodes	Bilateral pheochromocytoma
	Diarrhea	Marfanoid habitus
		Intestinal ganglioneuromatosis
Ultrasound of the thyroid gland	Nodular goiter	May be normal
Scintigraphy of the thyroid gland	Cold nodules	May be normal
Screening	Calcitonin ↑, carcinoembryonic antigen (CEA) ↑	*RET* mutational analysis; calcitonin and CEA may be normal
Follow-up	Looking for:	Looking for:
	Recurrence of MTC	Recurrence of MTC
		Pheochromocytoma
		Primary hyperparathyroidism

CEA carcinoembryonic antigen

Table 20.3 Survival rate and tumor stage in patients suffering from medullary thyroid cancer (MTC)

				5-Year survival rate[a]	10-Year survival rate[a]
Stage I	T1 (<1 cm)	N0	M0	98%	98%
Stage II	T2–4 (<4 cm)	N0	M0	94%	90%
Stage III	Each T	N1	M0	84%	79%
Stage IV	Each T	Each N	M1	46%	46%

Based on the pTNM classification (postsurgical classification) of the International Union Against Cancer (UICC) for thyroid carcinoma
[a]Data derived from the German register for medullary thyroid carcinoma, October 1997

20.3 Sporadic Form of MTC

Most MTC patients, i.e., 88%, suffer from the sporadic form of MTC. After exclusion of a germline mutation in the *RET* proto-oncogene, the patient can be diagnosed as having sporadic MTC, and there must be no regular testing for manifestations of primary hyperparathyroidism or pheochromocytoma in the follow-up.

20.3.1 Calcitonin as Tumor Marker During Follow-up

By determination of calcitonin, the adequacy of surgery can be assessed. During follow-up, calcitonin serum levels reflect the tumor burden very well over a wide extent of the disease.

20.3.2 Testing the Result of the Primary Operation

The primary operation procedure should comprise at least a total thyroidectomy and a systematic lymph node-dissection of the central compartment of the neck. During the operation all carcinoma cells and all normal C-cells should be removed. The result of the primary operation has to be tested by measurement of calcitonin and carcinoembryonic antigen (CEA). Due to its long half-life, CEA should be measured not earlier than 2–3 weeks after primary operation. If calcitonin and CEA are normal or not detectable, the possible cure of MTC has to be proofed by a pentagastrin stimulation test. If the pentagastrin test is negative, the patient is probably cured from MTC without the need for further examinations such as X-ray, ultrasound or CT scan, or further operation (Fig. 20.1).

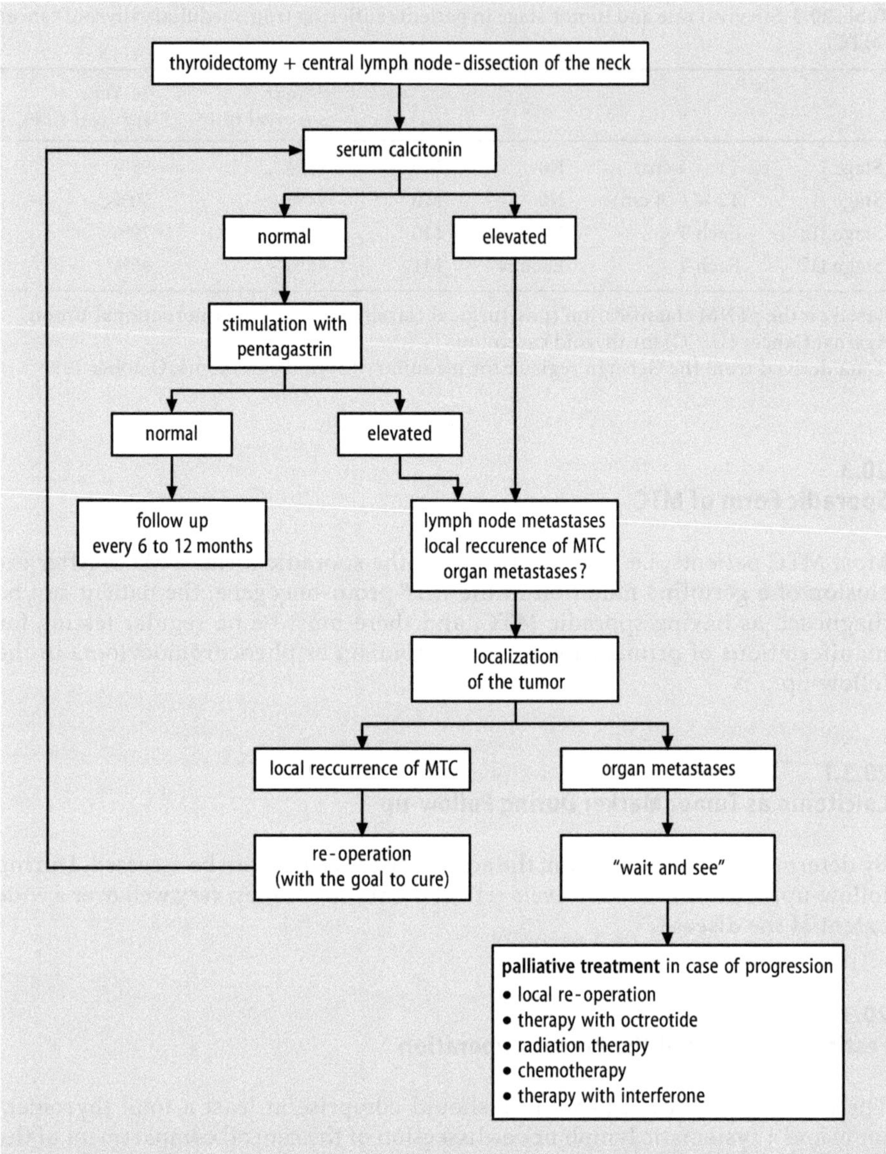

Fig. 20.1 Follow-up in patients with medullary thyroid carcinoma, either familial or sporadic

If calcitonin is still detectable after surgery has been performed, a de novo search to determine the exact localization of remaining tumor tissue is mandatory. A second "curative" operation attempt is only advisable if the remaining tumor tissue is localized in the regional lymph node area of the neck and if distant metastases of MTC to organs such as bone, liver, or lung are excluded. Thus at least X-ray of the chest (better CT scan), ultrasound of the abdomen, and bone scintigraphy have to be performed. After having excluded organ metastases, a second systematic microdissection of the affected lateral compartments of the neck should be undertaken in a specialized operation center. Systematic microdissection in patients with local lymph node metastases is able to normalize elevated calcitonin levels in up to 20–35% of patients [4, 10]. Whether the right, left, or both compartments of the neck are affected may be differentiated by CT scan, somatostatin receptor scintigraphy, and ultrasound. The most powerful tool for localizing the remaining tumor tissue is the selective venous catheterization of the neck. The diagnostic sensitivity of selective venous catheterization is nearly 90%, whereas the sensitivity of ultrasound is only 28% and that of CT scan is only 38% [1, 7]. Figure 20.2 gives an overview of the loci for blood sampling in the selective venous catheterization.

20.3.3 Follow-up in General

Postoperatively, patients are dismissed on lifelong levothyroxine replacement. Levothyroxine therapy is replacement and not suppressive therapy, in contrast to treatment of patients with differentiated thyroid carcinoma. Serum thyrotropin levels should be within the normal range. Radioactive iodine (^{131}I) has no place in the treatment of patients with recurrent or metastatic MTC [18].

20.3.4 Follow-up in Patients with No Detectable Calcitonin Postoperatively

Patients suffering from sporadic MTC with negative results of pentagastrin testing after operation are considered to be cured. Control examination of CEA and calcitonin by pentagastrin stimulation should be performed initially every 6 months. If the tests stay negative, the follow-up interval can be prolonged to 12 months. Without any clinical symptoms, there is no need in these patients for further examination [11].

20.3.5 Follow-up in Patients with Detectable Calcitonin Postoperatively

Patients suffering from distant metastases of MTC or from operatively incurable local lymph node metastases have to be surveyed every 6 months. If the tumor does not show a significant tumor growth, one should "wait and see" the further progression [20]. An intervention, either by reoperation or irradiation should only be performed when metastases provoke local complications by tumor growth (Fig. 20.1).

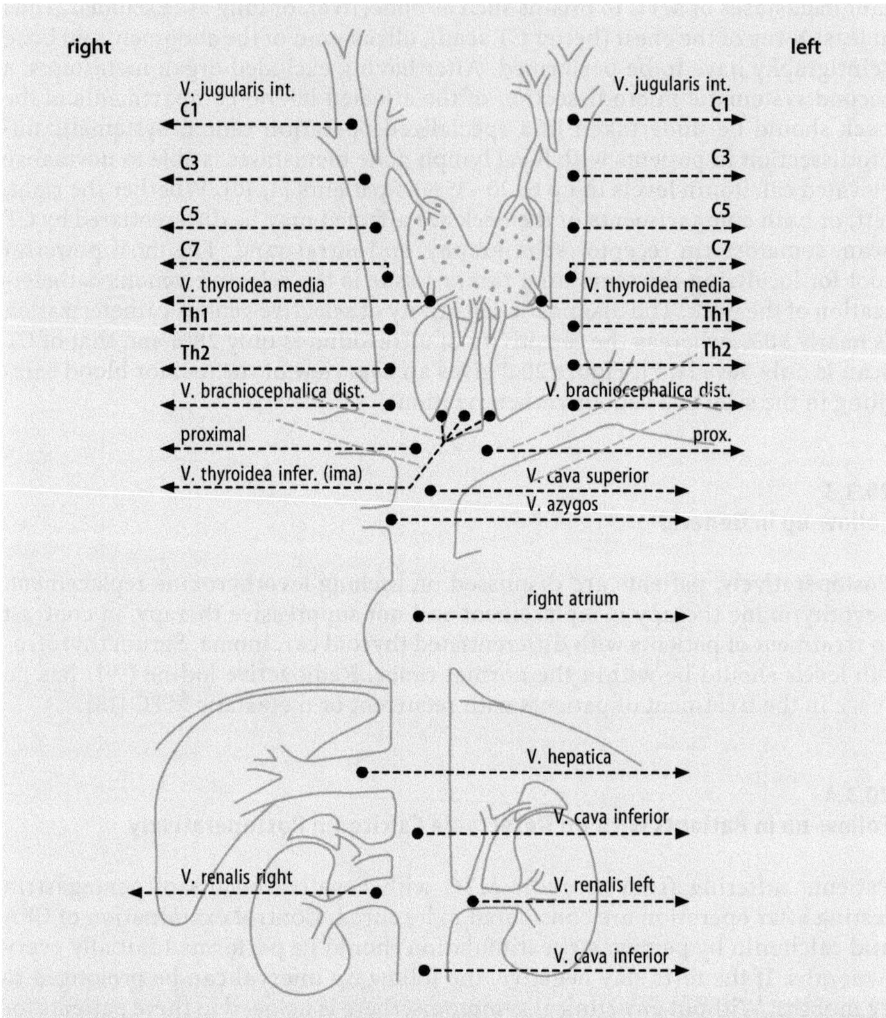

Fig. 20.2 Selective venous catheterization of the veins of the neck. Sequential analysis of calcitonin in the different blood samples is a powerful tool to localize medullary thyroid carcinoma tissue. Elevation of calcitonin in the vena azygos predicts lymph node metastases in the mediastinum. Elevation of calcitonin in the vena hepatica predicts liver metastases

20.3.6 Adjuvant Therapy

As mentioned above, external irradiation is used as palliative therapy for locally inoperable, recurrent MTC [3]. Most studies have been retrospective, and it is not clear whether radiotherapy is beneficial especially considering an improvement in overall survival [18]. In summary we suggest radiotherapy in patients with local neck recurrence that are not considered appropriate for surgical removal and symptomatic nervous system or skeletal metastasis.

Limited data are available on chemotherapy protocols for progressive MTC. In general, chemotherapy is of little help and is confined to patients with progressive recurrent MTC. Although many chemotherapeutic regimens have been tried, results are controversial, with no more than a 15–20% reduction in tumor size and probably no documented cures. Different chemotherapeutic protocols have included bleomycin, doxorubicin, cisplatin, cyclophosphamide, dacarbazine, fluorouracil, and vincristine [5, 6, 15, 21]. Antitumor drugs doxorubicin and cisplatin have been used to enhance the antitumor effect of ionizing radiation.

Long-term treatment with the somatostatin analog octreotide has not significantly improved morphological variables in patients with MTC, although there are case reports showing an antitumor effect of octreotide [8, 14]. Octreotide therapy may be considered for refractory diarrhea that commonly is associated with metastatic disease with high levels of calcitonin.

20.4 Familial Form of MTC (MEN 2)

Sporadic and familial form of MTC do not differ concerning diagnosis, treatment and follow-up of MTC. In patients with MEN 2, occurrence of pheochromocytoma and hyperparathyroidism has to be considered in addition to the diagnosis and treatment of MTC.

20.4.1 Screening for Pheochromocytoma and Timing Surgery

Patients suffering from MEN 2 should undergo yearly screening for pheochromocytoma. Available evidence suggests that 24-h measurement of urinary levels of catecholamines combined with selective use of thin-section, contrast-enhanced CT or MR imaging provides optimal screening for the asymptomatic patient at risk for developing MEN 2-associated pheochromocytoma [9, 12]. We recommend measuring urinary catecholamines yearly in asymptomatic MEN 2 gene carriers, and, if abnormal, CT should be performed. Scintigraphy using ^{131}I metaiodobenzylguanidine (^{131}I-MIBG) is the most sensitive measure of adrenal medullary hyperfunction [19]. The accumulation of ^{131}I-MIBG in the adrenal glands confirms the presence of bilateral hyperplasia even in the absence of clinical or biochemical abnormalities of catecholamine excretion or CT evidence of adrenal masses. Figure 20.3 summarizes the procedure for adrenal medullary screening. Similar to other neuroendocrine tumors, pheochromocytomas in these patients develop slowly and are unlikely to cause significant morbidity with adequate surveillance. Thus we do not recommend adrenalectomy for a positive ^{131}I-MIBG scan alone. Pheochromocytoma in MEN 2 is rarely malignant [13]; the patients are threatened by catecholamine crisis. Prophylactic bilateral adrenalectomy after early diagnosis of adrenal medullary hyperplasia

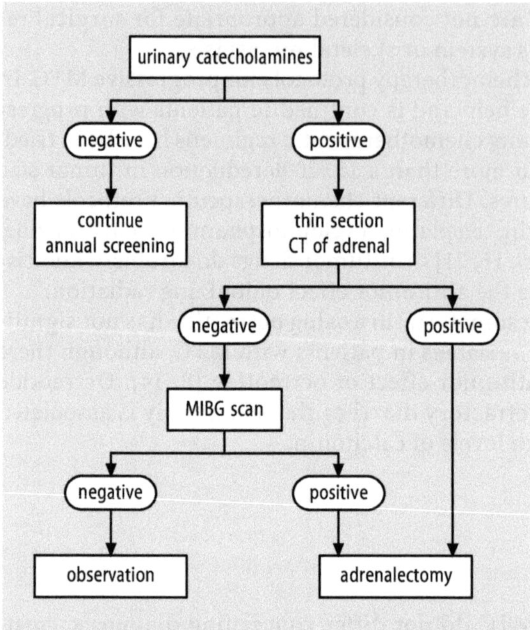

Fig. 20.3 Adrenal medullary screening in asymptomatic patients suffering from familial medullary thyroid carcinoma (MEN 2)

may carry significant morbidity, such as addisonian crisis, and have little oncological value. The goal of screening for pheochromocytoma is therefore to alert the physician to the need for adrenalectomy without putting the patient at risk for catecholamine crisis due to late diagnosis or for Addisonian crisis due to early, overzealous bilateral adrenalectomy. In the case of a unilateral adrenal abnormality in a MEN 2 patient, unilateral adrenalectomy is recommended [9]. Approximately one-third of patients who undergo a unilateral adrenalectomy will eventually require a second operation for a contralateral pheochromocytoma [13], but this may not occur for many years, during which time the patient will not be steroid dependent.

20.4.2 Screening for Primary Hyperparathyroidism

Primary hyperparathyroidism is the least common feature of MEN 2 and tends to develop usually after the third decade. Parathyroid hyperfunction seems to develop rarely in affected subjects who undergo total thyroidectomy at an early age after MEN 2 has been diagnosed [9]. This suggests either that removal of normal parathyroid glands during the total thyroidectomy reduces the incidence of parathyroid disease simply by reducing the number of parathyroid glands at risk or that removal of the C cells has removed a stimulus for parathyroid growth. Yearly measurement of serum calcium and if elevated of parathyroid hormone (PTH) is recommended for detection of hyperparathyroidism.

References

1. Abdelmoumene N, Schlumberger M, Gardet P, Roche A, Travagli JP, Francese C, Parmentier C (1994) Selective venous sampling catheterisation for localisation of persisting medullary thyroid carcinoma. Br J Cancer 69:1141–1144
2. Berndt I, Reuter M, Saller B, Frank-Raue K, Groth P, Grußendorf M, Raue F, Ritter MM, Höppner W (1998) A new hot spot for mutations in the *RET* protooncogene causing familial medullary thyroid carcinoma and multiple endocrine neoplasia type 2A. J Clin Endocrinol Metab 83:770–774
3. Brierley JD, Tsang RW (1996) External radiation therapy in the treatment of thyroid malignancy. Endocrinol Metab Clin North Am 25:141–157
4. Buhr HJ, Kallinowski F, Raue F, Frank RK, Herfarth C (1993) Microsurgical neck dissection for occultly metastasizing medullary thyroid carcinoma. Three-year results. Cancer 72:3685–3693
5. De Besi P, Busnardo B, Toso S, Girelli ME, Nacamulli D, Simioni N, Casara D, Zorat P, Fiorentino MV (1991) Combined chemotherapy with bleomycin, adriamycin, and platinum in advanced thyroid cancer. J Endocrinol Invest 14:475–480
6. Di Bartolomeo M, Bajetta E, Bochicchio AM, Carnaghi C, Somma L, Mazzaferro V, Visini M, Gebbia V, Tumolo S, Ballatore P (1995) A phase II trial of dacarbazine, fluorouracil and epirubicin in patients with neuroendocrine tumours. A study by the Italian Trials in Medical Oncology (I.T.M.O.) Group. Ann Oncol 6:77–79
7. Frank-Raue K, Raue F, Buhr HJ, Baldauf G, Lorenz D, Ziegler R (1992) Localization of occult persisting medullary thyroid carcinoma before microsurgical reoperation: high sensitivity of selective venous catheterization. Thyroid 2:113–117
8. Frank-Raue K, Raue F, Ziegler R (1995) Therapy of metastatic medullary thyroid gland carcinoma with the somatostatin analog octreotide. Med Klin 90:63–66
9. Gagel RF, Tashjian AH, Cummings T, Papathanasopoulos N, Kaplan MM, DeLellis RA, Wolfe HJ, Reichlin S (1988) The clinical outcome of prospective screening for multiple endocrine neoplasia type 2a. An 18-year experience. N Engl J Med 318:478–484
10. Gimm O, Dralle H (1997) Reoperation in metastasizing medullary thyroid carcinoma: is a tumor stage-oriented approach justified? Surgery 122:1124–1130
11. Giuffrida D, Gharib H (1998) Current diagnosis and management of medullary thyroid carcinoma. Ann Oncol 9:695–701
12. Jansson S, Tisell LE, Fjalling M, Lindberg S, Jacobsson L, Zachrisson BF (1988) Early diagnosis of and surgical strategy for adrenal medullary disease in MEN 2 gene carriers. Surgery 103:11–18
13. Lairmore TC, Ball DW, Baylin SB, Wells SA Jr (1993) Management of pheochromocytomas in patients with multiple endocrine neoplasia type 2 syndromes. Ann Surg 217:595–601
14. Modigliani E, Cohen R, Joannidis S, Siame-Mourot C, Guliana JM, Charpentier G, Cassuto D, Bentata PM, Tabarin A, Roger P (1992) Results of long-term continuous subcutaneous octreotide administration in 14 patients with medullary thyroid carcinoma. Clin Endocrinol (Oxf) 36:183–186
15. Orlandi F, Caraci P, Berruti A, Puligheddu B, Pivano G, Dogliotti L, Angeli A (1994) Chemotherapy with dacarbazine and 5-fluorouracil in advanced medullary thyroid cancer. Ann Oncol 5:763–765
16. Raue F (1998) German medullary thyroid carcinoma/multiple endocrine neoplasia registry. German MTC/MEN Study Group. Medullary Thyroid Carcinoma/Multiple Endocrine Neoplasia Type 2. Langenbecks Arch Surg 383:334–336
17. Raue F, Geiger S, Buhr H, Frank-Raue K, Ziegler R (1993) The prognostic importance of calcitonin screening in familial medullary thyroid carcinoma. Dtsch Med Wochenschr 118:49–52
18. Saad MF, Guido JJ, Samaan NA (1983) Radioactive iodine in the treatment of medullary carcinoma of the thyroid. J Clin Endocrinol Metab 57:124–128

19. Shapiro B, Copp JE, Sisson JC, Eyre PL, Wallis J, Beierwaltes WH (1985) Iodine-131 metaiodobenzylguanidine for the locating of suspected pheochromocytoma: experience in 400 cases. J Nucl Med 26:576–585
20. Van Heerden JA, Grant CS, Gharib H, Hay ID, Ilstrup DM (1990) Long-term course of patients with persistent hypercalcitoninemia after apparent curative primary surgery for medullary thyroid carcinoma. Ann Surg 212:395–400
21. Wu LT, Averbuch SD, Ball DW, Bustros A de, Baylin SB, McGuire WP (1994) Treatment of advanced medullary thyroid carcinoma with a combination of cyclophosphamide, vincristine, and dacarbazine. Cancer 73:432–436

Subject Index

U

V

W

X

MIX
Papier aus verantwortungsvollen Quellen
Paper from responsible sources
FSC® C105338
FSC
www.fsc.org

If you have any concerns about our products,
you can contact us on
ProductSafety@springernature.com

In case Publisher is established outside the EU,
the EU authorized representative is:
Springer Nature Customer Service Center GmbH
Europaplatz 3, 69115 Heidelberg, Germany

Printed by Libri Plureos GmbH
in Hamburg, Germany